DOC
OR
QUACK

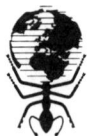

DOC
or
QUACK

Science and Anti-Science
in Modern Medicine

Sander L. Gilman

REAKTION BOOKS

For Kai, Hana, Bodhi and Quinn,

the next generation.

Published by

REAKTION BOOKS LTD

Unit 32, Waterside

44–48 Wharf Road

London N1 7UX, UK

www.reaktionbooks.co.uk

First published 2025

Copyright © Sander L. Gilman 2025

All rights reserved

EU GPSR Authorised Representative

LOGOS EUROPE, 9 rue Nicolas Poussin, 17000, La Rochelle, France

email: contact@logoseurope.eu

Printed and bound in Great Britain by Bell & Bain, Glasgow

A catalogue record for this book is available from the British Library

ISBN 978 1 83639 015 2

CONTENTS

Preface:
A Road Map

THIS IS A BOOK about shifts in the understanding of disease and illness that have taken place within modern ('scientific') medicine from when it arose towards the middle of the nineteenth century through to our present day. It is not primarily about 'quacks' in the sense of the confidence men and women who knowingly sell false promises to cure along with counterfeit nostrums in the marketplace, on the Internet and on TV. These do, however, make appearances throughout the book. They are the easiest cases to examine, as they sell nostrums that they rarely believe work for a quick profit and are simply looking to fulfil the desires of the purchasers for succour, no matter what! Rather, my take on quackery today was shaped by the debates about 'following *the* science', the mantra on the right as well as the left in all the debates about prevention, treatment and cure for Severe Acute Respiratory Syndrome Coronavirus 2 (SARS-CoV-2), later labelled COVID-19. Every time I type 'following *the* science' my autocorrect, which is insistent, directs me to write 'following science'. But that is, of course, *the* problem, as we learned after 2020, as the public's assumption that science was static, objective and value-neutral turned out to be wrong. When all sides claim to be 'following *the* science', where are we to turn?

This moment triggered my interest in the problem of docs and quacks. Throughout this debate, from 2020 to the time of writing, we have heard the accusation of 'quackery' echo on all sides of this issue, answered by the call to just 'follow *the* science'. Quackery and medical fraud, as well as medical malpractice, and 'science' itself, all became politically contested during the pandemic. Did these claims and interventions warrant even more state sanctioning, as all seemed to be labels for violations of the idea that health practices had to be in some manner authorized or at least tolerated by the state – as many of the practices that were labelled quackery came to be? Or were such debates not about quackery but about 'science' itself, held to be an objective intellectual space beyond state control, even if the results of 'following *the* science' were to be the tightening or the loosening of that control? 'Follow *the* science' was the mantra on all sides; but which science, or, perhaps more accurately, whose science? For, in the end, it was the question of who had or who was assumed to have had the power to define science that became the core of what defined quackery.

The cases recounted in this book reflect the debates and claims within mainstream allopathic medicine, the term used for contemporary, accepted scientific medicine (and state-sanctioned complementary and alternative medicine) about the origins of diseases and the therapies proposed for them. At some point in these debates, the accusation that one party or the other is a quack (or one of the many euphemisms) appears, echoing Godwin's Law that the longer an online discussion goes on (regardless of topic or scope), the higher the probability of a comparison to Nazis or Adolf Hitler. In this world, the more heated and confrontational the shifts within modern scientific medicine, and they are inevitable, the more likely that one player or the other will be attacked as a quack.

When early on in 2021 the British government decided to delay the second injection in a two-part vaccination programme, the British Medical Association wrote a furious letter to the then Health Secretary, Matt Hancock, as one report in the u.s. media outlines: 'In their letter they say that this plan undermines patient consent and that it fails to follow the science. Another developer of one of the vaccines, Pfizer, [is] also weighing in saying that there is no data, no evidence to back up this delayed strategy that the government is implementing.'[1] At the same moment a columnist for *The Telegraph*, Ella Whelan, bemoaned 'following *the* science', as '"Follow the science" is the favoured slogan among the COVID censors – but blind faith has never been scientific. We have been forced to give up all sorts of things in the last nine months, but we should never give up our freedom to question, call out and criticise those who think they have all the answers.'[2] In 2020, in his final year as president of the Royal Society, Sir Venkatraman 'Venki' Ramakrishnan (PhD, Physics, Ohio University, 1976; Nobel

Prize, Chemistry, 2009, 'for studies of the structure and function of the ribosome'), had already warned that 'there is often no such thing as following "the" science. Reasonable scientists can disagree on important points, but the government still has to make decisions.'[3] Following *the* science is hard, as it is always constrained by context, interpretation and ideology; even when the science is right, it is often wrong. And its political implications therefore seem always to be fixed and authoritative, if always based on tentative or partial or incorrect knowledge.

This was equally true at the very beginning of scientific medicine, as when in 1854 an anonymous reviewer critiqued a new book by Sir Thomas Spencer Wells – surgeon to Queen Victoria for four decades, baronet, president of the Royal College of Surgeons in 1883, and one of the pioneers of the use of anaesthesia in surgery – in one of the leading popular British magazines. No theories could be dismissed as mere quackery, the reviewer opined, in this new age of science, for as

> the knowledge of the materials of which man's body is formed increases, so views of diseases, their nature, and treatment, alter. Medicine is too far removed from the positive sciences for any practitioner to say that the theory which best explains the nature of disease, or the remedy which best cures a disease, to-day, may not be entirely supplanted to-morrow. Everyone, therefore, who has his wits about him, and comes with new views and new remedies, the result of cautious experiment and rational generalization, has a claim to be heard in the medical world.[4]

With the caveat, at mid-nineteenth century, that such claimants do no harm. By our age of biomedicine, another contemporary term for scientific medicine, that warning seems to be rare, given the claim that the practice of medicine is beyond grubby politics.

What I am examining here are the 'docs'. Let me note that I have been on the faculties at four distinguished schools of medicine as a tenured professor for over forty years. But I am not a 'doc'. I have a PhD, not an MD. Now that does make a real difference: I wore tweed jackets, not white lab coats. I know that in society, when I am introduced as a professor at a school of medicine, I have social capital that I have not earned, at least in the eyes of my interlocutors. I may *know* lots of things, but I am not invested with the same status. One of the jokes that circulate in every medical school class is 'What do you call the person who is last in their class?' The answer is obvious to the students: 'A doctor.' I'm a 'professor'. And that summarizes the cultural and social capital of the physician in our world, even beyond schools of medicine.

Nowadays the docs' status varies from time to place, from medical specialty to historical, geographic and physical location, just as working at a medical school today gives you more cachet than having a private practice or being in an NHS (UK National Health Service) clinic. In addition, such status is impacted by class, ethnicity, gender and race. But it is there always, for good or for ill, even if it is diminished in today's world by the simple fact that in the United States mega-healthcare systems and global pharmaceutical corporations often determine what is practised in the clinic. As was recently stated in the American press, '70 per cent of doctors work as salaried employees of large hospital systems or corporate entities, taking orders from administrators and executives who do not always share their values or priorities.'[5] In the UK, the NHS under Conservative governments simply substituted for the private or quasi-private American organizations, as indicated by the recent strikes by various organizations representing healthcare professionals, striking as if they were workers in factories or mines.

It is not that surprising that in 2016, well before our most recent global pandemic, the United Kingdom and the United States ranked next to last (UK) and last (USA) in access and quality of care among eight comparable healthcare systems in the Global North.[6] The claim for scientific medicine is that it was able to consistently raise the rate of life expectancy, at least in the Global North. But if the drop in life expectancy's rate of rise since the COVID-19 pandemic is an index, things have improved neither for healthcare providers nor the general population.[7] Indeed, once you break this down by group and deprivation status, women's rate of increase has fallen more than men's, and for the poorest 10 per cent of women, life expectancy has dropped across the Global North. It is this world and its inhabitants that my book wishes to portray, not simply to examine the idealized 'physician-healer' but rather to reflect on the wide range of individuals wrestling with the ever-changing and always contested world of what 'healing' is and what role the 'healer' plays in it, whether physician or nurse, public health practitioner, and so on.

I begin from a set of assumptions in this book: that the players are serious in their beliefs about their claims; that they have the imprimatur of colleagues or institutions or the state in their time to make their claims within the world of scientific medicine; and that scientific medicine is dynamic and ever-changing rather than inevitably moving towards the good or the perfect. Given that there is a wide-ranging spectrum of seemingly ancillary factors that play major roles in these shifts within allopathic medicine – from professional, social, ideological and economic status to more abstract notions of what is healing (and what is harm) – the notion that medicine simply 'follows *the science*' turns out to be at best incomplete, at worst deceptive. Patients, that is, individuals who understand themselves as ill, react to all these, labelling and relabelling themselves as well as responding in ever-shifting ways to healers as they seek succour. For some at any given time, succour is given, often influenced by the status of the healer and the reality shared with their patients, even when the science followed turns out to be spurious or ineffective. Sometimes, biomedicine can and does fulfil its promise and change the trajectories not only of individual lives but of entire communities. Therefore, science and medicine rhyme imperfectly.

I am beginning this book, however, with a first chapter that looks at the strictures and their histories in many settings as to what was understood to be 'good' and what 'bad' medicine. This is a relatively quick overview of the creation of several categories, such as the quack, standard of care, docs, non-medical practitioners, malpractice, indeed, even the patient, in a number of overlapping realms: the law, professional and state institutions, research communities and the creative arts. All mirror and distort the way we understand healthcare and its varied functions within these realms. These case studies draw on much existing research, yet I hope I have reconstructed each in ways that are new or at least unexpected in their juxtapositions of the slippery categories of doc and quack.

The cases, chosen precisely because they seem to be radically different, yet reveal the same underlying contradictions and problems that bedevil medicine today, are neither unique nor new. My first case (Chapter Two) deals with peptic and other ulcers of the digestive tract. Their history tracks each permutation in which clinicians applied the science of their time from the early modern era to the Anthropocene, each claiming that their predecessors were not merely wrong but did real harm to their patients. Naming a disease often meant diagnosing it surreptitiously and diagnosing meant engaging with specific therapies. The digestive system also provided ample examples about how all of these become linked to innovations in technologies, whether appropriate or not to the tasks at hand. Here we will see how the use of the case study as a micro-biography of healing is abandoned for statistical arguments about aetiology as well as therapeutic efficacy, and how notions of masculinity and femininity come to play ever greater roles in our discourses of scientific medicine.

In the second case study, Chapter Three, we see how the distinction between doc and quack becomes blurred as the question morphs over the past century to 'who is the scientist and who is the quack?' when we turn to surgical interventions. Surgery and pain are linked here in ever more complex ways. Our case study is ophthalmological surgery, with race science, eugenics and competition for funding and honours continuing to play a major role in defining scientific medicine. But 'seeing' is a complex concept, as we shall examine in detail here. Inherent in the rise of modern, scientific medicine was, as Michel Foucault has argued, the imposition of the 'clinical gaze' and vision, what he called 'the anatomo-clinical gaze', which provided the scientific evidence needed for the new medicine.[8] Looking comes to be separated from seeing – even in ophthalmology. Yet Foucault's overall argument about the rupture between the pre- and post-Enlightenment world in modern medicine did not seem to apply to surgery. Medical practice in Paris during the *Ancien Régime* saw an ever-narrowing social and professional gulf between innovative physicians and conservative surgeons, with the creation of what seemed to be a unified medical profession by the time of the French Revolution. This union proved to be less an abrupt rupture with the practices of the past than a slow and often halting 'gestation of the clinic'.[9] We shall observe this repeatedly as older models and attitudes persevere even while being actively replaced by ever more 'scientific' and therefore, it was assumed, better ones. Surgery, and the pain caused by the surgeon, thus becomes one more test case for the problems of transitions and how 'following *the* science' becomes ever more complex in the surgical theatre as surgeons replace physicians at the top of the social pecking order of healers.

My final study, in Chapter Four, turns our approach on its head. What we have been examining is how diagnostic categories and attendant therapies are created, amalgamated or restructured in response to innovations in science and technology. We will have seen how shifts in the claims of science change the expectations of both practitioners and patients in terms of efficacy in dealing with disease categories that seem always to be changing. Here our red line is a specific therapy, acupuncture, which can illustrate how therapeutic interventions become medicine or quackery depending on their claims on science – claims which are, as we shall see, always unstable. We will deal with it as an index of state-sanctioned alternative and complementary medicine, tracing the career of acupuncture, both positive and negative, through the other great historical wave that parallels the rise of scientific medicine: that of colonialism and its absorption into the clinical beliefs of the day. It is, therefore, a boundary case for biomedicine, as it has moved into mainstream medical practice (again, as we shall see) in the immediate past and has again been exiled to its margins. Here the question of not only *who* heals, but *what* heals comes into sharp focus again with an examination of placebos and nocebos. Given that one of the markers of healing and cure is the amelioration of pain, pain as a symptom of a disease process or pain as part of the process of cure, this case study also concludes our examination of healing and pain.

My conclusion – Chapter Five – provides a tentative set of counter-readings to some of the debates triggered by COVID-19 and indeed by the world of scientific medicine that I have sketched in these case studies. I hope this conclusion will further our goals of understanding the good, the bad and the ugly – as well as the brilliant, the original and the constructive – in medicine then and now.

What I am therefore going to illustrate in this book is that every movement of knowledge from the laboratory is transitory when it is applied to the clinic. Good science is always shifting, and even inappropriate applications of science can have a curative impact. All therapies cure some patients; no therapy cures all patients. This is a truism but one that our day-to-day expectations wish to exclude. 'Following *the* science' should be a magic bullet that, when science is found in the clinic, guarantees a return to health, so it does matter whether it can cure or not. The clinician is, as we shall see in my opening chapter, placed in a double bind: to achieve good outcomes, the patient needs to believe in the therapy, needs to be compliant; but the healer cannot offer such a guarantee, except implicitly. And this becomes ever more apparent in chronic diseases and, as we know now, in pandemics. The boundary between the belief in the healer and the healer's limitations is, as we shall see, one of the definitions of quackery in our age.

Who are the quacks; who are the healers? Does orthodoxy eclipse heterodoxy when the result is a euthanasia machine fuelled by graduates of the most praised medical schools in the world, as in the Third Reich?[10] Does heterodoxy eclipse orthodoxy when the cures are harmful or ineffectual but 'natural'? Perhaps the problem with Godwin's Law is not that in the end everyone calls everyone else a 'Nazi', but that there are times when that is true.[11] And, we need to add, sometimes it is inherently false. Thus we will examine the underlying claims that still shape our contemporary medical practice, beginning with the origins of the invention or discovery of a disease and then formation of the medical specialty that created it or that it created. As the reader will observe, each case is full of such digressions, looking at questions and problems that seem tangential to the cases I am describing, but which, although rarely evoked, are central to framing the debates that occur in 'following *the* science'. Who knew that our present fascination with 'fashion scrubs', worn by Gen X-ers on the bar scene (see Chapter Four), was intimately connected to one of the central factors often ignored in scientific medicine: our human need to believe that someone, representing some institution, can heal us, but also that our fear of their 'white coats' can harm us. All aspects played and play their roles in both medicine as a profession and the idea of medicine in the public sphere. For medical science is a blade that cuts both ways.

Innovation in medicine has always run up against human nature. The internationally renowned physician Sir William Osler (MD and CM [Master of Surgery], McGill University, 1872), in his 1906 lecture on William Harvey (MD, University of Padua, 1602) and the discovery of the circulatory system, noted that

> It is on this account that the man who expresses a new idea is very apt to be abused and ill-treated. All this is common among common men but there is something much worse which has been illustrated over and over again in history. How eminent soever a man may become in science, he is very apt to carry with him errors, which were in vogue when he was young – errors that darken his understanding and make him incapable of accepting even the most obvious truths. It is a great

consolation to know that even [William] Harvey came within the range of this law in the matter of the lymphatic system, it is the most human touch in his career.[12]

To remind you, Harvey got it wrong in that case because he incorrectly believed that the open lymphatic system was a closed circuit connected with arteries and veins. He had established that model through his own radical discovery of the circulation of the blood and he was simply wrong in the case of the lymphatic system. This is the dilemma that we address in this book, marking the relationship between science and the clinic, between shifts in science and those who follow them, honoured with rewards or condemned into intense obscurity, the ever-shifting boundary between good medicine and quackery.

Yes, what I am writing about are 'paradigm shifts'. Change but not necessarily progress. Thomas Kuhn (PhD, Physics, Harvard, 1949), after Hiroshima and Nagasaki had compromised the status of physics, was one of many who took Sir Karl Popper's notion of scientific progress in any field as questionable. Popper (PhD, Psychology, University of Vienna, 1928) had set forth in the 1930s and '40s a philosophy of falsifiability as a basic feature of those fields of science whose advances far outpaced development in other fields. 'Falsifiability' sees a scientific theory as capable of being true only if there is a means of testing whether it is false, a sort of Occam's razor of truth. However, a theory (as in the case of psychoanalytic theories – his example, not mine) that is consistent with all possible observations and therefore can *never* be disproven must be unscientific.[13] The ability constantly to test and retest the underlying evidence of a thesis reveals itself in claims about the progress of science; as Popper claimed, 'while we can never have sufficiently good arguments in the empirical sciences for claiming that we have actually reached the truth, we can have strong and reasonably good arguments for claiming that we may have made progress towards the truth.'[14]

In his *The Structure of Scientific Revolutions* (1962), Kuhn argued for the incommensurability of rival scientific paradigms, denying that science grows linearly through the accumulation of truths but radically through what he labelled 'paradigm shifts'. Yet his volume begins with a comment that disciplines live out their claims of progress in the institutions, such as schools of medicine, and the textbooks that codified that progress. He sees these claims as of little more value 'than an image of a national culture drawn from a tourist brochure or a language text'.[15] I take, in this volume, the opposite position: that medical journals, textbooks, popular, mass and high culture, the courts of law, indeed the public sphere in general, shape the relationship between bench science and clinical medicine and have, therefore, probative value in my writing of its history. Scientist-physicians from the nineteenth century to the present moment are simultaneously members of a guild of specialists as well as of the greater society in which they live and which has invested them with both status and professional identity, for good or for ill. That is, they function as doctors and citizens, scientists and authorities in a complicated jumble, sorted out by each generation in each culture of health and illness.

The astute reader will also recognize that in this book I am in a conversation with a ghost. No better understanding of the dilemmas of modern, scientific medicine is to be found than in the work of my late friend Roy Porter. Porter, who died in 2002, much too young, was a social historian whose focus was on medicine in all its complications. His point of departure was the British Enlightenment, and he authored many books on quackery. Since I am beginning with the results of Enlightenment science and medicine during the mid-nineteenth century, it is clear (and my references to Porter show) that I am indeed 'standing on the shoulders of a giant', a historical cliché to which we shall return in the course of our work. But what may give me some justification for returning to this set of questions is that my world after Roy's very untimely death saw a 'resolution' (not really) of the HIV/AIDS pandemic as well as a new global pandemic, COVID-19. The thinness of the air standing on Roy's metaphoric shoulders makes me gasp at how often he correctly described the complexity of healthcare, scientific medicine and the problematic social role of doctors and patients. Not that things have remained the same; they never do. But he left me a blueprint that I was able to follow and expand.

1

Confronting
the Problem

T ODAY'S SCIENTIFIC MEDICINE is complicated. For every
        intervention that is promising, there are many that are inef-
        fectual. Even therapies that prove to be efficacious in clinical
trials may well turn out not to be effective in the real world. When
some interventions are proposed, it may initially seem to society that
they are 'medicine'; when it is revealed that they have failed, they
become 'quackery'. Sometimes the obverse is true: new, innovative or
radical interventions are dismissed as 'quackery', only to be revealed
as 'real' when they are effective. Ironically, some of the failures may
be effective – at least for some. Diagnosis works only when it is tied
to prognosis; in healthcare we are ill-served to have a problem named
if that problem cannot be solved. It is a claim on the power to predict
that was granted to Apollo's oracle at Delphi and is today expected
when we go to the Mayo Clinic. All need to believe in these claims,
physician and patient. This is much more than claims made in the
1980s that 'deep in patients' unconsciousness, physicians are viewed
as miracle workers, patterned after the fantasized, all-caring parents
of infancy. Medicine, after all, was born in magic and religion, and the
doctor-priest-magician-parent unity that persists in patients' unconsciousness cannot be broken.'[1] It is also that the complexity of the
cultural structures of belief and trust in *scientific* medicine evokes such
a dependency.

Sometimes those who proposed such interventions are showered
with honours, as with the Nobel prizes. Some – we can think of Ignaz
Semmelweis (MD, University of Vienna, 1844), the physician who
advocated antisepsis in 1847 – were excoriated in their time. He was

committed to an asylum by his medical colleagues, who disavowed all that he found and called him a quack, only for him to be beaten to death there in 1865 by the warders, completely forgotten. Forgotten at least until antisepsis became the new dogma, if more in theory than in practice, during the first age of bacteriology, when Semmelweis was resurrected as the first martyr of modern scientific medicine.[2] And at such moments we need to draw into question any claim of the absolute efficacy of the universities and the state to differentiate, except in the moment, between helping and harming those seeking succour. Such claims are and have always been shifting over time.[3] Yet we necessarily rely on them at every moment.

The expansion of heterodox 'alternative and complementary medicine', from acupuncture to nutrition, as well as the concomitant expansion of those legally able to claim the mantle of state-recognized health practice, is only the most recent shift in 'boundary work', as defined by Thomas Gieryn.[4] He notes that late Victorian scientists, including physicians, demarcated 'science' from two of its competitors (theology and mechanics), as well as demarcating some scientists from those they wanted to exclude as 'pseudo-scientists'.[5] Remember that the term 'scientist' did not even exist until 1833, when it was coined by English polymath William Whewell, after the aged poet Samuel Taylor Coleridge challenged him that 'natural philosophers', as was then the term for those who studied what we might now broadly call 'science', were neither natural nor philosophers. We are going to think about such 'pseudo-scientists' as 'quacks', while understanding that such a status can change instantaneously and those scientists quite confident in their role judging their colleagues could just as easily become the 'quacks'.

Who Makes Physicians?

But who creates doctors in the first place? Schools of medicine, from the earliest age of Salerno (tenth century), Bologna (1088), Montpellier (1289) and Pavia (1361), made physicians by continuing the tradition of the Church that created priests through investing the individual priest with the power of the institution and, therefore, of God.[6] Whether it was the king, anointed by the priest, or the physician, anointed by his older colleagues in their role as the faculty of the university, investiture made a public promise that the powers of the collective would be transferred into the single figure – a figure then composed of both a human component, with all of its human fallibility, and a magical (or at least, in the case of the doctors, a competent) component, whose continuity was assured by the very existence of the institution itself. But those claims were shaken by the rise of modern science. From the secularized French 'grandes écoles', begun in 1794 when the National Convention created the 'école normale supérieure', to Wilhelm von Humboldt's 1810 Berlin University; from Thomas Jefferson's 'Report of the Commissioners for the University of Virginia', on 4 August 1818, to Jeremy Bentham's self-consciously secular London University of 1826 (soon to be renamed University College London): through such institutions theology became marginalized in the university and a new *secular* investiture of physicians came with promises of the efficacy of the new science.

In the course of the nineteenth century the notion of a laying-on of hands, physician creating physicians, came in conflict with the so-called scientific pragmatism of nineteenth-century science – a pragmatism mirrored in renewed state attention to certification and investiture. While the distinction between an individual and his pro-fession (in the exercise of which one is 'playing a certain role') had been carefully worked out by Scribonius Largus, the court physician to the Roman emperor Claudius, in the first century CE, the perhaps necessary blurring of this boundary in the service of healing made Enlightened physicians uncomfortable. Scribonius Largus observed that anyone, including the physician who 'practices any occupation[,] is playing a certain role. It may be one derived from chance circum-stances, the place in society to which he is born and by which his inclination toward a particular career and also his opportunities for it are conditioned; it may be one which he assumes through his own free decision, through a deliberate choice of an occupation.' It is trivial whether he (and they are all men) inherited the role or chose it freely, 'one must act one's part as the role demands it, just as in the two roles which nature, in addition, has assigned to everyone – as a human being who has the same duties as all other human beings, and as an indi-vidual endowed with specific intellectual and emotional gifts – one must live up to "the lines one has to speak".'[7] You are both a citizen and a physician, the latter a role handed down by those in the past, real or imagined, that sets you apart and that transcends your corporality.

Such a crisis of belief was articulated in professional circles and then in political ones in our age of scientific medicine. Indeed, in 1956 the exiled German-Jewish historian of medicine Ludwig Edelstein (PhD, University of Heidelberg, 1929) read Scribonius Largus as claiming that the profession of the physician is defined by 'sympathy and humanness in accordance with the will of medicine itself'. These are the obligations of the physician as a professional, and in fact Scribonius Largus calls being a physician a '*professio*', as opposed to the establishment quacks of his time. Edelstein retrospectively translates this as a 'calling', evoking the sociologist Max Weber's concept of '*Beruf*', in his 'Wissenschaft als Beruf' ('Science as a Vocation or Calling') – the lectures he held in 1919 on the nature of the professions, labelling them as a calling rather than a mere craft.[8]

Weber had set the bar defining the 'calling' of the physician in the new age of medical science. For him, reacting to the claims of scientific medicine, 'there are [today] no mysterious incalculable forces that come into play, but rather . . . one can, in principle, master all things by calculation. This means that the world is disenchanted . . . One need no longer have recourse to magical means in order to master or implore the spirits, as did the savage, for whom such mysterious powers existed. Technical means and calculations perform that service.'[9] And for Weber it is clear that this disenchantment is to be found in the claims of modern medicine, which is the 'greatest practical technology which is highly developed scientifically. The general "presupposition" of the medical enterprise is stated trivially in the assertion that medical science has the task of maintaining life as such and of diminishing suffering as such to greatest possible degree.' For Weber

> this is problematical . . . Yet the presuppositions of medicine, and the penal code, prevent the physician from relinquishing his therapeutic efforts. Whether life is worthwhile living and when – this question is not asked by medicine. Natural science gives us an answer to the question of what we must do if we wish to master life technically. It leaves quite aside, or assumes for its purposes, whether we should and do wish to master life technically and whether it ultimately makes sense to do so.[10]

And thus medicine, so long related to the power of belief, has been transformed into a reductive science. It no longer answers what Weber's core questions are – 'what shall we do? how shall we live?' That science, even when embedded in medicine, with its claim on the ethical calling of its practitioners, cannot answer questions of value and thus of meaning that lie at the heart of the complexities associated with medicine. This reflects the radical rethinking of the role and definition of the professional in modern science, which still plays a role in this debate today.

With the crisis of investiture during the age of scientific medicine, it was necessary radically to rethink who certified physicians and then who could recommend them to the state for licensure.[11] In spite of their qualms, the older model was maintained, with all of its complications, by assigning the qualities earlier invested by authority in an individual, but now defining that individual as the *scientific* practitioner, as 'the professional skills that are imparted and acquired in order to be applied (that is, exchanged and sold) are vested in individuals: the "impersonal" skills of the professional are therefore inseparable from his social and personal attributes, even though modern professionalization claims that skills can be separately and objectively evaluated.' And this was defined by the market, since 'the first professions to organize on a market basis – medicine and the law – provided services that were (and still are) "personal", immediately used or consumed by the buyer.'[12] Yet the conflict between the individual and the claims of the community led (and lead) often to instability in the definition of the practitioner: doc or quack?

Doubt about the 'efficiency of the master-figure' is what Eric Santner has called the 'crisis of investiture'. A crisis in the

> symbolic investiture whereby an individual is endowed with a new social status, is filled with a symbolic mandate that henceforth informs his or her identity in the community. The social and political stability of a society as well as the psychological 'health' of its members would appear to be correlated to the efficacy of these symbolic operations – to what we might call their *performative magic* – whereby individuals 'become who they are,' assume the social essence assigned to them by way of names, titles, degrees, posts, honors, and the like.[13]

For Santner, this results in the direct rule of experts legitimized by their knowledge, yet suffering simultaneously an excess of doubt, of permanent self-questioning. This becomes a central motivator for 'scientific medicine' and its re-creation of the 'quack' as being beyond science as part of attempting to resolve this crisis of belief. This is linked to the very notion of the expert and expertise as a legal and social category. The physician is now given the certainty of the scientific expert even though the practice of medicine was and remains unstable. This was very much felt in the 1930s, when the blame for quackery was laid at the feet of the new medical science and its alienation from the patient:

> We little Asklepiads are not Aesculapius himself. An effectual preventive of death is not yet ours. Nature, the great healer, makes no distinction betwixt quacks and experts, but the quack never omits to claim the credit when his merciful ally effects a cure. Moreover, the higher medical science has risen, the more it has, in its pride, estranged the public from the doctor. When medical art moves from the sick-bed to the laboratory, when we treat diseases rather than diseased people, there slips from our grasp a powerful instrument, the personal influence of one man on another, which the quack knows how to handle in a masterly way.[14]

For Santner, such claims of a crisis of science and medicine heighten what he describes as 'the site of an excess of power, a signifying stress'. Both power and the concomitant stress came to be invested in the institutions that arose in the wake of the Enlightenment. The transformation of theological models of continuity, those institutions which guaranteed the transition from one ruler to the next in the age of the 'divine right of kings', in our age of radical secularism is most clearly presented in 'their modern avatars among men of science and medicine – the ultimate biocrats – who work to isolate and protect the charismatic "stuff" or "matter" of general equivalence enjoyed by members of the race'.[15] While Santner, here paraphrasing the German-American social philosopher Hannah Arendt, is looking at 'Race Science', a red thread in scientific medicine as we shall see, this is of course true of scientific medicine in general.

In his groundbreaking study of the 'two bodies of the King', which becomes the model for professional investiture, Ernst H. Kantorowicz quotes Seneca about the distinctions created by professional identity: '*Duas personas habet gubernator* – Two persons are combined in the pilot: one he shares with all his fellow-passengers, for he also is a passenger; the other is peculiar to him, for he is the pilot. A storm harms him as a passenger, but it harms him not as a pilot.'[16] This is the presumed 'two bodies' of the physician. Our contemporary biopolitical condition, Santner seems to suggest, is the result of the continuity of that very investiture, and, we can add, its perceived failure a century earlier. For if the ship sinks, the pilot, no matter what his professional role, also drowns, and is quickly labelled as a failure, as the maritime equivalent of a 'quack'.

If we are serious about Eric Santner's evocation of Max Weber's notion of 'charisma', which for Weber is that 'personal quality that makes an individual seem extraordinary, a quality by virtue of which supernatural, superhuman, or at least exceptional powers or properties are attributed to the individual', which inhabited the king once anointed and crowned, then this is charisma second-hand, now given to the physician by the institutions in the state.[17] Weber had noted already in his 1919 lectures on the nature of the professions that such charisma, in the modern age, could be attained by egalitarian means, by sitting examinations, such as had been the case in imperial China, not purely by the elites' laying-on of hands, perpetuating their status:

> The 'special examination', in the present sense, was and is found also outside of bureaucratic structures proper; thus, today it is found in the 'free' professions of medicine and law and in the guild-organized trades . . . Special examinations, on the one hand, mean or appear to mean a 'selection' of those who qualify from all social strata rather than a rule by notables. On the other hand, democracy fears that a merit system and educational certificates will result in a privileged 'caste'. Hence, democracy fights against the special-examination system.[18]

The set examination allows anyone to acquire the charisma of the professional and thus become part of the elite, which Weber experienced in the new status of an elite, scientific medicine. Weber notes that there is a 'broad range of "great" heroes, prophets, and healers that a value-free sociology considers as equally endowed with charisma'. This is now accessible through the investiture of the state and is the 'calling' ascribed to the physician in the modern world.

Reinforced by the claims of the physician carrying out the truths of science at the bedside, the disenchantment of science replaces the charisma of the '"shamans", that is, sorcerers who, in the pure type, were subject to epileptic seizures before falling into trances'.[19] Weber had a rather nostalgic fantasy about the charismatic healer in his undefined past. If I can add a counterfactual moment to his example: one Neolithic denizen watching the shaman fall into his prophetic seizure turns to another: 'The old shaman was much better. He gave us mushrooms before he prophesied, and we too shared in his vision.' His friend scoffs: 'You're never up to date. Mushrooms are so last year. He was such a quack!' (Maybe not so hypothetical. In 1736 Philip Johan von Strahlenberg, a Swedish prisoner of war in Siberia during the Great Northern War between Sweden and Russia, described the use of such mushrooms by the local elites. The mushrooms were rare and expensive, so the poor waited for the rich to relieve themselves and drank their urine so they too could have some of the psychotropic effect.[20]) No science, only enchantment, wherever you turned.

Weber assumes that such figures had a power that shaped and moved the world through their very presence, their charisma, for a leader was then 'the charismatic leader of the hunt and war, the sorcerer, the rainmaker, the medicine man – and thus the priest and the doctor and finally, the arbiter. Often, yet not always, such charismatic functions are split into as many special holders of charisma.'[21] Today, the elite healer, while granted charisma through his or her investiture, seems to be merely a technocrat, isolated from the meanings of things. The reality is, of course, that such claims echo back through every age leading to that of scientific medicine. There were always golden ages when men truly believed the shaman as opposed to us poor fools relying on the innovations of the moment, beset by both science and quackery.

The Wavering Border Line between Quacks and Docs

'Quackery' is thus a concept that is useful and perhaps even necessary, since the drawing of such boundaries is never absolute. For years I had always assumed that the very word 'quackery' (in German *Quacksalberei*) came from a quack cure, 'quicksilver' (*Quecksilber*): mercury treatment for syphilis. But I was simply wrong: indeed, the term comes from the seventeenth-century Dutch *kwaken*, modern German *quaken* – shouting out one's 'salves' (*zalven*; *Salbe*) in the public market. The louder one shouts, the more attention is brought

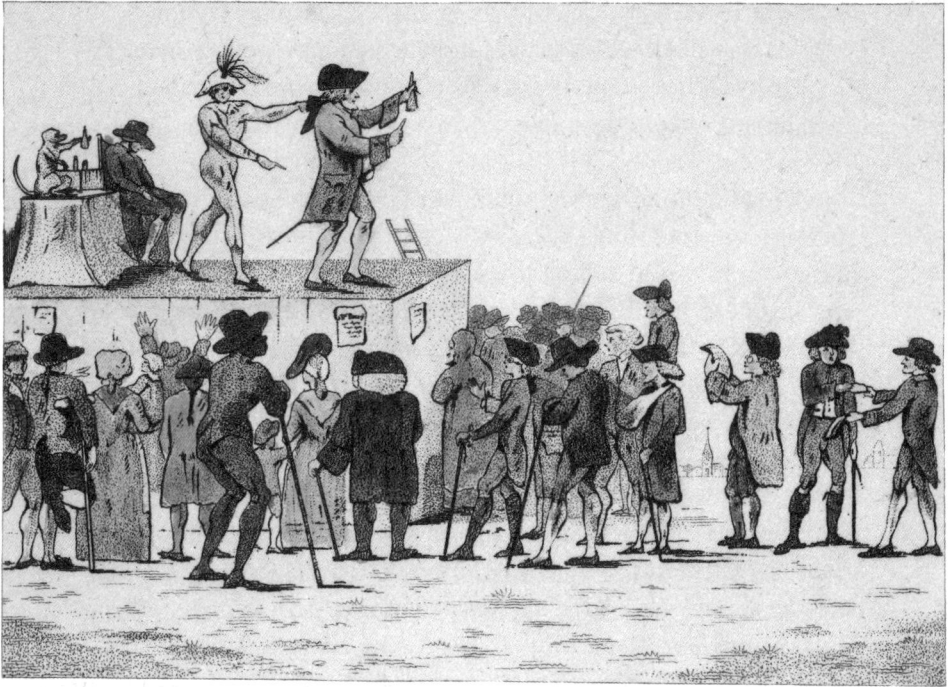

W. Birch, after A. van Assen, *Dr Bossey and the People Taken from the Life*, 1792, engraving; the last of the London itinerant quack-doctors who hawked medicines on a stage.

to one's views. As Daniel Defoe notes in his (semi-fictive) *Journal of the Plague Year* (1722), the desperate go to those 'who fed their Fears, and kept them always alarm'd, and awake, on purpose to delude them, and pick their Pockets: So, they were as mad, upon their *running after Quacks, and Mountebanks*, and every practising old Woman, for *Medicines and Remedies*, storeing themselves with such Multitudes of Pills, Potions'.[22] So too those who defined themselves as physicians, such as Augustin Belloste in 1701, who laments in his book on the art of surgery that it is 'indeed a notable Shame, that a wounded Person should go from under their Hands, to be cur'd by a Quack, a Clown, or a simple Woman'.[23] Such quacks exist across all national boundaries, drawing on fear and discomfort, for the quack is

> generally equated with charlatanry: it is said that one Latan, a famous quack, used to go about Paris in a splendid charabanc, in which he had a traveling dispensary. A man with a horn announced the approach of this magnate, and the delighted sightseers used to cry out 'Voila le Char de Latan!' In Italian,

the term is ciarlatano, a babbler or quack. And 'mountebank'?
This was the bank or bench on which shopkeepers of yore
displayed their goods – street vendors used to mount on their
bank to patter to the public.[24]

William de Meij, in 1834, continued Defoe's charge that the 'quack
... wants external show: instead of addressing himself to competent
judges, he refuses to submit to their judgement, accuses them often
of exaggerated severity, nay, even of envy, and injustice. He appeals to
the multitude; the public papers establish the ephemeral theatre of his
fame, praise his pretended discoveries, and afford him opportunities
to boast and vent them out with impunity.'[25] De Meij's true scientists
avant la lettre are Francis Bacon and René Descartes, neither one of
whom shied away from public celebrity and honours.

We need to be careful about such charges as they mask judgement
calls that look more at output than outcome. Some folk remedies of the
'practising old Woman' led to pharmaceuticals; what at one moment
is efficacious treatment, think blood-letting or massive use of antibiotics, turns out to be fatal; and 'orthodox medical science has at times
examined herbal and other remedies of unorthodox medicine and has
sometimes found useful medicines in this way. Orthodox medicine
has, however, retained its illness-oriented therapy and has continued
to ignore the patient-oriented therapy of the deviant medicine from
which the treatment was obtained. The history of mesmerism in the
nineteenth century may be viewed as another example of this kind of
vindication.'[26] Mesmerism was condemned by the French state – in
1784 – and its promulgator Franz Mesmer (MD, University of Vienna,
1766) was labelled a dangerous quack who endangered the virtue of
its female citizens, a view strongly supported by Benjamin Franklin,
the leading celebrity scientist of the day and a member of the Royal
Commission that condemned Mesmer. In 1841 James Braid (Licentiate,
Royal College of Surgeons of Edinburgh, 1815) changed mesmerism's
name to 'hypnotism', adding it to the repertory of psychotherapy, where
it remains today. No one's virtue seemed to have been at risk any longer
in the new age of scientific medicine.

So too the notion that only charlatans 'shout their wares in the
marketplace', as a surgeon bemoaned in the 1890s: 'the physician and
surgeon allow professional work of the most sacred character to be
heralded though the columns of the daily press as a consequence of

reporters being present at operations, or of bulletins being issued daily.'[27] Scientific medicine has successfully competed in the public sphere from at least Louis Pasteur to the latest TV programmes about CRISPR (Clustered Regularly Interspaced Short Palindromic Repeats) and gene editing.[28] American periodicals, at least seemingly all of those that you find on board aeroplanes, list the '10 BEST Aesthetic Surgeons/Internists/Allergy Doctors in New York/Phoenix/Los Angeles'. These lists are high-powered advertisements underwritten by the docs themselves.

Publicity is and always has been part of the selling of scientific medicine, no matter how reluctant professional organizations are to acknowledge this and how active they are in dismissing this as unprofessional. Thomas Percival (MD, Leiden University, 1765) writes in 1803, in the first widely adopted Anglophone manual of medical ethics, that being a medical professional meant hewing to the values of the collective, for 'every man who enters into a fraternity engages, by a tacit compact, not only to submit to the laws, but to promote the honour and interest of the association, so far as they are consistent with morality, and the general good of mankind. A physician, therefore, should cautiously guard against whatever may injure the general respectability of his profession.'[29] Even among heterodox thinkers this remained gospel. In the 1920s Erwin Liek (MD, University of Königsberg, 1902), a radical German physician demanding a rethinking of modern scientific medicine, still argued, now in the age of mass communication, that 'we doctors should shun propaganda by film and wireless and such-like publicity.'[30] We are not to shout in the marketplace if we want our patients to trust us. Paul Starr, in what has become the classic account of the rise of American scientific medical practice, observed:

> Medicine and other professions have historically distinguished themselves from business and trade by claiming to be above the market and pure commercialism. In justifying the public's trust, professionals have set higher standards of conduct for themselves than the minimal rules governing the marketplace and maintained that they can be judged under those standards only by each other, not by laymen. The ideal of the market presumes the 'sovereignty' of consumer choices; the ideal of a profession calls for the sovereignty of its members' independent, authoritative judgment. A professional who yields too

much to the demands of clients violates an essential article of the professional code: Quacks . . . are practitioners who continue to please their customers but not their colleagues.[31]

As scientific medicine infiltrated clinical practice and the physician became an extension of the laboratory, the ethical difference between the newly redefined role of the physician and their antithesis, the quack, became more and more necessary.

The reality is that medicine was always part of the marketplace, even in those halcyon days of the rise of scientific medicine in the mid-nineteenth century, when essays by and about noted Harley Street practitioners and leading medical scientists regularly appeared in high-brow publications as well as gossip rags. Mass advertising in daily newspapers by patent medicine manufacturers producing potions sold by quacks (and others) in the nineteenth century gave way to mass advertising on TV in the United States that features pharma-ceuticals that only licensed physicians can prescribe. Thus they are advertisements for the docs as well as the drugs. And, certainly, any Google search for certain specialties, globally, will turn up websites that are just as flagrant in hawking their products as the loudest and most officious quack in the early modern marketplace – and with a much wider reach. We too shall run after these 'quacks' in this book, but with another purpose. We shall try to understand the implica-tions of the charges of being beyond the bounds of state or culturally approved healthcare treatment, and how often, but not always, such labels reveal more about those undertaking the labelling than those who are so labelled.

Medicine Is Never Value-Neutral

The ever-shifting line between medicine and quackery is drawn and redrawn with multiple intentions and contradictions in the public sphere in modernity. And that seems to be irrespective of the systems of medicine – ancient, alternative, complementary, TCM (Traditional Chinese Medicine, an invention of the twentieth century, which we will discuss in some detail in Chapter Four) or modern allopathic medi-cine in what we label as the first age of biology, the latter half of the nineteenth century. This distinction between allopathic and alterna-tive therapy, ironically, is one first made by Samuel Hahnemann (MD,

University of Erlangen, 1779), the early nineteenth-century founder of one of the competing medical sects, homeopathy (which will feature throughout this volume), who differentiated medical doctors who subscribed to a homeopathic philosophy from those who did not.[32] Hahnemann believed that '*similia similibus curentur*' ('like cures like'), creating symptoms analogous to those generated by the disease in the least virulent way possible by diluting his ingredients until unmeasurable. It was the opposite of the 'heroic medicine' of the time, medicine that by its excesses killed as often as it cured.[33] Ironically, homeopathy becomes the touchstone for quackery in debates occurring early on in the era of scientific medicine.

Allopaths, then as now, were also called 'regular' doctors, but were then only one of several medical sects trying to establish themselves professionally during the pre-scientific age and, as we shall discuss below, acquired monopolistic control over medical practice by the early part of the twentieth century. Structural factors contributed to the demise of most of the competing sects, among them educational reform, medical regulation and control of the medical marketplace. Those sects not eliminated were co-opted, subsumed or marginalized, and allopathy became legally established as the standard for the medical profession.[34] 'Allopathic' medicine then became orthodox medicine became scientific medicine, and any practice not sanctioned by the orthodoxy became heterodox practice and was dismissed as quackery.[35]

Michel Foucault observed that clinical medicine did not qualify as a science in post-Revolutionary France 'not only because it does not comply with the formal criteria, or attain the level of rigour expected of physics, chemistry, or even of physiology; but also because it involves a scarcely organized mass of empirical observations, uncontrolled experiments and results, therapeutic prescriptions, and institutional regulations'.[36] He described the production and diffusion of biomedical knowledge in the late eighteenth century as reflecting the emergence of a 'collective consciousness'. This can be seen as a process that entails 'all developments which favored positive attitudes to health, illness and science-based medicine in conjunction with the spread of rationalist value-systems and forms of behavior, particularly in private life, the displacement of traditional behavioral orientations fixed in subcultures and the adoption by society in general of bourgeois norms'.[37] And it moved the focus of healthcare simultaneously onto newly defined secular professional structures authorized by the state as well as onto a greater reliance on notions that science replaced or at least competed with theology in popular belief.

With the rise of modern scientifically oriented medicine typified by Germanophone schools of medicine in the mid-nineteenth century, the presumption about the relationship between the acquisition of scientific knowledge and its application to medical therapies came to be based on an image of empirical science that evolved as much in physics and chemistry as it did in biology. Indeed, Jeremy Bentham, at the very beginning of the nineteenth century, when organic chemistry begins to come into its own defining the new science, uses this analogy when he writes that 'as chemistry extends itself, the quack is injured. So as Utilitarianism spreads, the political and ethical quack is exposed.'[38] Thus one of the central questions we need to confront is whether the ever-shifting standards of evidence in the so-called bench sciences are appropriate when applied to the amorphous field of 'medical science'.

Wilhelm von Humboldt, Prussian academician and statesman, created the model of the modern research institution in Berlin in 1810. He envisaged a *universitas litterarum* uniting teaching and research under the same roof. This concept of a university devoted to creating and transmitting knowledge (*Bildung*) spread throughout the German-speaking world during the nineteenth century and served as a model for universities over the next century and a half. But he also insisted that it be a moral force. Humboldt was influenced by the reform ideas of the philosopher Johann Gottlieb Fichte, first vice chancellor of the university in Berlin, and by the theologian and philosopher Friedrich Schleiermacher. Both wished to break with the institutions of the past that perpetuated older views rather than questioning them. From the outset, the university had the traditional four faculties of Law, Medicine, Philosophy and Theology. But it was claimed that these faculties were radically different from the traditional university, with its medieval origins, its notions of investiture and its exclusive concern with the passing on of received knowledge rather than the *generation* of knowledge.

Research had been undertaken – if at all – in the academies. This was especially true in the new 'natural' sciences, such as biology. When Johannes Müller (MD, University of Bonn, 1822) came to Berlin in 1833 as a full professor of anatomy, physiology and pathology, he pioneered the idea of the modern laboratory, even though he undertook his research in his own rented rooms. He created a research group, apportioned aspects of each of his projects and encouraged his students to undertake research. Müller strongly encouraged his students to branch off and conduct further work on their own and in collaboration with other young scientists. Among these students numbered the founders of modern neurology, including Robert Remak (MD, University of Berlin, 1838) (Remak's fibres) and Friedrich Henle (MD, University of Bonn, 1832) (Henle's sheath). Another of Müller's students was Hermann von Helmholtz (MD, University of Berlin, 1842), well regarded as a physicist, physiologist, physician, biologist, mathematician, philosopher, engineer and inventor – a polymath who made important discoveries in physiology, optics, electrodynamics, mathematics and meteorology.

These students and others, such as Rudolf Virchow (MD, University of Berlin, 1843), the father of modern cellular pathology, were the cream of nineteenth-century medical science, and their students included physicians such as Sigmund Freud (Dr. med., 1881; habilitation, 1885, Neuropathology, University of Vienna, with advanced studies in Paris), a student of the polymath Ernst von Brücke (MD, University of Berlin, 1842), who had been a student of Müller. All saw collaborative research as the core of natural science and the university as the appropriate place to undertake this. The reform of the Viennese university and the creation of the so-called Second Viennese School of Medicine in the 1830s, under the aegis of the pathologist Carl Rokitansky (MD, University of Vienna, 1828), with its emphasis on laboratory research and its application to human medicine, took place in the shadow of Humboldt's reforms.[39] Indeed, Rokitansky became the first freely elected rector of the University of Vienna in 1852. This resulted in the concomitant development, in Vienna and elsewhere, of ever more specialties and sub-specialties. Vienna saw the first clinics in the world for dermatology, as well as for conditions of the eye and also of the ear, nose and throat; these, and many others, were quickly paralleled across the teaching institutions and their practice of medicine. Does ever greater specialization not mean a system of merit based on scientific accomplishment and ability? Is not elite, objective medical science, proven through examination, separate from all the tawdry aspects of the quotidian, as Max Weber had imagined?

This was certainly not true in scientific medicine, where race, gender and class were seen as disqualifications for medical training. At

the close of the nineteenth century, Sigmund Freud found those within
Vienna's medical education and practice establishment increasingly
hostile to psychoanalysis because he and most of his early followers were Jews. The great surgeon Theodor Billroth (MD, University
of Berlin, 1852) had already warned about such eastern Jews as the
Moravian Sigmund Freud, who studied with Billroth in 1876–7, and
who were already present (in his estimation) in overly great numbers
in the Viennese medical school exactly at that moment, in 1876:

> the Jews are a sharply defined nation, and . . . no Jew, just like
> no Iranian, Frenchman, New Zealander, or African, can ever
> become a German; what they call Jewish-Germans are simply
> nothing but Jews who happen to speak German and happened
> to receive their education in Germany, even if they write litera-
> ture and think in the German language more beautifully and
> better than many a genuine Germanic native. Therefore [we
> should] neither expect nor want the Jews ever to become true
> Germans in the sense that during national battles they feel the
> way we Germans do.

Those Jews who had emigrated from the eastern Marches of the Austro-
Hungarian Empire, he argued, were lacking 'our German sentiments',
which were based on 'medieval Romanticism'. Not mere chemistry, as
the Jews were accused of reducing medicine to. Billroth admitted that
inside, 'even though I have reflected about this a great deal and do like
some of them individually', he still felt 'the gap between purely German
and purely Jewish blood to be just as wide as the gap a Teuton may
have felt between himself and a Phoenician'.[40] Billroth, who later in
the century became an *opponent* of political antisemitism, spoke from
the metaphoric lectern of the new scientific structure of the European
medical school, where race science was ubiquitous.

It was little different in Berlin in 1884. For when the then Montreal-
based Sir William Osler returned to Berlin he found that

> the modern 'hep, hep, hep' [yelled in the streets by antisemites
> hounding Jews] shrieked in Berlin for some years past has by
> no means died out . . . I hope to be able to get the data with
> reference to the exact number of professors and docents of
> Hebrew extraction in the German Medical Faculties. The

number is very great, and of those I know, their positions have been won by hard and honorable work; but I fear that, as I hear has already been the case, the present agitation will help to make the attainment of University professorships additionally difficult. One cannot but notice here, in any assembly of doctors, the strong Semitic element; at the local societies, and at the German Congress of Physicians, it was particularly noticeable, and the same holds good in any collection of students.

He concludes: 'All honor to them!'[41]

In the United States Theodor Billroth's views became dogma in the age of scientific medicine as William H. Welch (MD, Columbia College of Physicians and Surgeons, 1875; postgraduate work with, among others, Rudolf Virchow in Berlin), the founding dean of the school of medicine as well as the school of public health at Johns Hopkins, introduced a translation of Billroth's screed in 1924, half a century after it was published. There he described the book as a work of enduring value, characterized by a breadth of view as sound and as needful today as when it was first published in 1876, as it heralded 'the centrality of a liberal and scientific training in preparation for the study of medicine'. And he characterized Billroth's overt antisemitism as 'his remarks concerning the lack of cultural, family background and the dire effects of penury on many of the medical students'.[42] Something, of course, the American Brahmins of the new scientific medicine would try to avoid. No hunting Jews down in the streets of Cambridge, Massachusetts, crying 'hep, hep, hep!' Rather the president of Harvard, A. Lawrence Lowell, in 1926 quietly instituted the creation of quotas for Jews in all aspects of university life and education after the percentage of Jewish students, however defined, rose to uncomfortable levels (for him) in Ivy League institutions. This was quickly adopted in elite medical schools across the country.

Is Medicine Ideological?

One needs to add that Jeremy Bentham's assumptions about the age of Enlightenment science (biology and chemistry at least) and the concomitant reforming of the practice of medicine into medical science were not merely a response to the innovations and thus revised status of 'science' but a reaction to the mid-century claims that medicine, rather than being apolitical, was *very* political. Transparency is the key word for Bentham's Enlightenment: 'How many are the dangerous remedies – nay, actual poisons – sold boldly by quacks as a secret and wonderful cure, as to which it would be easy to disillusion the most credulous mind by simply disclosing their composition?'[43] And that too is the physician's task. In the great year of revolutions, 1848, Rudolf Virchow, who became a leading figure both in the radical innovations within biology and medicine (through his focus on 'cellular pathology', the title of his 1858 book) and (as a longtime member of the German parliament) in his political opposition to Bismarck, stated in the preface to his new – and sadly short-lived – medical journal:

> Medicine is a social science and politics is nothing else but medicine on a large scale. Medicine as a social science, as the science of human beings, has the obligation to point out problems and to attempt their theoretical solution; the politician, the practical anthropologist, must find the means for their actual solution . . . Science for its own sake usually means nothing more than science for the sake of the people who happen to be pursuing it. Knowledge which is unable to support action is not genuine – and how unsure is activity without understanding . . . If medicine is to fulfil her great task, then she must enter the political and social life . . . The physicians are the natural lawyers of the poor, and the social problems should largely be solved by them.[44]

The echoes of Jeremy Bentham can still be heard here: 'what the physician is to the natural body, the legislator is to the political: legislation is the art of medicine exercised upon a grand scale.'[45] That Virchow sees the true physician as an advocate, not merely as a scientist, leads him to place his understanding of the potential of a new social medicine in opposition to the quacks, whom he sees as a product of ignorance rather than its exploiter: 'Laws should be made, not against quacks but against superstition.' (Echoing Enlightenment opposition to 'theology', not religion.) For, he notes, 'Imprisoned quacks are always replaced by new ones.' Within or without the established medical system.[46] And that system too has its innate problem, one Virchow knew better than most as he was also a powerful advocate for social reform. Scientific medicine in its infancy was unstable in its claims, for following *the* science often meant being left in the dust by the next wave of science. In an age when eugenics was as important a science as bacteriology, the implications for the application of any given science could lead to consequences that would have shocked Virchow, as was evident in Nazi Germany only a few generations later.[47] And he overlooked something that became evident as scientific medicine evolved, that 'certain features of doctor-patient encounters "medicalize," and therefore depoliticize, the social structural roots of personal suffering.'[48] Something that will also be a red thread in this volume.

Virchow's British contemporary, the economist and essayist Walter Bagehot, observed that 'It is, as people say, so upsetting; it makes you think that, after all, your favourite notions may be wrong, your firmest beliefs ill founded; it is certain that till now there was no place allotted in your mind to the new and startling inhabitant; and now that it has conquered an entrance you do not at once see which of your old ideas it will not turn out, with which of them it can be reconciled, and with which it is at essential enmity.'[49] Disconcerting in an age demanding a new scientific verity for diagnosis and predictability. But not a new dilemma in modern medicine. The newly invested George Cheyne (MD, King's College, Cambridge, 1701), the noted Scottish physician and friend of Isaac Newton, had asked in 1702 'whether one who practises by a certain demonstrable Theory, be not to be esteem'd a truer Physician, than one who practises by a false Precarious and Contradictory one; Or (seeing a False Theory is worse and more Prejudicial to Practice than none at all) whether an able Physician, be not to be trusted too rather than a meer [*sic*] Quack.'[50] That in an age where theories gave way to theories, all well founded, and all contradictory, and all capable of healing or harming.

We need to remember that the conflict between France and Germany, after France loses the Franco-Prussian War in 1870–71 and the king of Prussia is crowned emperor of Germany in Versailles, continues to be played out in the fields of medical science. French schools of medicine that had dominated its very beginnings gave way to the model of the new, integrated Germanophone universities. The 'German Problem' of the late nineteenth century – as the newly unified Germany increasingly gained scientific, technological and industrial dominance – fed tensions among European nations during this age of scientific medicine. Germ theory's applications were embedded in the heightening quest by France, Germany, Britain and Italy to colonize Africa and Asia with the aid of a new medical (and scientific) specialty, that of tropical medicine. In 1883 a massive cholera epidemic broke out in Alexandria, Egypt. Both Louis Pasteur (Doctorate, Chemistry and Physics, École normale supérieure, Paris, 1847) and Robert Koch (MD, University of Göttingen, 1866) were sent on missions vying to identify its cause. Koch returned victorious, whereupon Pasteur switched research direction and began the development of a rabies vaccine. And German medicine became the world's norm. Meiji Japan, when it sought to modernize, brought imperial Germany in to create modern, scientific medical training (and a modern armed forces). Germs may be 'apolitical', but scientific medicine is not.

Science in Medicine

The idea that there could be absolute boundaries for the new scientific medicine is perhaps best exemplified by the model ascribed to Robert Koch, who was believed to have defined the evidence one needed to correlate infectious agents with resulting disease processes. Koch had identified the bacteria that were causal for cholera and would later win the Nobel Prize for Physiology or Medicine in 1905 for his 'investigations and discoveries in relation to tuberculosis'. The microscopic organisms that cause the disease, he was claimed to have postulated in the early 1880s, should be found in those presenting with the disease; they should be able to be cultured in the laboratory outside of the host; they should cause the disease when reintroduced from the bench sample, and should then be able to be harvested from the newly infected patients. This was evidence that evoked the assumptions of the science of the day.

We need to note that Koch seems never to have made these radical claims in defining the parameters of scientific medicine. They were first presented in a rough and ready way in 1884 in a paper on diphtheria by the University of Greifswald-based bacteriologist Friedrich Loeffler (MD, University of Berlin, 1874), who in 1898 identified the *virus* that caused foot-and-mouth disease. The scientific method was attributed to Koch because of his prominence, even though Koch, like Pasteur, was often much looser with his claims about evidence in his laboratory practice. Indeed, the debates about Koch's postulates 'proving' causality in infectious disease is based more on anecdote than actual clinic practice. As Christoph Gradmann writes: 'Koch's postulates do not stand for any particular methodology. They depict instead a world view that lends itself to be represented in numerous methodologies.'[51] Koch quickly realized that there were asymptomatic patients with the cholera bacillus, one of the diseases he studied, and we now know that there were causal agents (eventually identified as viruses) that could not be grown on a petri dish, and most importantly that not all infectious agents caused disease in everyone exposed.[52]

Still, today 'Koch's postulates' remain an article of faith in the transfer of the claims defining evidence in nineteenth-century bench science to human medicine.[53] And in public health, the field that deals with the definition of infectious diseases in its day-to-day activities and which was the focus of much of Koch's research, his attempt to provide a working definition of causality failed. In 1965 Sir Austin Bradford Hill (BSc, Economics, London University, External, 1922), who had created the first modern randomized study, that of the efficacy of streptomycin in 1948, trying to rethink what he thought were 'Koch's postulates', argued that a much wider range of criteria needed to be employed to understand causality of disease transmission within and between collectives: strength, consistency, specificity, temporality, biological gradient, plausibility, coherence, analogy and perhaps even reversibility. Hill noted that one could perhaps, *might*, appeal also to experimental evidence as another criterion.[54] At the rise of our age of genetics, more attention was paid to molecular identification of the causation of pathology. New criteria for causation were developed by the microbiologist Stanley Falkow (PhD, Microbiology, Brown University, 1961) in 1988 as 'Falkow's postulates', which linked a specific phenotype with a negative outcome, the ability to 'turn off' the link to eliminate the pathology, and to reverse or replace the gene to restore pathology.[55] By 1996, David N. Fredricks (MD, Case Western Reserve University, 1990) and David A. Relman (MD, Harvard Medical School, 1982) had upped the chain of proof to seven guidelines for establishing genetic causation.[56] Each scientific model of efficacy and evidence is succeeded by new ones as the very models of science change, moving from the cell to society, from the race to the gene.

Underlying the problem of defining modern medical science was and is the question: what is being treated by allopathic medicine? One of the great revolutions of the nineteenth century was the abandonment of the Cartesian claim that the mind and the body were two distinct and separate entities. The German Romantics had already taken on Descartes (as well as his Platonic predecessors), who argued that there was an inherent dualism between – and here lies the problem of nomenclature – psyche/mind/soul and our physical self, however defined. Yet Descartes' concept of the reflex arc and the postulation of the body as a machine responding to the immediate environment, and the mind as seat of the soul and passions, quite separate from the body, opened up the possibility of animal models of bodily function, whether appropriate or not, and gave rise to modern experimental medicine that still needed to distance the soul from the body.

By the nineteenth century these aspects of the human being were seen as marginally interactive with each other, but only with the rise of scientific medicine over the nineteenth century did this relationship come to be understood as cutting both ways: that the mind could impact the body just as much as the body could impact the mind. The relationship of these two aspects of the human still gave prominence, however, to the physical. The mental was seen as an epiphenomenon even when labelled as intrinsic. This was the age of a clearly biological psychiatry, as Wilhelm Griesinger (MD, University of Tübingen, 1838) wrote in 1868: 'The so-called mental illnesses are found in individuals suffering from brain- and nerve illness.'[57] Griesinger and neurologist Carl Westphal (MD, University of Berlin, 1855) led a school proposing a materialistic theory of mental diseases. They argued early on that psychiatric diseases were diseases of the brain and soon would support this view with scientific data obtained from detailed microscopic studies stained to reveal evidence via the newest chemical innovations. These methodological and related scientific innovations gained importance in the practice of medicine towards the end of the nineteenth century and led to a mutual enhancement and eventual merging of science and medicine. Today we still struggle to think about human beings as a single entity. We no longer assume the existence of mind *and* body or brain, mind *and* body or soul, brain, mind *and* body, but rather, as the field of Disability Studies has proposed, as a 'bodymind'. That there are *no* boundaries between these categories we acknowledge, but we still seem to be unable to imagine ourselves without such boundaries. Scientific medicine cannot escape boundaries even where no boundaries could possibly exist.

Medical Degrees and Nobel Prizes

As the reader has seen and will continue to see throughout this book, I have noted both the academic degrees and the specific honours, especially the Nobel Prize in Physiology or Medicine, given to a range of medical scientists: the puzzle of this book is that some of these individuals are now seen as 'quacks'. Investiture is defined by status and status by titles and awards. Degrees matter, as we shall see: in Great Britain by the end of the nineteenth century the core degree to practise medicine as a licensed physician was the BM or BS (Bachelor of Medicine or Bachelor of Surgery); the MD (*Doctoris Medicinae*, or Doctor of Medicine) was a research degree, gained by thesis; in the USA the degree needed to practise medicine is the MD or the DO (Doctor of Osteopathy); in Germany, the basic examination needed to practise is a three-part examination in medicine given by the state, and only about 60 per cent of those who pass go on to the MD (with the title Dr med., or Doctor of Medicine) – this is technically a research degree, as there is a formal need for a thesis, but the true research degree is the habilitation in medicine.

One can note that in Great Britain people could qualify as practitioners without a university degree up until the 1980s by gaining the conjoint diplomas from the Royal College of Physicians and the Royal College of Surgeons (designated MRCS, or Member RCS) and LRCP (Licentiate of the RCP), or until the 1990s with the LSA, Licentiate of the Society of Apothecaries. Eligibility to sit for these diplomas was based on having had a recognized university-based education. Likewise in the USA, until the end of the nineteenth century, it was possible to achieve licensure in some states through an apprenticeship with a licensed physician.

All of these are the prerequisites for state licensure. In all cases it is the state that grants the right to practise medicine, but the university that grants the degree. What is also given is the status of the physician in the estimation of the patient, for whom a degree (and the attendant state licensure) proves the bona fides of not only the individual but the claims of the therapies and underlying science. The stature of the institution seems to add a guarantee of its products, however well or poorly prepared they seemed to be. A doc from a prestigious university (Harvard or Oxford) already has a level of believability, of charisma, baked into their degree.

The status of surgeons as opposed to physicians has shifted over time: in the early modern period, while their skills were recognized, they were considered different from the doc, who also covered the role of the pharmacist. The British tradition of calling surgeons 'Mr' rather than 'Dr' – which arose in 1745, when surgeons could be self-certified by the Company of Surgeons (later the Royal College of Surgeons) but not invested as physicians – made a distinction, which after the introduction of anaesthesia and antisepsis attributed a higher, rather than lower, status. Indeed, there remains a certain snobbism in the United Kingdom and the Republic of Ireland associated with surgeons calling themselves 'Mr' or 'Miss' (or indeed 'Ms') rather than 'Dr'.[58] This never caught on in the United States, where the title 'Dr' always provided higher status, whatever the specialty, even though in 1765 John Morgan (MD, University of Edinburgh, 1763), newly returned from Great Britain, advocated for the separation of surgery from 'physic',[59] as well as the state licensure of physicians – to great opprobrium from his fellow physicians, all of them doctors. Of course, Morgan and his colleagues could not have imagined certifying a female physician!

One needs to note that the limitations of the use of the title 'Dr' remain arbitrary. Today California has the most stringent control of this appellation, as only licensed physicians or surgeons, that is, MDs or DOs, can be a 'Dr'. In a recent case a local district attorney fined a nurse with an 'earned doctorate degree in nursing practice', who 'began promoting herself as "Doctor Sarah Erny"', almost $20,000. 'While in most instances Ms. Erny indicated that she was a nurse practitioner, she failed to advise the public that she was not a medical doctor and failed to identify her supervising physician'.[60] Certainly, alternative healthcare approaches, such as chiropractic practices, also fail this test, even if the individual has earned a doctorate. As one commentator noted, 'if you read the law literally, it appears to prohibit even PhDs and university professors from using the title'.[61] Never mind medical school professors without an MD.

The Nobel Prize remains the most sought after and most prestigious award in scientific medicine. Yet there are always outliers. Here we can mention the Portuguese neurologist António Caetano de Abreu Freire Egas Moniz (MD, University of Coimbra, 1899), who was awarded the 'Nobel Prize in Physiology or Medicine' in 1949 'for his discovery of the therapeutic value of leucotomy in certain psychoses'. In other words, for the development of the lobotomy, the most controversial of all surgical interventions for mental illness. I was raised with the horrific image of the transorbital lobotomy in Ken Kesey's novel *One Flew over the Cuckoo's Nest* (1962) and Miloš Forman's film of 1975. Indeed, when I wrote my *Seeing the Insane* (1982), a cultural history of how the mentally ill were portrayed, I concluded with the patients of Ward 81 – a high-security, locked psychiatric facility for women photographed by Mary Ellen Mark at the Oregon State Hospital in Salem, where the film was shot. Yet almost fifty years later, we could argue (but won't here) that the plethora of contemporary technologies such as the responsive neurostimulator and deep-brain stimulation are the bastard children of the lobotomists, who were so convinced that mental illness was a structural brain malfunction that they felt only a physical, not a psychological or pharmaceutical, intervention was necessary.

Moniz was one of only two psychiatrists ever to win the Nobel Prize for Physiology or Medicine. The first was Julius Wagner-Jauregg (MD, University of Vienna, 1880) in 1927 'for his discovery of the therapeutic value of malaria inoculation in the treatment of dementia paralytica'.[62] Wagner-Jauregg's contribution, the treatment of tertiary syphilis ('general paralysis of the insane') by infecting patients with malaria, seems just as much a form of quackery today as does the lobotomy, if we do not recognize that it was the forerunner of a wide range of 'shock therapies' for mental illness – including the Italian neurologist (MD, University of Rome, 1901; trained also in Turin, Paris and Munich) Ugo Cerletti's development of electroconvulsive therapy (ECT) in 1938. ECT was initially scientific medicine, then it was cruel quackery; today, with many tweaks, it is again scientific medicine.

Some of the Nobel Prize winners were and are seen as medical pioneers but sometimes did not completely understand the implications of their innovations, while others, ignored in their own times by such honours, were true pioneers. I have also mentioned when and where physicians received their medical qualifications as far as I could uncover this information, as this too is an index of status and provides a roadmap to the trajectory of scientific medicine. Such social indexes measure the status and visibility of medicine and its practitioners in our world in the light of what Jacalyn Duffin calls the 'Secular Religion of Science':

> The Prizes celebrate discovery. But the concept of a 'Eureka-like' discovery is unfashionable among historians or philosophers

– and with good reason. Every important discovery arises from another. New observations rarely turn out to be as original as they first seem; most are reformulations of old ideas. Moreover, many discoveries emerge simultaneously by different workers in different places. Scientists are all chipping away at the same coalface. Second, the prizes assign priority to individuals, sometimes undeserved, often contested, and frequently political. Yet – just as historians doubt the originality and singularity of discoveries, they have also become skeptical of celebrating individual actors of the past. Rather, they emphasize external forces that conspired to place a person in position to observe (or proclaim) something seemingly new.[63]

The medical sociologist Robert K. Merton wrote of the 'instructively ambiguous' categories of 'excellence' and 'recognition' that feature in the Nobel Prize as an example of 'excellence as performance/ recognition as honorific'.[64] Alfred Nobel's three famous criteria for a prize-worthy achievement ('recency', 'benefit to mankind' and 'discovery') seem to not only shift during the twentieth century, the age of scientific medicine, but waver between what Merton sees as the key to the prize, the single achievement, and a lifetime's work.[65] In the end the Nobel Prize is an index that creates public awareness of scientific medicine rather than tracking it.

We shall be focusing for obvious reasons on the Nobel Prize for Medicine or Physiology. This was first awarded in 1901 to the German physiologist Emil Adolf von Behring for his discovery of serum therapy in the development of the diphtheria and tetanus vaccines that put 'in the hands of the physician a victorious weapon against illness and deaths'. In this book, as I have noted, I often identify the academic position, training and degrees that individuals acquired. Behring, for example, did not come out of the fabled medical school of Humboldt's University of Berlin, where it was claimed laboratory science and clinical medicine were first merged, but rather the very marginal Kaiser-Wilhelm-Akademie, the training school for military physicians. He received his degree from what was a trade school in 1878 and achieved his status in the academy only in 1895, with a professorial appointment at Marburg. Behring's award sets the tone for many of the later prizes, as it is seen as a weapon in the struggle to overcome the vulnerabilities of the human condition through science. It is always an account of the laboratory presenting to the clinician the necessary tools of science and therefore is always, as Jacalyn Duffin concludes, a case of 'inspiration in narratives of overcoming obstacles and conquering problems. These are optimistic stories for a world that is skeptical of saints and unbelieving in God, and ready for the secular religion of science.' This too is part of our story, for those who fail to fulfil this role often wind up over time becoming 'quacks'.[66]

Our Age of Quackery

Our modern sense of quackery seems to be a reflex of the first age of biology, of the age of Robert Koch and Louis Pasteur, with its often contradictory claims about scientific objectivity. It rests on the claim, hotly debated during the late nineteenth century, that science 'unveils' nature. That is, what science does is to examine a reality separate from

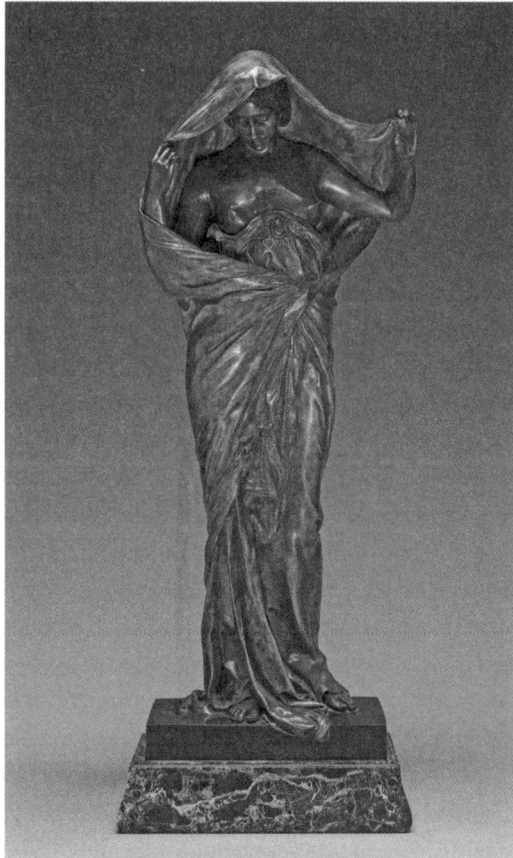

Louis-Ernest Barrias, *Nature Unveiling Herself before Science*, model 1895–9, cast *c.* 1900, bronze with silvering and malachite.

all ideology and perception. This anti-Kantian notion shapes science
and demands an absolute and demonstrable distinction between science and 'quackery'. It is no accident that this Enlightenment trope
becomes realized in Louis-Ernest Barrias' sculpture, often reproduced
at the time, of *Nature Unveiling Herself before Science*, which 'blends
the ancient trope of the veil of Isis, interpreted as nature's desire to
hide her secrets, with the modern fantasy of (female) nature willingly
revealing herself to the (male) scientist, without violence or artifice'.[67]
What is central to our interest is that it was commissioned in 1889
to decorate the new scientific faculty of medicine created during the
1880s at the medieval university at Bordeaux, which had been founded
in 1441.

The first anti-quackery society, the Vereniging tegen de Kwakzalverij
(Society against Quackery), was founded in the Netherlands in 1881 and
has published its magazine *Nederlands Tijdschrift tegen de Kwakzalverij*
(Dutch Magazine against Quackery) ever since. In imperial Germany it
took two decades until the Deutsche Gesellschaft zur Bekämpfung des
Kurpfuschertums (German Society for the Repression of Quackery)
was founded at Berlin in 1903, primarily by physicians.[68] Its goal, never
completely fulfilled, was to encourage better hygiene – and therefore
less reliance on quack medicine. It also wanted to further new legislation defining quackery and limiting those who could practise healing
to those with formal medical training, rescinding a law passed in
1869 granting *Kurierfreiheit*, the right of anyone, no matter what their
training or lack of it, to treat. These limiting measures were never
realized.

The focus of such claims on the part of the new medical science
was against those drugs and therapies that did 'harm', which many
certainly did, for this new age of scientific medicine in the early nineteenth century rediscovered the ancient Hippocratic oath and added
to it the admonition, missing in the Greek, to 'do no harm'. But then
again it was Euripides, author of a string of ancient Greek tragedies,
who made the claim that 'blessed is he who has gained the knowledge
of science. He has no impulses to harm his fellow men or to do unjust
deeds; he contemplates the ageless order of deathless nature, how it
came to be formed, its manner, its ways. Such men have no care for
deeds of shame'.[69] A claim to be found more frequently even among the
Greeks in the world of fantasy than in reality.[70] Few in the first age of
scientific medicine asked loudly about efficacy, for that demanded the

sort of claims that were much weaker than 'do no harm'. Thus, the law quickly realized that the legal term for quack in German – *Kurpfucher*, or 'to botch a cure' – could apply even to those with medical training and licensure, who 'did harm'.

The British surgeon and antiquarian Thomas Inman (MD, University of London, 1844) did understand this. It is to Inman that the modern introduction of the phrase 'to do no harm' has been regularly attributed.[71] He in turn attributes the phrase *primum es tut non nocere* (first of all do no harm), in a historicizing gesture, to the noted seventeenth-century physician Thomas Sydenham (BM [Bachelor of Medicine], University of Oxford, 1648), in whose works it is not to be found. Inman employs it to give a basis to his own claim that using colchicine to cure gout was a useless and painful intervention if dosed in such a way as to produce violent physical symptoms, as, paraphrasing the Latin, 'we believe that the principle of doing evil to the constitution that good may come is as false in medicine as it is in theology'.[72] Colchicine, while long used as a natural therapy, was isolated in 1820 by the same chemists who had isolated the active ingredient in quinine. It was part of the new biochemical science in the employ of scientific medicine. Inman does not dismiss colchicine as an effective therapy for gout even with its potential to cause death, but he rejects a sort of reversal of the homeopathic notion of 'like curing like', which he dismissed as it was claimed that only when the dosage of the medication created violent symptoms was it efficacious. But efficient it is. Following *the* science had to be mediated by clinical experience.

The age of science defined the new quack in a political context. For this was also the age of European literary naturalists, who examined the impact of poverty and alienation (Émile Zola, Henrik Ibsen, Gerhart Hauptmann), and their North American cousins, the so-called Muckrakers, from Upton Sinclair to Jacob Riis, who focused on poverty and capitalism. Social inequality was marked to no little extent by the state of the people's health and the invidious role played by state structures to undermine it, as in Ibsen's *An Enemy of the People* (1882) and *The Jungle* (1905/6) by Upton Sinclair. These were followed up by the Muckraker journalist Samuel Hopkins Adams's widely read 1905 essays in *Collier's Weekly*, later circulated by the American Medical Association (AMA) as a pamphlet entitled 'The Great American Fraud'. The result is that there was a demand for some type of intervention to help assure the health of the most vulnerable. The USA's Pure Food and

Drug Act of 1906 seemed to ban quack medicine, though it turned out only to demand a listing of ingredients with no proof of efficacy (other than the puffery of the manufacturer). In 1912 the Act was amended to require that labels must not 'bear or contain any statement, design, or device regarding the curative or therapeutic effect of such article or any of the ingredients or substances contained therein, which is false and fraudulent'.[73] Who was to judge what was false and/or fraudulent was left up to the u.s. Department of Agriculture's Division of Chemistry, which had published a series of pamphlets from 1887 to 1902 on food adulterants. The state defines and then determines efficacy for the clinician.

In the United Kingdom, the British Medical Association (BMA) began publishing a series of articles from 1904 to 1909 (later collected as *Secret Remedies: What They Cost and What They Contain*) that exploded the claims of a wide number of products and their purvey-ors.[74] Subsequent to the passage of the American Pure Food and Drug Act, British and European laws based on it were passed. With the passage of the amendments to the American act, eventually the Division of Chemistry morphed into the Food, Drug and Insecticide organization in 1927. Its name was eventually shortened to the Food and Drug Administration (FDA) in 1930. Science all, defining the clinic through its power to prohibit or promulgate specific forms of medical intervention, from pharmaceuticals to devices. And as you shall see, such state structures continue to play a major role in this debate, for good or for ill, until today.

Making Scientific Physicians

The labelling of docs either as physicians or as quacks seemed ever more fixed during the first ages of scientific biology. In the United States the proliferation of medical teaching institutions, the ability to self-certify as a physician by having been 'in pupillage' to a physician, and the relatively loose state certification, radically different from state to state, had meant that many who claimed the title 'doctor' (and practised some form of healing beyond the puffery of the title in advertising 'patent' medicines) were the subject of little oversight. In France, as early as 1778 rigorous state control over medical training and practice had been introduced, a system copied widely in continental Europe by the early nineteenth century. The Société royale de médecine policed

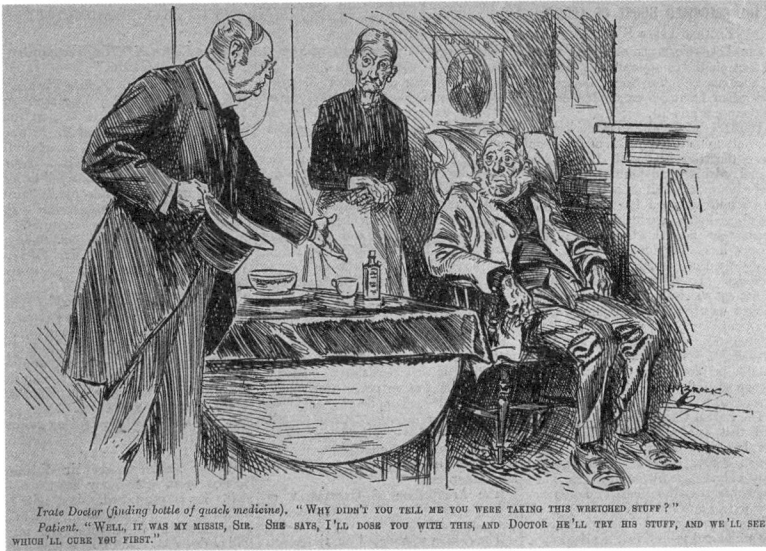

Irate Doctor (finding bottle of quack medicine). "WHY DIDN'T YOU TELL ME YOU WERE TAKING THIS WRETCHED STUFF?"
Patient. "WELL, IT WAS MY MISSIS, SIR. SHE SAYS, I'LL DOSE YOU WITH THIS, AND DOCTOR HE'LL TRY HIS STUFF, AND WE'LL SEE WHICH'LL CURE YOU FIRST."

A doctor angry with his patient for trying quack medicine as well as his own
prescription, engraving by H. M. Brock from *Punch; or, The London Charivari*
(20 October 1909).

both the practice of medicine and the sale of cures, as physicians were
often the source of the latter. It defined who and where one could
practise and what could be sold.[75] Quacks were thus those beyond the
system or who abused the system and the definition of both were left
to the state to enforce. Yet it was evident that 'untrained' (or at least
uncertified) practitioners, known as 'feldshers', could be as, or perhaps
even more, competent than those trained at universities.[76]

Great Britain, which had had a much looser set of structures, with
medical treatment reflecting Adam Smith's fantasy of the hidden hand
of the marketplace more than the science of the time, still defined and
acted upon notions of quackery. Yet Smith, ever aware of the fallibility
of human beings, paraphrases Epictetus in his other great book, *The
Theory of Moral Sentiments* (1759), in saying that medicine relies on
belief, for when we listen to the physicians' prescriptions 'we ought to
say that nature, the greater conductor and physician of the universe,
has ordered to such a man a disease, or the amputation of a limb, or the
loss of a child. By the prescriptions of ordinary physicians, the patient
swallows many a bitter potion – undergoes many a painful operation.
From the very uncertain hope, however, that health may be the consequence, he gladly submits to all.'[77] The Enlightenment, or at least
Adam Smith, recognizes that 'hope', belief, defines medical practice

47

of all stripes. This explains, as he says, 'the frequent, and often wonderful success of the most ignorant quacks and imposters'.[78] For him, the core of all human responses to interventions in disease is belief, linking both doc and quack.

The British medical historian Roy Porter put his finger on this when he wrote that the real question was not heterodoxy versus orthodoxy, as the state (at least in Great Britain in 1815) 'elevated medicine on to a more professional, more ethical plane, in part through erecting a tighter cordon sanitaire between it and what it abhorred as money-mongering quackery'.[79] But rather it was the case that medical practitioners 'of all sorts were competing for custom, recognition and reward. Each in his own way – top physician, humble general practitioner, empiric, folk healer – made his bid to seize the moral high ground in the medical arena in which the law was acknowledged to be dog-eat-dog.'[80] The world was not so 'divided neatly between physicians and surgeons practising their vocation, and disreputable businessmen selling their proprietary pills to a gullible public'. Porter also gestures at the difference between pre-modern (let us read this as pre-scientific) and modern (allopathic medicine in the age of laboratory science), as the profession itself created a distinction 'between the ways in which the "typical" itinerant, and the "typical" regular practitioner – both mythical beasts – drummed up custom and turned a penny: or whether the differences were as much matters of manner as of substance'. Porter demanded that we must 'examine the careers of quacks and regulars in tandem, rather than, as traditional, distinctly in separate genres of study'.[81] The dichotomies between 'popular' and 'elite' medicine, between 'popular' and 'professional' medicine, between 'school' medicine and 'traditional' medicine, or 'scientific' and 'alternative' medicine, were and are boundaries, seen as fixed and unchanging, among various schools and approaches. Yet wobbly they were and are.

The age of scientific medicine is therefore the age of medical professionalization. There are two models of professionalization following Max Weber: one proposed by the Harvard sociologist Talcott Parsons in his 1939 essay 'The Professions and Social Structure', where he described professionalization as a process characterized by self-regulation, technical expertise, disinterestedness and association among professionals; and the other, rooted in criticisms of Parsons's model, informed most concretely by Michel Foucault, which posited that the driving force of professionalization was to create and consoli-date power.[82] These complement each other in the rise of scientific medicine, as Parsons noted there was little difference between the 'altruism' ascribed to the profession of medicine and the 'egoism' that defined the businessman.[83] Indeed, in our discussion of stomach ulcers in the next chapter both models can be seen to be elided in medical praxis. Among the professions, medicine 'and possibly . . . medicine alone' was able to create 'a clear pattern of occupational dominance (or hierarchical organization of functional areas) . . . in a specific area of the social division of labor'.[84] *Sui generis* in all ways.

Parsons's work gave the political economist Eliot Freidson space to question the process of becoming a physician, of who could and can have access to schools of medicine, and the central role in scientific medicine of state licensure, of economic power and status acquisition within that now self-defined but not completely self-governing arena.[85] In other words, medicine was little different from all other professions except in its own account of its 'calling', as Max Weber labelled it. This concentration of power was accomplished, to no little degree, by ever greater levels of certification or investiture until physicians formed a 'community within a community', in the words of William J. Goode.[86] All still evoking and employing the magic of 'charisma' associated with healing even in the age of science.

In the United States in the mid-nineteenth century there were 150 American medical schools and more than 25,000 students attending them. Many of these medical schools were proprietary – run for profit by the physicians who owned them. Amazingly, almost half of the world's medical students were in this age of scientific medicine study-ing in American institutions. And on top of this it was still possible to practise medicine after a 'pupillage' (an apprenticeship with little or no formal medical study) or by having gone to the reformed medical schools of Europe, where the training was certainly much better than in the United States.

The typical American medical school curriculum consisted of two years of study, comprising text-based anatomy, physiology, chemis-try, pathology and 'materia medica' (pharmacology); the second year repeated the same lectures. This was followed by a pupillage for as long as four years. And most of the 'materia medica' was suspect, as a note in a medical journal in 1896 stated:

[The Columbus Pharmacal Co.] also furnishes prescription blanks on which the physician is requested to state whether the prescription is to be refilled or not, and the direction of the physician will be followed in this respect. It also announces that no proprietary or quack nostrums will be kept in stock and no cure-alls will be advertised or sold out of its store, its aim being to run a strictly first class pharmacy and to protect the physician and his patient from some of the abuses that have grown up in the drug business in the past few years.[87]

By the end of the nineteenth century, you could no longer simply shadow senior physicians as an apprentice and become a physician. Formal certification was demanded even when you shadowed them, yet over and over again the AMA, beginning with its founding in the 1840s, refused to require a formal medical school education for certification. Professional organizations, recognized by the state, were created for credentialling and the state accepted these, having acknowledged them as necessary for state certification. As early as the 1870s 'states began passing licensing laws in the hopes of raising standards. Medical progressives – hygienic optimists and therapeutic pessimists – agitated for them to prevent disease as well as "quackery".'[88] All that resulted was the proliferation of state-certified, but otherwise fly-by-night, schools of medicine that basically produced 'certified' quacks.

The line between quack and doc was often seen as an arbitrary boundary. The American novelist Caroline Lockhart moved as a working reporter to the West, to Cody, Wyoming, in 1904, exactly as the AMA finally began its work to regulate scientific medical training and thus certification. She authored a bestselling autobiographical novel reflecting life on the Western frontier that gives a sense of how medicine at this moment was seen to function, at least in the eyes of the lay public. In the novel, her protagonist comments to someone newly arrived at the frontier on the flexible ethical standard of physicians and their training:

'Of course there are high-brows who set the standards for themselves and others pretty high, and if I acted, or failed to act, in violation of all recognized methods of procedure, and with fatal results, they *might* make me trouble. But you can bet,' she finished with a grin, 'the ethics of the profession have saved many a poor quack's hide . . . Oh, they may have diplomas. A diploma doesn't mean so much in these days of cheap medical colleges where they grind 'em out by the hundreds; you need only know where to go and have the price . . . What difference does it make where your diploma's from to jays like these? . . . A little horse sense, a bold front, a hypodermic needle, and a few pills will put you a long way on your road among this class of people. I'm talkin' pretty free to an outsider, but,' she looked at him significantly, 'I know we can trust each other.'

The implication irritated him, but he ignored it for the present. 'Do you mean to tell me,' he demanded, 'that there are medical schools where you can *buy* a diploma? Where *anybody* can get through?'

She laughed at his amazement.[89]

Indeed, it did seem that 'anybody' could and did become a physician. And that, as at least one American-trained British physician at mid-century claimed, no such doctor can be a quack. The British physician in question had been condemned as a 'quack' by a professor at the University of Edinburgh for peddling a homeopathic, but seemingly effective, cure for 'cases of cancer, lupus, and ulcers'. His defence was, in 1854: 'the doctor, however, is not a quack; a term legitimately applied to those who, without a professional education, or a regard to the rules of science, make experiments with medicines . . . [He] was, for ten years, actively and extensively engaged in surgery in the United States. He obtained his diploma in the University of New York.'[90] This physician was John Pattison (MD) and his degree had been granted in 1843. His compound of the plant goldenseal (*Hydrastis canadensis)* and zinc chloride had long been recognized as having therapeutic value beyond the allopathic medicine of the time. By 1851 the pharmacologist Alfred A. B. Durand reported having isolated goldenseal's active ingredient: the alkaloid crystal $C_{22}N_{23}NO_6$. So much for that, as American medicine became the target of organized academic medicine, and its demand was that medicine hew to new standards, not of care, but of science, at least the science of which it approved.

But this was also the age of Arts and Crafts, a reactionary modernism that preached a return to the simpler forms for art and architecture, and also a radical reaction to such reforms and their claims. Its anti-industrial stance extended to the new scientific medicine. One of the most important American innovators of this school was the American Elbert Hubbard, a self-educated follower of William Morris, who published his screed against modern medicine in drama form, *The Doctors: A Satire in Four Seizures*, in 1909.[91] The plot of his drama is familiar: Mrs X is sent unconscious and in chains to the State Hospital asylum by her minister husband Rev. Cecil Kelrusey, whose family is distraught that he has married an 'actress'. Seizing their young child, he wants his wife declared permanently incompetent. Hubbard's satire echoes the life of Mrs Elizabeth Packard, which had made headlines in the 1860s when her minister husband had her committed for disagreeing with his theology. She was released only after a widely publicized court case recounted in her *Marital Power Exemplified; or, Three Years Imprisonment for Religious Belief* (1864).

The doctors who undertake to treat Mrs X in Hubbard's play use all the modern techniques of the time, such as the 'rest cure', described as a means of torture, in which the patient was strapped to a bed for weeks at a time. The names of the doctors, such as the head of the asylum Agnew Weir (based on S. Weir Mitchell [MD, Jefferson Medical College, 1851], the neurologist and creator of the 'rest cure') and his assistant Jean Charlcot (a satire of the Parisian neurologist Jean-Martin Charcot [MD, University of Paris, 1853], the major proponent of the diagnosis of hysteria), echo those of prominent 'alienists', the by then antiquated term for those dealing with pathologies of the mind. By the early twentieth century they would have been called psychiatrists. Despite the doctors and with the help of the workmen at the asylum Mrs X becomes a force for good in the lives of the patients, introducing 'healthy' activities such as gardening and exercise. She eventually converts Weir to her cause. And Weir admits:

> The science of medicine is an exploded science. It is founded on the idea that man's physical economy is not automatic; that it needs an engineer and also demands as much tinkering as a gasoline-engine. The doctors have called in the police to protect them in a monopoly under the pretense of protecting the people. That is, they have passed laws making it a misdemeanor for anyone to practice medicine save as the individual practices as they did [*sic*] . . . The irregulars have doubtless cured just as many patients as the orthodox doctors, and always you were safer in the hands of an ignoramus who

knew that he didn't know, than in the hands of an allopath who was sure he did.[92]

Mrs X is given a divorce, reclaims her child and marries Weir, who will run the asylum on heterodox principles, as 'this woman taught me truth. And hereafter I will practice the science of health, not the science of disease . . . No more violence – no more coercion – no more drugs.'[93]

The new asylum avoids modern, invasive therapies and relies on healthy food, exercise and fresh air, like American John Harvey Kellogg's Battle Creek Sanitarium, created by the vegetarian Seventh-Day Adventist Church. Indeed, this is the age in which 'Dr John' (MD, Bellevue Hospital Medical College, 1875) became a national figure advocating for what today would be called alternative and complementary therapies (such as his invention of the perfect breakfast, Corn Flakes) to be part of the new scientific medicine.[94] 'Be moderate in all things save the use of water, fresh air, & sunshine,' reads one of Hubbard's aphorisms in the play. All the 'scientific' doctors quit in disgust. Hubbard's critique of the evolving predominance of scientific medicine is that it is inhumane and unethical. For Hubbard, it is the docs who are the real quacks, treating the healthy and the ill for their own gain; being cruel and exploitative of the gullibility of their patients and refusing to acknowledge the 'natural' pathways to health.

An acid remark in 1906 by Hubbard's contemporary, the Irish vegetarian-naturopath George Bernard Shaw, echoes this discomfort in his drama *The Doctor's Dilemma* (1906), pitting the new medical science against public morality — and public morality loses when the physician-researcher in question excludes a subject from a trial of a new treatment for tuberculosis because he wishes to seduce the patient's wife. Shaw begins his very long preface to the drama by stating boldly that 'I presume nobody will question the existence of a widely spread popular delusion that every doctor is a man of science . . . the rank and file of doctors are no more scientific than their tailors; or, if you prefer to put it the reverse way, their tailors are no less scientific than they. Doctoring is an art, not a science.'[95] Shaw's Nobel Prize for Literature (1925; awarded 1926) was 'for his work which is marked by both idealism and humanity, its stimulating satire often being infused with a singular poetic beauty'. That year Johannes Fibiger (MD, University of Copenhagen, 1890) was awarded the prize for Physiology or Medicine, after ten years of being nominated annually, for his claim that he had discovered a causal link between stomach cancer and nematode (roundworm) infections, when in fact the non-cancerous tumours he observed were the result of his lab rats having been deprived of vitamin A. Not only was this simply wrong but it was one of the biggest blunders ever perpetrated by the Karolinska Institute that awards this Nobel Prize, according to one of its officials.[96] We know nothing about Fibiger's tailor.

Remaking American Medical Schools

In 1904 the AMA created the Council on Medical Education, which commissioned a report on the 150 medical schools then operating. By 1900 its constituency comprised fewer than 7 per cent of American 'healers'. Its membership had moved from the 1840s, where many of their members were themselves the product of the catch-as-catch-can system, to include more and more elite physicians who had had postgraduate training in Europe and many who were affiliated with university hospitals as researchers and educators. Allopathic physicians had begun to refer to their type of practice as 'scientific medicine' to differentiate themselves from 'quacks'.[97]

The AMA's Council on Medical Education, lacking both expertise and perceived neutrality, turned in 1908 to the Carnegie Foundation for the Advancement of Teaching to undertake a survey of the wide range of medical schools and then redefine who and what made a physician. The president of the Carnegie Foundation, Henry Pritchett, a staunch advocate of medical school reform, chose the schoolmaster and educational theorist Abraham Flexner (BA, Classics, Johns Hopkins University, 1886) to head the project. Flexner, who was to reform American medical education, was born in 1866 in Louisville, Kentucky, to German Jewish parents, and was the first of his family to attend university. Among his eight siblings, Simon Flexner (MD, Louisville Medical College, 1889; postgraduate studies at Johns Hopkins), whose studies Abraham funded through his teaching, became a bacteriologist and pathologist and later the first director of the Rockefeller Institute for Medical Research.

Abraham Flexner, who by 1904 was running a for-profit 'college' in Louisville, Kentucky, was funded by the Carnegie Foundation to examine the (implied: poor) state of American medical education. The report reflected its author's educational philosophy; it also reflected his obsession with the model of education that he had experienced as an undergraduate at the newly founded Johns Hopkins University. He had had the luck to study at the first American version of Humboldt's reformed university. His report institutionalized the claims of the first generation of modern bacteriology, of Robert Koch and Louis Pasteur and their followers: laboratory science was to be the basis for allopathic medicine. Bench science defined good medicine; everything else was quackery.

For Flexner, *The* Johns Hopkins University (its official name), established in 1876 in Baltimore, where he had gained his BA, was to be the model. Johns Hopkins was the first German-type research university in North America, which meant that its medical training combined bench science with the practice of medicine. Daniel Coit Gilman, founding president of Johns Hopkins, broke with the British 'college' model to create the first American research university. 'I think', Flexner wrote, 'it is a modest claim to say that the founding of the Johns Hopkins University by President Gilman was the starting point of higher education, in the modern sense of the term, in the United States.'[98]

The philanthropist Johns Hopkins had hired Gilman, the head of the Sheffield Scientific School at Yale prior to taking on the presidency of the University of California, as its first president. Gilman in turn brought in exponents of scientific medicine, such as the public health missionary and authority on hospital management John Shaw Billings (MD, Medical College of Ohio, 1860) to build the medical centre; and the pathologist and public health specialist William H. Welch, whom we have already met, as the medical school's first dean. Billings chose the Canadian Sir William Osler in 1893 to be the teaching hospital's physician-in-chief. All were exponents of scientific medicine, even at the bedside.

Flexner saw Osler, the physician who had returned from studying in imperial Germany, as 'a clinical scientist versed in both bedside medicine and the application of the knowledge and techniques of the fundamental sciences to the study of human diseases.'[99] *For Flexner,* 'progress in chemical, biological, and physical science was increasing the physician's resources, both diagnostic and remedial. Medicine, hitherto empirical, was beginning to develop a scientific basis and method. The medical schools had thus a different function to perform:

it took them upwards of half a century to wake up to the fact.'[100] Among the authorities that shaped his argument was Theodor Billroth's virulently antisemitic text of 1876, that, as we have seen, came to shape the accessibility of Jews, such as his brother, to American medicine. These new scientific medical schools, Flexner stated, were intended to dislodge only poorly trained doctors, not outright quacks:

> Already in 1907, 903 of the doctors graduated in that year held academic degrees; that is to say, fully one-half of the number the country actually needed could conform to the standard that has been urged, or better. There is at this moment absolutely nothing in the educational situation outside the south that countenances the least departure from the scientific basis necessary to the successful pursuit of modern medicine. For whose sake is it permitted? Not really for the remote mountain districts of the south, for example, whence the 'yarb doctor', unschooled and unlicensed, can in no event be dislodged.[101]

Regarding 'the medical dissenter: now, the primitive belief in magic crops up in his credulous respect for an impotent drug. Again, all other procedures having failed, what is there to lose by flinging one's self upon the mercy of chance?'[102] Here Flexner articulates the claims of the new scientific medicine that it is not a closed system, but rather an experimental one, like the bench sciences:

> We may then fairly describe modern medicine as characterized by a severely critical handling of experience. It is at once more skeptical and more assured than mere empiricism. For though it takes nothing on faith, the fact which it accepts does not fear the hottest fire. Scientific medicine is, however, as yet by no means all of one piece; uniform exactitude is still indefinitely remote; fortunately, scientific integrity does not depend on the perfect homogeneity of all its data and conclusions. Modern medicine deals, then, like empiricism, not only with certainties, but also with probabilities, surmises, theories.[103]

This, however, with verifiable, empirical data, and not subjective evaluation. Sir William Osler could claim in 1902 that

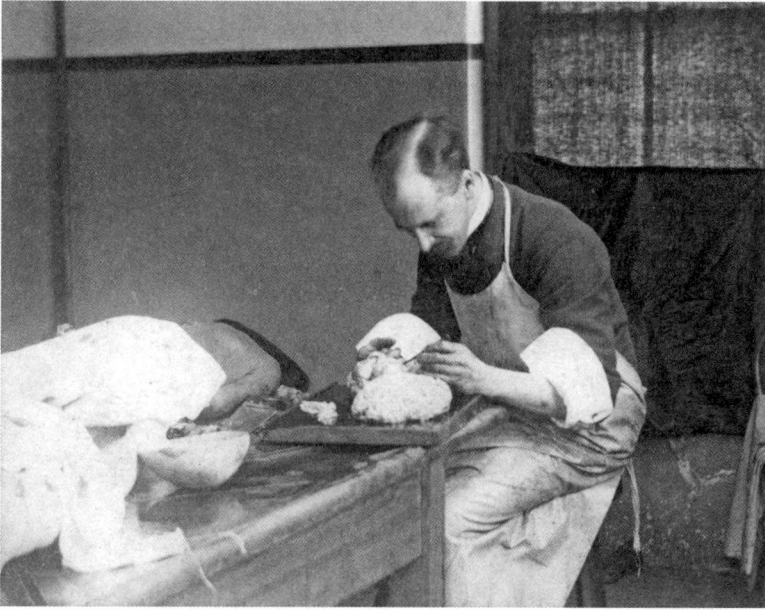

William Osler performing an autopsy at the Blockley Mortuary in Philadelphia, 1886, photograph by Samuel McClintock Hamill. Osler was appointed an official pathologist at Blockley Hospital soon after his arrival in Philadelphia, where he was Chair of Clinical Medicine at the University of Philadelphia from 1884 to 1889.

in the fight which we have to wage incessantly against ignorance and quackery among the masses and follies of all sorts among the classes, diagnosis, not drugging, is our chief weapon of offence. Lack of systematic personal training in the methods of the recognition of disease leads to the misapplication of remedies, to long courses of treatment when treatment is useless, and so directly to that lack of confidence in our methods, which is apt to place us in the eyes of the public on a level with empirics and quacks.[104]

We need to create an absolute boundary between them and us.

The result of Abraham Flexner's reforms in the United States, however, was a massive restructuring of who could provide medical education, who could certify and who could undertake the provision of healthcare. Medicine would not be a meritocracy, for who could be invested as physicians was still clearly delineated by race, class and gender. In the world of Jim Crow, race also defined the boundaries of good medical training and thus the line between physician and quack. Of the seven 'Negro' medical colleges only two – the federally funded Howard University in Washington, DC, and Meharry School of Medicine in Nashville, Tennessee – remained open by the First World War. In the age of medical segregation, the consensus was that white medical personnel should not treat African American patients, thus the exceptions. And as Flexner stated, it was important that these schools focused on hygiene (not surgery) to mitigate those diseases that could reach beyond their community 'to their white neighbors'. Specifically, because the scientific medicine of the time labelled African Americans as at greater risk for the widest range of disorders. But also because African American physicians were, for the most part, labelled as quacks, as their patients, as Flexner observed, were 'perhaps, more easily "taken in"'.[105] Even W.E.B. Du Bois, in his 1903 *The Souls of Black Folk*, his coming to terms with the impact of Jim Crow on the emancipated African Americans of his day, observed:

> By the poverty and ignorance of his people, the Negro minister or doctor was tempted toward quackery and demagogy; and by the criticism of the other world, toward ideals that made him ashamed of his lowly tasks. The would-be black savant was confronted by the paradox that the knowledge his people needed was a twice-told tale to his white neighbors, while the knowledge which would teach the white world was Greek to his own flesh and blood . . . This waste of double aims, this seeking to satisfy two unreconciled ideals, has wrought sad havoc with the courage and faith and deeds of ten thousand thousand people, – has sent them often wooing false gods and invoking false means of salvation, and at times has even seemed about to make them ashamed of themselves.[106]

On the contrary, as I argued decades ago, African American allopathic physicians, in rejecting 'white' medicine during the age of Jim Crow, often adapted a religious (or better said biblical) rhetoric that would appeal to their patients.[107] Thus they distinguished their practice from the world of plantation allopathic physicians, many of whom, such as the gynaecological surgeon J. Marion Sims (MD, Jefferson Medical College, 1835), the president of the AMA in 1871, had exploited them as research subjects during and after slavery.[108] Defending Flexner in eliminating 'bad' 'Negro' medical schools meant recognizing that alternative forms of *allopathic* medicine, for whatever reason, in the first age of biology, had to be defined as quackery.[109]

Women and Jews were likewise systematically excluded from medical education (after they had acquired greater access both in the United States and in Europe).[110] A number of hospitals affiliated themselves with teaching institutions and winnowed their faculty based on the claims stated by Flexner and the unspoken removal of those deemed not to fit the model of the scientific physician. As a result of the Flexner report the practice of medicine in the United States became primarily white, male and educated (read: upper class); everything else was quackery. Flexner's view was reformist, but it was not democratic. Like Daniel Coit Gilman, he saw education as a vehicle not of social transformation but for improving the generation and transmission of knowledge. All these presuppositions turned out to be at least partially wrong.

Flexner's views closed schools of electrotherapy, while colleges of homeopathy and osteopathy were seen as violating his norms. And as women had become a force in these fields it meant that most women were excluded from the system. Prior to the report a mixture of allopathic and homeopathic schools and nine medical schools had admitted women.[111] Afterwards access was limited to the new scientific medical schools, which were radically less welcoming. At the same time as heterodox therapies such as osteopathy were adopting the Flexner model of science and therapy, they also limited the intake of their students. All other therapies became quackery overnight. Flexner and the AMA knew where quackery lay, and it was in a world defined as antithetical to science. Yet even subscribing to the model of scientific medicine was never truly sufficient. As Morris Fishbein (MD, Rush Medical College, 1913), the long-time (1924–50) editor of the *Journal of the American Medical Association* (*JAMA*), could still write in the 1930s: 'In the practice of medicine as a whole an osteopath cannot compete with a properly trained physician. When he tries to compete, he indulges in claims which mark him as a quack and a charlatan . . . osteopaths merely dilute the quality of medical care available to the people of this country. The people should weigh well the question of whether they care to submit themselves and their families to substandard medical care.'[112] By then the control of who was a doc had been passed into the hands of a professional organization by the state, and there it remained.

Abraham Flexner's views about science and medicine had already been widely debated in Great Britain. In 1900 the distinguished dermatologist and medical educator Philip Henry Pye-Smith (MD, University College London, 1863; studied in Berlin with Virchow) would note the pernicious effects of such unscientific systems from earlier in the century as the '"iatrochemical" and "iatromechanical", the Brunonian with its "indiscriminate use of corroborants or tonics", and the still present concept of homeopathy "of which the theoretical absurdity is somewhat concealed by the mere obvious nonsense of infinitesimal doses."' Such systems seemed to persevere even in the light of modern science.

Amorphous theorizing blended for Pye-Smith into the new world of statistical reasoning, advocated by the life insurance industry and the new claims of Public Health: 'we must never allow theories, or even what appears to be logical deductions, or explanations however ingenious, or statistics however apparently conclusive, or authority however venerable, to take the place of one touchstone of practical medicine, experience.' In the end it is the new scientific medicine that will heal: 'If . . . medical science without art is inefficient, medical art without science is not only unprogressive but almost inevitably becomes quackery. As soon as we treat our patients by rule of thumb, by tradition, by dogmas, or by metaphysical axioms we do injury to ourselves as well as to them.'[113] But this is true across the new medical disciplines. The professor of pathological anatomy at the University of Aberdeen, David James Hamilton (MB, University of Edinburgh, 1870, FRCSE (Fellow of the Royal College of Surgeons, Edinburgh), FRSE (Fellowship of the Royal Society of Edinburgh)), in his address on the study of pathology in 1882, would make a similar criticism of the various 'schools of pathology' that had dominated thought in the past, noting that 'the foundation of . . . [their] teaching were the various theoretical notions of the structure and mechanism of the animal body, held by different sects of speculative philosophers. Thus, the humorists, solidists, Methodists, and dogmatists represented different schools, each founded upon a hypothesis whose truth could not be experimentally demonstrated.'[114] Science is defined by consensus; all need to agree about the definitions of method and all evidence brought forth to define its parameters. QED: everything else is quackery.

Caroline Lockhart's previously mentioned account of medicine on the frontier at the cusp of Flexner's reforms reflected the tenuous relationship between science and medicine in the popular culture of the twentieth century. Sinclair Lewis (Nobel Prize for Literature, 1930) published his *Arrowsmith*, mentioned in his Nobel award, in 1925, a work that he stated he had co-written with the microbiologist Paul de Kruif, whose bestselling *Microbe Hunters* appeared the next year. In many ways Lewis's novel and de Kruif's non-fiction were the popularization of the claims of Abraham Flexner's pre-First World War reforms of American medical education, well underway by the 1920s, and the moral dilemmas of the clinician in that new world.

Arrowsmith tracks the inner conflict of a young researcher, Martin Arrowsmith, between striving for public recognition for his world in the laboratory – hunting a microbe killer ('microphages' or perhaps today 'bacteriophages', viruses which were an important precursor to antibiotics) – and his role as a caring physician dealing with the ill and the infirm. Microphages were the cutting edge of science and have regained importance in our age of growing antibiotic resistance. The climax comes after he has discovered a cure for bubonic plague, which has broken out on an island in the Caribbean. The standard of research demands that he cannot use his discovery until it is thoroughly tested, even at the expense of lives that might be saved. Only after his wife, Leora, and all the other people who came with him from the institute where he works to the island die of plague does he reluctantly abandon rigorous science and begin to treat everyone on the island with the microphage. This so destroys his sense of what it is to be a medical scientist that he eventually flees into a hermit-like existence in Vermont, shunning all his relationships, to devote himself to pure medical research.[115] The 1931 film, directed by John Ford, won the Academy Award for Best Picture. Such works of fiction problematized the conflict between the objective science of medicine and the realities of clinical work, the difference between an objective scientific stance and what is designed to be the empathetic response of the doc.

An echo came in the UK in 1937 with A. J. Cronin's *The Citadel*, which is reputed to have created the popular demand for what came to be the National Health Service a decade later. Cronin (MB ChB with honours from Glasgow University in 1919, awarded his MD there in 1925 after getting a diploma in public health two years earlier) contrasted the claims of scientific medicine and the quotidian experiences of a young physician, Andrew Manson. Manson, an idealistic, newly qualified doctor, arrives from Scotland in 1924 to work in the small (fictitious) Welsh mining town of Drineffy. Manson is confronted there with a radical choice. Would he have a practice in the town treating those whose lungs had been destroyed by silicosis from working in the mines or would he turn to research, looking for a future cure for silicosis as an employee of the 'Mines Fatigue Board'? That was a field in which Cronin had worked in the 1920s, reporting on 'black lung disease' among the Welsh miners. The clinic or the laboratory? In the novel a 'quack' appears in the form of the American Richard Stillman, who does not have a medical degree, even though one of Manson's patients had been successfully treated at his tuberculosis clinic. Stillman's treatment, that of pneumothorax, which involved collapsing an affected lung with nitrogen, works, but sending a patient to him almost gets Manson struck off.[116] Yet Stillman's approach was the best medical practice of the day. In the science of medicine versus its art, who then is the 'quack?'

Medicine in Flexner's Germany

Now, one of the great ironies of the claims about science and medicine in imperial Germany was that while the model of the integration of research and teaching espoused by Johannes Müller in Humboldt's reformed universities, including in schools of medicine, was an ideal, the reality of the allopathic physician's role in Germany was even more complex than in the United States. And the status of the 'quack' – heterodox healers – even more so, especially after the creation of the German Reich in 1871.

Until the 1880s German physicians did not form a unified occupational group but fell into a series of extremely heterogeneous groups. Given the different competing groups offering health services, the lack of verifiable established expert knowledge prevented the formation of professional autonomy for the small subgroup of academically trained physicians. In imperial Germany the medical scientist achieved this autonomy only in the late nineteenth and early twentieth centuries, in the age of Flexner. The reason was that their professionalization was stimulated by uniting against one of Bismarck's great social innovations: statutory health insurance, introduced in 1884. This had been introduced as a measure against the programmes offered by the parties on the left for social security and the improvement of the public's health. As Rudolf Virchow, co-founder and member of one of those parties, the German Progressive Party (*Deutsche Fortschrittspartei*), in the Reichstag from 1880 to 1893, said in 1848, all medicine is at its core political.[117]

Germany defined the boundary between allopathic and heterodox medicine but permitted both. Flexner notes in his later account of the model for the restructuring of American medical certification that in Germany, as he writes, quacks must register as quacks. They cannot claim to be physicians, but they do continue to practise within the law. The *British Medical Journal* (BMJ) tabulated them in 1902, sounding a bit like Leporello's 'catalogue' aria from *Don Giovanni* enumerating the protagonist's seductions:

> 476 quacks, male and female, the number of legally-qualified practitioners being about 2,000. Of the male 'healers' 20 per cent. have been servants or workmen, 40 per cent. artisans, and 16 per cent. tradesmen. Among 125 'lady healers' only one has had more than the most elementary education, while 58 per cent. are of the servant class, 24 per cent. shopgirls, 10 per cent. factory hands, and 4 per cent. sick nurses. The number of illegal practitioners in Saxony in 1900 was 1,578. This does not include a number of quacks who ply their trade without the knowledge of the police authorities.[118]

The numbers rose spectacularly through the beginning of the century; by 1909 it was claimed that 21,014 lay practitioners of medicine existed in Germany.[119] But quackery is not merely a question of fraud or malpractice, for 'some of it is intra-professional and thus escapes prosecution . . . some of it burrows underground and thus escapes detection.'[120]

In Germany heterodox medicine – Flexner's quacks – was also organized in institutions that looked like those of allopathic medicine because of the professionalization of allopathic medicine. In imperial and then Weimar Germany alternative practitioners were organized in associations like the Kneippbund, the Priessnitzbund (both advocating competing forms of hydrotherapy), the Reichsbund für Homöopathie (traditional homeopathy) and the Biochemischer Bund (a spinoff of homeopathy, first developed in 1873, claiming to incorporate the newest biochemical discoveries), all of which stood for competing alternative approaches. Such societies also provided the organizational and moral backup for non-medically qualified practitioners. It has been estimated that in 1933 the number of these lay therapists was roughly equal to that of physicians registered in Germany. Perhaps this was proof of the social historian Reinhard Spree's argument that the combined efforts of professional organizations and medical administrations to define the quack was a way of protecting old-style guild privileges in a changed medical marketplace by attempting to exclude from this market non-licensed healers as well as licensed outsiders.[121] But the response was that heterodox healers simply mirrored the institutional structure of investiture, now up for debate in the courts of law.

In 1894, the German Supreme Court had endorsed the legal view that medical interventions constituted physical injuries no matter what medical theories the practitioner advocated. This meant that any therapy (except in medical emergencies) required the patient's consent. In Germany ethical views were expressed in late nineteenth- and early twentieth-century writings about doctors' duties, considering especially the issues of truth-telling, euthanasia and abortion. As a result, the famed dermatologist Albert Neisser (MD, University of Erlangen, 1877), who was responsible in the age of scientific medicine for the discovery of *Neisseria gonorrhoeae*, the causative agent for gonorrhoea, went on trial for medical malpractice. In 1895 he injected young prostitutes with a syphilis serum, hoping to confer immunity; many instead contracted a full-blown case of the disease, prompting a widespread debate on the ethics of human experimentation and the development of the world's stiffest restrictions against experimental abuse – Prussia's famous 1900 Code.[122] The psychiatrist Albert Moll (MD, University of Berlin, 1885) published his *Ärztliche Ethik: Die Pflichten des Arztes in allen Beziehungen seiner Thätigkeit* (Medical Ethics: The Obligations of the Physician in Relationship to their Practice) in 1902 at the moment the science of medicine had all but succeeded in defining the scope of modern medical practice. For him the real problem was not the presence of the heterodox healer but the wobbly ethical standards of the physician. Indeed, he views the attraction of the quack as a result, more of less, of the poverty of ethical norms in allopathic medicine.

Beginning in the 1920s German allopathic physicians were also the largest professional group to join the NSDAP (Nazi Party), with its clearly defined programme of eugenics and race theory, both helping to bring them to power and then fighting turf wars over who got to make the 'selections' at the Nazi death camps. They all 'followed *the* science', believing that, as Virchow had naively claimed in the 1840s, a benign politics would carry out the science of medicine, a belief shattered in the Third Reich. As a 2001 study asked, 'Why is it that we hold physicians in high moral regard, rather than viewing them as any other sort of contractor – some better, some worse – instead of considering immoral or marginal practices particularly heinous when engaged in by physicians? It cannot be denied that some of these expectations are rooted within our particular culture.'[123] And here I would comment that the link may well lie between a culturally acceptable moral code and the claims of a neutral, objective scientific stance that enhanced the status of the physician in the twentieth century. The Third Reich abandoned the ethical stance of imperial Germany as well as reinterpreting the scope of scientific medicine early on when they created a new racial and collective 'Path to Health'. As the deputy Reichsärzteführer (chief medical officer) Friedrich Bartels (MD, University of Munich, 1921) wrote in 1936: 'each is required to seek for the collective's health based on his racial and hereditary ability and health.'[124] He was simply 'following *the* science'. By then Jewish physicians, as defined by the Nazis, had already long began to be removed from positions in the medical faculties.

Flexner believed that the triumphs of scientific medicine in the nineteenth century replaced folk or traditional healing in Germany. He knew the claim that the new state of Germany had become one of the centres of scientific innovation. And while medical researchers were increasingly able to identify disease-causing agents, licensed physicians in Germany (and we can add the United States) were slow in replacing traditional humoral and environmental perceptions of disease with bacteriological ones. (Although that was also true of the introduction of antisepsis into surgery.) The reality was that there was a real disjuncture between the basic science of the time and a medical education that was ineffective in preparing doctors for practice.

Moreover, local political conditions and bureaucracies as well as religious affiliations prevented physicians from applying public health measures, whether based on older 'environmentalist' models of disease or on the latest bacteriological knowledge. As a study of pre-First World War southwest Germany has shown, 'shared or disparate concepts of disease could influence patients' views of physicians; patients most frequently associated doctors, especially government employed district physicians, with undesired state intervention into their traditional ways of dealing with health and disease.' In collapsing all forms of state-sanctioned, scientific medicine, both public and private, 'patients projected their negative experiences with district physicians onto private physicians, and thereby impeded the rise of scientific medicine in general. At the turn of the century, most patients had not yet developed trust in "scientific" physicians, a prerequisite for successful doctor-patient relationships.' But the clinical applications of the new biological discoveries remained, for this population, quite distinct from its popular image of bench science, as 'people seem to have developed more quickly a faith in laboratory-test results rather than physicians. Many people did not associate practicing physicians with the scientific medicine represented by bacteriological laboratories. On the contrary, patients and relatives frequently rejected physicians' clinical diagnoses until they saw bacteriological test results.'[125] For Robert Koch, and in France Louis Pasteur, had become ideological heroes of German and French politics and science, well publicized in all the daily papers. The laboratory, if not the clinic, was blessed with that public cachet.

The compartmentalizing of science and medicine, at least in imperial Germany, led to a more permissive acceptance of folk medicine that took on the institutional trappings of scientific medicine. Indeed, 'for most of the late nineteenth and early twentieth century a doctor's academic title and his scientific training played a minor role in physicians' differentiation from unlicensed practitioners. Until the 1910s, it appears that physicians also accepted other healers, as long as they contributed to the well-being of patients.'[126] And the scope of these other healers, the quacks or *Kurpfuscher*, was wide ranging, from barbers to unlicensed midwives and herbal and natural healers – 'naturopaths'. The rule seemed to be that all had to avoid 'doing harm'; otherwise, all were tolerated.

Back in the United States Abraham Flexner had become the founding director in 1930 of the Institute for Advanced Studies in Princeton, where he could watch what was happening in the world of German scientific medicine with the rise of National Socialism. In the 1920s the department store magnate Louis Bamberger had wanted to create a medical school in New Jersey that would allow Jews to study medicine unencumbered, but Flexner persuaded him that a stand-alone research institute, separate from any instruction, would better serve the purpose of furthering knowledge, as there needed to be clinics in addition to research labs for a modern medical school. Flexner had remained quiet as admissions of Jews to American elite medical schools were sharply curtailed in the 1920s, as he believed that American Jews had to maintain a low profile, and thus was hesitant to become engaged with the ever more onerous quota system in his reformed schools of medicine.[127] Unlike his Zionist brother Bernard, he did not publicly espouse 'Jewish' causes. As a result, Flexner was *quietly* involved, after 1933, in the rescue of scientists from Nazi persecution because they were Jewish, as a founding member of the board of the Emergency Committee in Aid of Displaced Foreign (originally called 'German') Scholars.

As director of the Institute for Advanced Studies at Princeton, Flexner confronted its most famous Jewish member, Albert Einstein, in the late 1930s over his allegiance to 'Jewish' causes. While Einstein had arrived in the United States before the Nazis came to power in January 1933, Flexner was anxious thereafter about being seen furthering 'foreign scholars' over 'real' Americans after Jews were forced out of German universities. Flexner preferred a more assimilationist approach much in keeping with the anxiety of being seen as not scientific. One example from the 1930s will have to suffice: although he was actively involved in luring Einstein to Princeton, Flexner did not share his activist approach to fighting persecution of the Jews, whether at home or abroad. In discouraging Einstein from having anything to do with the press regarding a proposed violin performance by the famous scientist meant to raise money for Jewish refugees, Flexner lectured Elsa Einstein, 'I know America far better than you or he.' Flexner, a staunch believer in quiet (indeed almost silent) diplomacy, feared that 'such publicity was certain to continue and would in the long run harm her husband's work and that of the institute.'[128] Being quiet about 'Jewish' questions, he still believed, would enable Jews to function within the ideal university as Flexner imagined it, not the way it became in the United States and Germany. Flexner died in 1959, well after the consequences of elite German medicine had been revealed at the Nazi Doctors' Trial at Nuremberg.

In Germany, what Flexner had bemoaned, the toleration of heterodox medicine in imperial and Weimar Germany, became state policy in 1933 (after the Nazi assumption of power in January 1933), when German alternative and complementary medicine was reorganized under the banner of the 'New German Therapeutics' (*Neue Deutsche Heilkunde*). Nazi officials created a new profession, the *Heilpraktiker* ('health practitioner') – a profession which was meant to become extinct within one generation, as heterodox medicine would be seamlessly merged with allopathic praxis. The competing pre-1933 allopathic physicians' organizations, the Hartmannbund, created in 1900 as a professional advocacy organization by the Leipzig physician Hermann Hartmann (MD, Würzburg, 1885) and the Ärztevereinsbund (Physicians' Association), created in 1873 from regional medical organizations, were *gleichgeschaltet* (merged) by the state in 1936 into the Reichsärztekammer (Reich Medical Association). The move was under the banner of reinvigorating the moral calling of all, as was a claim that the more scientific medicine had become, the less it reflected the 'soul' of the nation (and the race).

While these changes promoted greater use of heterodox drugs, both folk medicine and homeopathic formulas, by the medical community, the pharmaceutical industry, which was manufacturing allopathic drugs, gave little space to producing these medications. Indeed, I. G. Farben completely ignored the 'New German Therapeutics', suggesting that the large chemical-pharmaceutical manufacturers did not take this new, state-mandated policy very seriously. Those that did, such as the medium-sized manufacturers Knoll and Schering, worked towards obtaining a scientific basis for the treatments and to do so they employed conventional methods of chemical analysis and proof of activity. There were, of course, long-standing companies manufacturing alternative medications, but even though the new state approach favoured them, they seem to have expanded their production only slightly over what had been the case before 1933.[129]

The 'New German Therapeutics' was aimed at ensuring the dominance of the Aryan race, as race science was at the core of Nazi medicine. Gerhard Wagner (MD, University of Munich, 1914), the first Reichsärzteführer (chief medical officer), and a strong advocate of heterodox practices, wrote in 1935: 'If today we want to construct a new German healing practice, then its basis cannot be that formed by the exact sciences, but its basis must be our national socialist world view.'[130] In October 1933, Wagner had published an appeal in the medical journal *Deutsches Aerzteblatt* (German Physicians' Journal) calling 'all German physicians who engage with biological medicine' to come together. He wrote, among other things, that there were therapies which were not in line with mainstream medicine but still proved successful, if not superior, to the medicine taught at universities. Little wonder, then, that the editors of the leading homeopathic journal, which also served as the homeopathic association's mouthpiece, happily embraced Wagner's appeal, and indicated their willingness to cooperate. In an open letter addressed to Hitler, the long-term editor of the *Allgemeine Homöopathische Zeitung* (General Homeopathic Journal), Hans Wapler (MD, University of Leipzig, 1895), director of the Homeopathic Clinic in Leipzig, emphatically concludes: 'There can be no National Socialist physician who – if made aware of it – would not recognize the crucial importance that Hitler's political evaluation of the *Similia similibus* [the homeopathic 'like cures like' principle] has had for Germany.'[131] Wapler had, as early as 1919, argued for a rapprochement between scientific medicine and heterodox approaches to healing in order to create a new 'German self-consciousness' in medicine.[132] That this was desired by the political leadership defined it as good medicine.

So, the state wanted a unified, race-based heterodox medical praxis and the 1935 founding of the Arbeitsgemeinschaft für eine Neue Deutsche Heilkunde (Working Group for the 'New German Therapeutics') was created to lump all strains of 'alternative' healers together, much as the Nazi state had simply unified all youth groups, all sports groups and all social activity under the banner of the party (*Gleichschaltung*).[133] Homeopaths, spa doctors, folk medicine practitioners and anthroposophical healers were joined together as *Heilpraktiker*, needless to say with the exclusion as of 1933 of Jewish practitioners, such as Otto Leeser (MD, University of Berlin, 1912), who advocated for a rapprochement between allopathic practice and homeopathy. The goal, as the spa doctor Wilhelm Spengler wrote in 1936, was to create a 'German, that is, a strong, heathen practice, full of strength and conscience, sympathy and soul [*Seele*]' in order to 'heal the German Volk through hardening and fulfilment'.[134] The practical result was that any alternative therapist could become a physician as of 1939 by simply adopting the title 'physician of natural healing'. And some could even enter medical schools without any of the required prerequisites, based on their experience with heterodox therapies. Even those who were not singled out in this manner could continue to practise if they collected no fees.[135]

But the merger never took place in healthcare; by 1937, the attempt to merge all these organizations had failed, never to be attempted again. The reason was clear. By 1936 the 'Four Year' economic plan

was moving towards rearmament and eventually war, so that allopathic medicine was seen as a vital field and further investment in
the university training of allopathic physicians was mandated. Also,
the heterodox fields remained quite heterogeneous, unable to seek
common goals or find any 'ideological ability' to permeate with their
therapeutic claims the shield of 'scientific medicine' upheld by the
state allopathic medical institutions. The *Heilpraktiker* remained an
alternative profession just as it had been in imperial Germany. But
allopathic medicine could not abandon its distinction from heterodox medicine, even when the ultimate totalitarian state demanded it.
Maybe Germany was not the very best model for scientific medicine,
as 'following *the* science' had radically different meanings when 'race
science' became dominant.

Chemistry Becomes Medicine

What is clear is that the official and cultural response to quackery is
parallel to the rise of the scientific model within medicine. Organic
chemistry was the model science for the medical profession. It too
had grown out of the earlier metaphysics of alchemy to free itself (it
believed) from all superstition and claimed reliance on observation
and experimentation. Chemistry, cure and commerce were as inter-
locked within the rise of modern medicine as to make them in their
origin part of the same anti-quackery enterprise. Modern, scientific
medicine thus was interchangeable with modern, scientific chemistry,
which sought to explain the chemical and physical actions underpin-
ning every human and animal physiological mechanism, as an answer
to the divine vitalism of human beings. As the American medical
historian Karl Ludmerer has written, 'The clinician's diagnosis was
equivalent to the scientists' hypothesis; both diagnosis and hypothesis
needed to be submitted to the test of an experiment. In the clinician's
case, the experiment might be the results of a laboratory test or the
response to a particular treatment.'[136] The goal was creating 'scientific practitioners' as an answer to quacks. For the official responses to
quack medication were triggered by the risk such medications (and
we can extrapolate also to include procedures and theories) presented
to the ill. Not their efficacy.

This was already implicated in what the disability studies scholar
Eli Clare describes as the 'ideology of cure'. Such a cure 'saves lives;

cure manipulates lives; cure prioritizes some lives over others; cure makes profits; cure justifies violence; cure promises resolution to body-mind loss.'[137] Aspirin follows this trajectory. Acetylsalicylic acid was created in 1853 by the French organic chemist Charles-Frédéric Gerhardt (Doctorate in Chemistry, University of Paris, 1841), who compounded the widely used medicine sodium salicylate, a non-steroidal anti-inflammatory agent, with acetyl chloride to produce acetylsalicylic acid for the first time. (Salicylic acid was part of the classical Greek pharmacopoeia, which used the bark of willow trees for various forms of relief.) The movement to industrial production came about because of the rise of interest in coal dyes, such as aniline, at mid-century.

Primarily, coal-tar dyes were a new spectrum of colours to dye fabric for the newest fashions, and one of the newly invented colours, 'mauve', defined an epoch. But they quickly replaced even the most widely grown natural colours, such as indigo, one of the colonial system's primary crops, with new, inexpensive, commercial dyes. German chemist Adolf von Baeyer (PhD, Chemistry, University of Berlin, 1858; Nobel Prize, Chemistry, 1905, 'in recognition of his services in the advancement of organic chemistry and the chemical industry, through his work on organic dyes and hydroaromatic compounds') manufactured an artificial version of indigo, to dye Levi Strauss's jeans.

While first discovered in the pre-industrial world of the early Enlightenment as an undesired by-product of iron production and coking plants, coal tars came also to be central to the new study of cellular anatomy, as they dyed various types of cells different tints.[138] First used by William Henry Perkin, trained in 1853 at London's Royal College of Chemistry, they quickly became the basis for the modern pharmaceutical industry and its intimate relationship to the rise of modern scientific medicine.[139] (Today they are on the World Health Organization's 'List of Essential Medicines'.) Coal dyes enabled at least two Nobel Prize winners in medicine to 'see' the causes of the diseases they were able to describe: in 1879, Paul Ehrlich (MD, Leipzig, 1878; Nobel Prize, Physiology or Medicine, 1908, together with Ilya Ilyich Mechnikov, 'in recognition of their work on immunity') published his technique for staining blood films and his method for differential blood-cell counting using coal tar dyes; he used Eosin, a bright red synthetic dye discovered in 1874 by Heinrich Caro, the director of the German chemical company Badische Anilin- und Soda-Fabrik. In

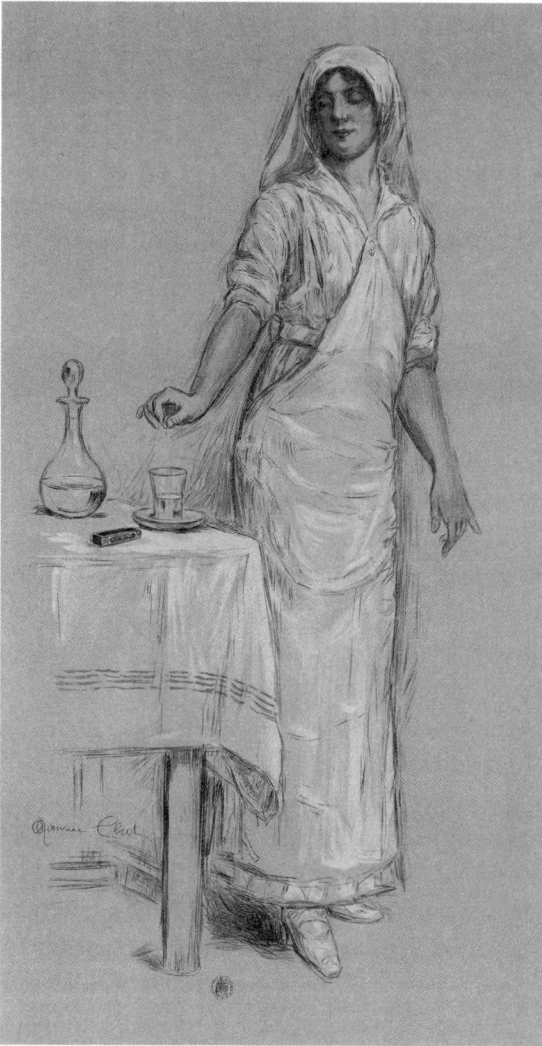

A nurse dropping an aspirin pill into a glass of water, advertising soluble aspirin. Lithograph by Maurice Cliot, Paris, c. 1910.

1882 Robert Koch (Nobel Prize, Physiology or Medicine, 1905, for his work on tuberculosis), using the new staining technique, employed methylene blue to stain the tubercular bacillus and distinguished it from other background tissue that he had stained with the vesuvin dye, which turned brown. In 1884 Hans Christian Gram (MD, University of Copenhagen, 1883) noted the differences in the way bacteria react to stains. Those bacteria (pneumococci) that retained a deep purple stain, even after they were washed, were termed 'stain positive'; those that did not were 'stain negative'. Today we speak of gram positive and gram negative.

The Nobel Prize winner Paul Ehrlich, the creator of chemotherapy with his treatment for syphilis, also found that some of the dyes had the ability to reduce malarial fever; indeed, they came to be used when quinine was unavailable during the First World War. From this accidental discovery of the physiological impact of ingesting coal-tar derivatives came the move to the first anti-psychotic drugs decades later, such as chloramine, and eventually our comprehension of the mechanisms by which paranoia was created in the brain through pathways analogous to the shaman's magic mushrooms. All seemed to be nature revealed through chemistry and evinced a pragmatic but also a programmatic relationship between industrial chemistry and the evolving science of medicine. But coal-tar derivatives were also employed early on as a food additive, to create the illusion, not of health, but of tastiness and attractiveness, a form of mass delusion still present in our own foodstuffs and, by the way, in all of our pharmaceuticals – orange being a particularly attractive colour for children's medication.[140]

Coal dyes were a lucrative source of income as they were quickly connected to the production of modern medication. By 1900 Paul Ehrlich had been able to describe how the stains worked, by attaching themselves through what he called 'poison receptors' to the cells. The idea of the 'receptor' seemed to him limited to the process by which the dyes attached themselves to the receptors in the cell. By 1907 he came to understand that this was how he could explain the pharmacological actions of synthetic drugs, which could attach themselves to 'chemoreceptors' and enter the cell, initiating biological effects or inhibiting cellular functions.[141] Organic chemistry and pharmaceuticals were of one piece.

The dye firm of Friedrich Bayer and Company hired Friedrich Hoffmann in 1894, who, as part of a larger research group, in 1897 began studying acetylsalicylic acid as a less irritating replacement medication for common salicylate medicines.[142] The legend, perpetrated by the public relations firms of the company, later claimed that he had had a personal and a compassionate source for his interest: to relieve the rheumatic pains experienced by his father. No profit motives to be found here, only altruism. By 1899 Bayer had tested and patented its product as 'Aspirin' and sold it around the world as an 'ethical drug', meaning it was made available only through state-sanctioned pharmacies to distinguish it (and other ethical drugs) from the world of quacks. One other drug generated by Bayer was 'heroin', so labelled because it made those who tested it feel 'heroic'. When the Pure Food and Drug Act of 1904 banned the listing of trademarked drugs, assuming that all were, on one level or another, quack medicine, Bayer sold its pills (featuring its company logo, an embossed cross) by the chemical name, but made sure that everyone used the name 'Aspirin' when ordering the drug. At least that was the case until the First World War, when the United States seized the American patent as enemy goods and made it and the name available to Allied manufacturers.

To heal also could harm. The Greeks knew well that the *pharmakon*, the drug or cure, was also a poison. The *pharmakon* may 'pursue a kind of phenomenology of drugs as embodied processes, an approach that foregrounds the productive potential of medicines; their capacity to reconfigure bodies and diseases in multiple, unpredictable ways'.[143] It is in the unpredictability of the drug that harm may lie. As Socrates notes in Plato's *Phaedrus*, 'one man is able to give birth to the elements of an art, but it takes another to judge what measure of harm and benefit it has for those who are planning to use it'.[144] In complex ways this has always been the obligation of the healer.

Big Pharma arrives in the nineteenth century aware of this duality: that is, the potential dangers of vaccines and opioids, but even that of aspirin. Aspirin was seen as potentially deadly, for 'the practising physician knows that any simple and reputedly harmless drug, such as aspirin . . . can be taken in quantity till the limits of its compatibility with nervous health are overstepped; the individual becomes a drug-taker, and his morbid state a disease . . . From the medical viewpoint, there is no difference whatsoever between addiction to aspirin and addiction to morphia'.[145] Suicide by aspirin became a global anxiety.[146] Thus, in the United Kingdom it came to be so dispensed that an overdose was harder to take; in the United States, where this is not the case, suicide by aspirin remains a permanent fear.[147] Wherever cure resides, so does harm.

But harm also was present in the world of organic chemistry, because suddenly medicine, the healing art, was reduced to mere mechanical science – and who was at fault? Too materialistic by far, this was the result of the Jewish infiltration into the very idea of scientific medicine. For it is the Jews who focus on the dead, the inert. Hermann Schneider (MD, University of Heidelberg, 1898) remarked that the Jew today 'as a physician adopts those natural laws and material experiences which he could not have created; once he acquires them, he knows how to apply them and to expand them logically and empirically but only in details.'[148]

Erwin Liek, the Danzig surgeon and strong advocate of homeopathy, coined the phrase 'Crisis in Medicine' and bemoaned the *Entseelung* (un-souling) of medicine through the strictures of scientific, laboratory-based innovations. Medicine had become more chemical formulae than clinical practice, according to Liek, who blamed the Jews for overvaluing exactitude and for bringing a certain superficiality and 'showmanship' into science.[149] Beware the reduction of the medical clinic to the laboratory and to the business of drugs. Yet he also labelled himself a self-styled heretic, identifying with Louis Pasteur *and* Sigmund Freud, so that he knew the limits of his position both professionally and in the public sphere.[150] One of Freud's Jewish students, Otto Weininger (PhD, Philosophy, University of Vienna, 1902), thus saw the Jews as natural chemists, which explains why medicine has become biochemistry: 'The present turn of medical science is largely due to the influence of the Jews, who in such numbers have embraced the medical profession. From the earliest times, until the dominance of the Jews, medicine was closely allied with religion. But now they make it a matter of drugs, a mere administration of chemicals . . . The chemical interpretation of organisms sets these on a level with their own dead ashes.'[151] This Weininger labels as a 'Jewification' of medicine, a view and a term that echoed among physicians well after his suicide in 1905 in the room in which Beethoven had died. The 'naturopaths' of the 1920s and '30s such as Karl Strünckmann (MD, University of Leipzig, 1897) saw the same disenchantment, also knew who was at fault. Strünckmann's take on this was not only *völkisch* but clearly antisemitic, seeing scientific medicine as a perversion of Aryan (read as heterodox) medicine by 'Jewish-bolshevist scientific medicine.'[152] All led to the rationale of why pharmaceuticals, and the world they defined, became ever more contested even by those who advocated for them.

The new medicines may have worked better than the quack medicines, or indeed the medications compounded by the local, state-certified pharmacists, but the means of selling them still relied on claims of belief. Sir William Osler, lecturing to the medical students at the University of Pennsylvania in 1889, saw the risks inherent in the scientific claims of the new medicines, since much of it is advertisements of notions foisted on the profession by men who trade on the innocent credulity of the regular physician, quite as much as any quack preys on the gullible public . . . A still more dangerous enemy to the mental virility of the general practitioner, is the 'drummer' of the drug house . . . No class of men with which we have to deal illustrates more fully that greatest of ignorance – the ignorance which is the conceit that a man knows what he does not know; but the enthrallment of the practitioner by the manufacturing chemist and the revival of a pseudo-scientific polypharmacy are too large questions to be dealt with at the end of an address.[153]

All aspects of the merger of bench science, of organic chemistry in all its various manifestations, with the rise of modern clinical medicine, learned at the bedside, contain exactly such quirks. In the twenty-first century these quirks remain with us, given our contemporary debates about efficacy, cost and risk. American television viewers are nightly bombarded by advertisements for the newest, most effective drugs to treat the widest range of diseases, at least those with the largest possible market share. Osler would not have been surprised by their presence, but might well have been amazed by their cost.

Science Shapes Evidence-Based Medicine

What vanishes with the restructuring of medical practice as an offshoot of bench science is the ambiguity that should reside at the heart of medical practice – especially when the boundaries of 'evidence' harden and become rigid in the twentieth century. C. David Naylor (MD, University of Toronto, 1978), professor of medicine at the University of Toronto and later its president, wrote in 1995, regarding the by then established field of evidence-based medicine, that 'the limits to medical evidence continue to limit the ambit of evidence-based medicine. The craft of caring for patients can flourish not merely in the grey zones where scientific evidence is incomplete or conflicted but also in the recognition that what is black and white in the abstract may rapidly become grey in practice, as clinicians seem to meet their individual patient's needs. To paraphrase [Sir William] Osler let us agree that good clinical medicine will always blend the art of uncertainty with the science of probability.'[154] That Naylor and Osler qualify statistical reasoning, with all its claims for scientific rigour, with the 'uncertainty' of medical practice is central to my argument. If basic premises are false or incomplete or simply misread, then all the claims for rigour fall by the wayside. Thus, the responsibility lies not only with those making the claim, but with those accepting or rejecting the verity of the science.

The greater notion of what the social sciences call 'transferability' plays a major role in determining how either case studies or evidence-based studies were employed in the debates concerning 'following *the* science' during COVID-19. For it is 'the readers of case study reports [who] must themselves determine whether the findings are applicable to other cases than those which the researcher studied'.[155] This is true of all presentations of evidence, statistical or not. It is what links the process of interpretation in law, the very notion of selecting and then generalizing from precedent, to the function of evidence in scientific medicine. The key is always that we must question the validity of all generalizations. Yet a claim that it is 'the researcher's liability . . . to afford sufficient contextual information to facilitate the reader's judgment as to whether a particular case can be generalized to a specific field of practice' does not lead to one author's conclusion that 'we could regard such views of generalization as empowering or democratizing'.[156] Or autocratic and disempowering, depending on the reader, the reader's ideology, the reader's intent, the reader's setting. It is no wonder that it is to the law that the questions of scientific medicine and quackery constantly turn to resolve this ambiguity. And then this becomes part of a never-ending process of adjudication.

By the mid-twentieth century evidence-based medicine (EBM) had evolved, initially examining only the seeming efficacy of any given intervention, using randomized, double-blind studies of cohorts rather than individual cases. Such studies using the principle of alteration were already present in the first age of scientific medicine and continued, as randomized trials, well into the twentieth century. But it was Austin Bradford Hill's randomized trial of streptomycin for pulmonary tuberculosis in 1948, as we mentioned earlier in this chapter, that created the benchmark for what became, by the 1960s, evidence-based medicine anchored in the world of statistical reasoning. The case study, in the age of the dominance of psychoanalysis from the 1920s to the 1960s, seemed to bench-science-trained physicians at mid-century always too limited and too patient-analyst specific, especially for studies of pathophysiology (which studies the effects of disease on physiological processes). For, they argued, 'even if one isolates the therapeutic variable in a given client through a rigorous single case experimental design, critics have noted that there is little basis for inferring that this therapeutic procedure would be equally effective when applied to clients with similar behavioural disorders (client generality) or that different therapists using this technique would achieve the same results (therapist generality).'[157]

Science seemed easily translated into statistics – and had potentially been so from the late nineteenth century – as statistics seemed to be objective, not bound to the researcher, in their representation of a generalizable claim of efficacy. Ambiguity was the enemy of evidence-based biomedicine. Statistical reasoning, as Nikolas Rose argued, was a means of taming an 'unruly' population and reducing it to a form that lent itself to oversight, whether by the state or the state's agents, the physician.[158] The biologist Peter Medawar (DSc [Doctor of Science], University of Oxford, 1947; Nobel Prize, Physiology or Medicine, 1960, 'for discovery of acquired immunological tolerance') acknowledged in 1979 that 'exaggerated claims for the efficacy of a medicament are very seldom the consequence of any intention to deceive; they are usually the outcome of a kindly conspiracy in which everybody has the very best intentions. The patient wants to get well, his physician wants to have made him better, and the pharmaceutical company would have liked to have put it into the physician's power to have made him so. The controlled clinical trial is an attempt to avoid being taken in by this conspiracy of good will.'[159] And thus further meta-analyses, consisting of compilations of randomized controlled trials, seemed to be necessary to document overall efficacy. Each stage of analysis receded from the actual complexity and difference of each case, often overlooking meaningful differences because of a lack of nuance.

The rise of rigorous bench-science-based models of medicine was, at the close of the twentieth century, labelled 'evidence-based medicine or practice' because of the work done at McMaster University in Canada in the 1980s. Gordon Guyatt (MD, McMaster University, 1983) coined the term 'evidence-based medicine' in 1990, defining it as 'the conscientious, explicit, and judicious use of current best evidence in making decisions about the care of individual patients.'[160] But in the end it was simply the application of newer bench-science standards to medical practice that had been in place by the beginning of the century[161]

– large, double-blind studies with clearly defined methodology that were subjected to rigorous peer review in recognized professional journals and could thus be replicated by other researchers. We will see in the course of this book how each and every claim that defined EBM was potentially a trap for the physician. Guyatt built upon work in the 1970s by researchers such as Archibald 'Archie' Cochrane (MB, BS, King's College, Cambridge; medical qualification, University College Hospital, London, 1938) in the United Kingdom, Alvan Feinstein (MD, University of Chicago, 1952; long-term editor of the *Journal of Clinical Epidemiology*) in the United States and David Sackett (MD, University of Illinois, 1960), Guyatt's colleague at McMaster. Sackett recounted his conversion to *the* science of medicine at the bedside:

> By 1959, I had become a final-year medical student, and I once found myself responsible for a teenager who had been admitted to a medical ward with hepatitis. After a few days of enforced total bed rest – the standard management of the condition – his spirits and energy returned and he asked me to let him get up and around. I felt I needed to have a look at relevant evidence to guide my response to his request. I went to the library and came across a remarkable report for which the lead author was Tom Chalmers. A meticulously conducted randomised trial had made clear that there was no good evidence to justify requiring hepatitis patients to remain in bed after they feel well. Armed with this evidence, I convinced my supervisors to let me apologise to my patient and encourage him to be up and about as much as he wished. His subsequent clinical course was uneventful. That report of a (factorial) randomised trial challenging the validity of two standard treatments for hepatitis – bed rest and low fat diet – helped to change my career.[162]

What Sackett experienced was seeing *the* science as necessarily prior to received bedside wisdom. But over time *the* science comes more and more to be driven not only by the experimental mode, but by the increased availability of specific technologies during the latter twentieth century – from imaging techniques to genetic screening. The gold standard became randomized trials but, as Sackett continued, 'randomised trials are not always possible for investigating putative effects of treatment: but numerous actual examples show that they are more often an option . . . than many people believe. The main precondition seems often to be the professional humility to admit that, on the basis of the evidence available, we are uncertain whether a treatment is more likely to do good than harm, and the need to use reliable research to identify its effects.'[163] Do no harm is the magic formula that warns us against quackery, even in the realm of evidence-based medicine. We need to stop here and remind you that the so-called 'Hippocratic Oath', introduced in the age of scientific medicine, originally did not claim that the physician should first and foremost 'do no harm.' And yet even Gordon Guyatt and David Sackett recognized that 'clinicians must be ready to accept and live with uncertainty and to acknowledge that management decisions are often made in the face of relative ignorance of their true impact.'[164] As does everyone else.

Yet we know what is lost here: the patient. EBM is hollow as we can see 'the need for clinicians, staff, and health care systems to shift focus away from diseases and back to the patient and family'.[165] Indeed, what is evidence during laboratory and double-blind studies makes sense only in the reception, correctly or falsely, within the world of those treated, as 'the status of scientific data as evidence rests not only in the research itself, but in the diverse communities of physicians who interpret and use them.'[166] Moving from evidence to practice is complicated as it demands an awareness of the limitations, some institutional, some economic, some moral, that colour all such shifts from one sphere to another. This is the distinction, mentioned at the opening of the chapter, between efficaciousness in the laboratory and effectiveness in the clinic. They often do not overlap.

Patient autonomy may well limit the ability of the physician to make, what is from their point of view, the best choice.[167] The specificity of *the* patient needs to be very local. It is of no use to have the absolute best treatment available if a single individual does not have access to it because of local conditions – not only the difference in funding structures (as between the United States and Canada) but geographic differences. We know well that American patients who live close to the Canadian border often cross it to access pharmaceuticals unavailable or, more frequently, unaffordable in their home state. It is also of no use to find oneself in a nation-state that claims to give access to all citizens for healthcare, if your cultural presuppositions are not understood as 'medical', as in the decade-long struggle to persuade the NHS to cover infant male circumcision as a medical procedure and not as a religious one.[168] Repeatedly, new and complex interventions were and are needed to include the patient in the context of culture, religion, family, class, gender, sexual identity and ethnicity that enters into the medical mix. The claim has been made that such framing of the medical experience results in quicker recuperation times and fewer negative outcomes.[169]

In the 1970s what differed over time was the technology, not standards of evidence. Sidney Shapiro, at Laurentian University, at that moment was able to access computerized data to link drugs to health effects in some of the first case-control studies using 'big data'. For 'the social and cultural milieu of North American medicine in the early 1990s, into which EBM made its debut, was overall ripe for the new methods. Quantification practices, the use of statistics and epidemiology, the introduction of computers and online digital databases, and new clinical research methodology saturated the medical environment of the time.'[170] And this model spread quickly across all medical disciplines, without hesitation, as it claimed for itself a type of objectivity. Such trials came to be seen as '"tombstone trials" – (randomize and count the dead) as [they] have sufficient statistical power to permit reliable subgroup analyses, provided the analyses are limited in number and sensibly motivated a priori by epidemiological or biological arguments. However, many of the outcomes that matter to patients making clinical decisions are subjective and expensive to measure in large-scale trials. In sum, individualised decision analysis seems contingent on either unusually strong evidence or lots of educated guesswork.'[171] A contingency seemingly underwritten by the cutting-edge technology that shaped it:

> So, while the technocentricity of medicine has allowed an extended lifespan with chronic disease, it is only nominally prepared to address the personal consequences of illness. The reason for this inaptitude lies in the fact that the technological model has been bastardized; the relative ease that was to be gained through the application and use of technology was supposed to allow greater temporal latitude for humanitarian pursuits: in medicine, technology was to empower the physician-patient relationship . . . This is consistent with the investiture of medicine as a techno-economic deliverable:

technology is instrumental to the good of medicine, therefore techno-centric medicine becomes seen as an instrumental
good. As such, the practice of medicine assumes an increasingly business ethos, and the patient assumes the role of
consumer.[172]

Not only practice but even the patient role shifted as scientific
medicine became less focused on the individual case as it deemed
itself to become more scientific. What was lost was the ambiguities
of individuals; by eliminating the nuanced differences among those
studied, the evidence seemed to be predetermined. The claims that
scientific medicine deals with *cura personalis* – care of the whole
person – become less and less imaginable. But it simultaneously drew
a line between real evidence and mere suppositions or assumptions.
And thus, the definition of quackery came to be radically apparent – quackery violated the fixed claims of scientific evidence even
if it was efficacious in the clinic. And this debate about boundaries
changed radically when it moved from the clinic to the law courts,
the space in which contemporary society adjudicates what or what
is not real medicine.

In the end, as Edzard Ernst (MD, University of Munich, 1978), the
first professor of complementary medicine in Great Britain, observed:
'The quack is always someone else. The modern physician has become
so confident in his or her guesswork that a danger exists of confusing
personal opinion with evidence, or personal ignorance with genu-
ine scientific uncertainty. Opinions in medicine shift as new evidence
emerges.'[173] But that is equally true of the nature of quackery, in
Ernst's sense.

Quackery, Medicine and Law

In the 'Common Law for Dummies' compiled by the eighteenth-
century jurist William Blackstone, the charge of quackery is a problem
of someone shouting in the marketplace. Calling someone a 'quack'
is slander: 'As if I can prove the tradesman a bankrupt, the physician a quack, the lawyer a knave, and the divine a heretic, this will
destroy their respective actions; for though there may be damage sufficient accruing from it, yet, if the fact be true, it is *damnum absque
injuria*; and where there is no injury, the law gives no remedy.'[174]

We are confronted with the basic problem of science as a reflection of society, with truth as absolute or as relative. In the age of the early Enlightenment, science still had an aura of immutability; but medicine was not quite yet understood by Blackstone and his contemporaries as science. Who draws the line, even before the court, and whether as in Blackstone's examples, all drawing of lines is equal. For I may be able to 'prove' the bankruptcy of the tradesman through documentation; so too (perhaps) the heresy of the divine. But, unlike the banker, the physician was bound, by *law* as a professional, by an implied contract requiring him to practise his profession skilfully, carefully and properly. Blackstone wrote of the early common law 'that everyone who undertakes any office, employment, trust, or duty, contracts with those who employ or entrust him, to perform it with integrity, diligence and skill. And, if by his want of either of those qualities any injury accrues to individuals, they have therefore their remedy in damages by a special action on the case.'[175] Thus calling a physician a quack seems to be an analogous claim.

We now find ourselves in the world of civil lawsuits: one individual accusing another of representing themselves as a competent judge of the course and treatment of disease but causing damage or at least not fulfilling the promise of their professional identity. If they cause injuries or violate the belief that the patient has in the physician, as Blackstone stated,

> affecting a man's health, are [*sic*] where by any unwholesome practices of another a man sustains any apparent damage in his vigour or constitution . . . by the neglect or unskillful management of his physician, surgeon, or apothecary. For it hath been solemnly resolved, that mala praxis is a great misdemeanor and offence at common law, whether it be for curiosity and experiment, or by neglect; because it breaks the trust which the party had placed in his physician and tends to the patient's destruction. Thus also, in the civil law, neglect or want of skill in physicians and surgeons.[176]

Is this 'bad' medicine in this age of heroic medicine or is it physician incompetence that is at stake here?

By the Enlightenment Adam Smith, praising the new, scientific medical school in Edinburgh in a 1774 letter to William Cullen, observes that it is the very medical establishment that generates quacks, at least south of the border: 'The great success of quacks in England has been altogether owing to the real quackery of the regular physicians. Our regular physicians in Scotland have little quackery and no quack accordingly has ever made his fortune among us.'[177] At least not to his knowledge, as the 'resurrection men', the grave robbers and murderers William Burke and William Hare and their employer, the racist anatomist Robert Knox (MD, University of Edinburgh, 1814, FRSE, FRCSE) at the Royal College of Surgeons, lurk just a bit in the future:

> Up the close and down the stair
> In the house with Burke and Hare
> Burke's the butcher, Hare's the thief
> Knox the man who buys the beef.

For we need to remember that it was Robert Knox who claimed self-righteously that any doctor who lacked training in pathological anatomy was a '*quack*', no matter how he attained it.[178]

In our modern world, there are civil laws concerning malpractice. Are you 'mainstream' enough in your training and investiture to practise medicine and what happens when this stream is polluted? What must you as a practitioner do to be mainstream enough? We speak blithely of 'standard of care' but that does not mean that this is ever clearly defined, or is it always dynamic and situational? The courts note that you can digress from a majority view if you agree a 'respected minority ascribing to the standard of care'. Here one's peers determine appropriate care, not the patient irrespective of the outcome, and indeed not the state, at least directly. 'Unlike any other group of persons or professionals, physicians enjoy the somewhat inexplicable privilege of establishing the legal standard to which they are answerable through their own behavior.'[179] At least when there is a single course of action. But as this is rarely if ever the case, the courts ask whether the physician acted competently in making a choice and whether the choice was so judged by his or her peers, who had to have equivalent credentialling by the state and the profession in the same field. All are defined as 'reasonable men' who would not be negligent, for 'negligence is doing what a reasonable and prudent man would not have done or not doing what such a man would have done.' Regarding any particular act under consideration, the 'question . . . [is] whether, considering how people generally act and the ordinary exigencies of life, it will generally be reasonable to act in that way . . . The test of reasonableness is what would be the conduct or judgment of what may be called a standard man in the situation of the person whose conduct is in question.'[180]

As early as the beginning of scientific medicine, reasonableness came to be a standard for medical practice. 'What usually is done may be evidence of what ought to be done . . . but what ought to be done is set by a fixed standard of reasonable prudence, whether it is complied with or not.'[181] Or in this case the reasonable physician is not the sum of medical practice, as one jurist in Australia found in 1980 that 'it is not the law that if all or most of the medical practitioners in Sydney habitually fail to take an available precaution to avoid foreseeable risk of injury to the patients that none can be found guilty of negligence.'[182]

But who is this reasonable man now robed in the investiture of his profession as a physician. The law thus assumes that the reasonable physician is the medical equivalent of the 'man on the Clapham omnibus', aka the American 'man on the street', the Australian 'man on the Bondi tram', the Canadian 'person on the Yonge Street subway' who defines Reasonable Man. Where is the 'Reasonable Physician' to be found: in medical societies, in medical schools, in the offices of state that license and thus technically control them? What is their 'Clapham omnibus'?

Reasonable man and therefore the reasonable physician is 'a mythical creature of the law', as Justice James Laidlaw of the Ontario Court of Appeal aptly described him in the 1950s.[183] He cited the original definition of 1856 by Justice Edward Hall Alderson, who created the reasonable man thus furnishing the world of common law with a 'natural' definition of negligence: 'Negligence is the omission to do something which a reasonable man, guided upon those considerations which ordinarily regulate the conduct of human affairs, would do, or doing something which a prudent and reasonable man would not do. The defendants might have been liable for negligence, if, unintentionally, they omitted to do that which a reasonable person would have done, or did that which a person taking reasonable precautions would not have done.'[184]

In fact, the legal satirist A. P. Herbert, in his caricature of the reasonable man, goes further in attributing a personality – and perhaps neuroses – to the man who navigates the world with a self-conscious awareness of the implications of his every action, 'who invariably looks where he is going, and is careful to examine the immediate foreground before he executes a leap or bound; who neither star-gazes nor is lost in meditation when approaching trap-doors or the margin of a dock; who never mounts a moving omnibus, and does not alight from any car while the train is in motion'.[185] Is this not the idealized physician of nineteenth- and twentieth-century fiction? It is vital, however, following Blackstone's notion that the claim of quackery must be proven based on a lack of knowledge, that they do have their professional competence. As Herbert writes:

> To say of a doctor that he had no knowledge of medicine, of a solicitor that he knew nothing of the law, or of a banker that he did not know his business would without doubt be defamatory, however honestly the opinion was held and however moderately that opinion was expressed. Nothing but the strongest proof that the assertions were true in substance and in fact would be sufficient excuse for them in an action of defamation; yet it is undeniably a matter of public interest that our doctors, our solicitors, and our bankers should know their business.[186]

Should they not?

And that means clearly and rigorously identifying the scope of practice of the medical professional as defined by the state when they received their medical licence to practise, a definition that is malleable and shifts according to need and responds to the ever-changing boundaries of every medical field. Indeed, the very first case of medical malpractice defined thus was in the reign of the English king Henry IV (1399–1413), when a 'decision arose from the burgeoning doctrine requiring persons who practiced a "common calling" (meaning, probably, a skilled profession) to act as would any reasonably competent person practicing under like conditions or be liable for an action in trespass on the case'.[187]

After the Second World War and the creation of the NHS, 'malpractice' in Great Britain, where the concept originated, came to be seen as the 'American Disease'. In 1980 it was judged as 'that quite horrifying picture of what is happening in the United States of America and for the thought that, subject to taking heed of the warnings, something similar might happen here.'[188] Malpractice seemed to be seen in that light as a problem purely of the judicial and not the medical system. The 1980 article stated: 'I think that the most significant ones are those in which judgments are moving towards automatic compensation without regard for the strict standards of proof of negligence and those in which there are very high awards. If we do think these things are developing, the time to do something about it is now. If we do not do anything, we shall only have ourselves to blame.' But that means that consensus medicine in the NHS was not to be immune from the liability of malpractice, even if, as the eminent jurist Alfred Thompson 'Tom' Denning, Baron Denning, noted in a compensation case of a doctor who suffered brain damage after an anaesthetic: 'we have in this country a National Health Service. But the Health Authorities cannot stand huge sums without impeding the service to the community. The funds available come out of the taxpayers' pockets; they should not be dissipated by paying more than fair compensation.'[189] He goes on to argue that only overt and truly egregious acts (quackery one removed) will be punished, and in those cases the question was not the act itself but the court's compensation to the victim. He says:

> Every one of us every day gives a judgment which is afterwards found to be wrong. It may be an error of judgment but it is not negligent . . . Likewise with medical men. If they are to be found liable whenever they do not effect a cure, or whenever anything untoward happens, it would do a great disservice to the profession itself. Not only to the profession but to society at large. We must say, and say firmly, that, in a professional man, an error of judgment is not negligence.[190]

For the professional man is also a 'reasonable man'.

In British law today, negligence can be judged so gross, that is, so bad, as to raise an action in criminal negligence. 'Grossness' in this respect answers to some notion of criminal action as evidenced by recklessness, which was tested in the case of *Regina v. Adomako* ([1994] 3 All ER 79). The question was whether the conduct of a defendant was so negligent as to amount to a criminal act or omission when it resulted in the risk of death or severe injury. The litmus test remained 'reasonableness,' as demonstrated by 'circumstances that a reasonably prudent person in the defendant's position would have foreseen a serious and obvious risk of death or severe injury arising from the act or omission and the breach of duty is so reprehensible and falls so far below the standards expected of a person in the defendant's position with their qualifications, experience and responsibilities that it amounts to a crime'.[191] John Adomako was a British anaesthetist in charge of a patient during an eye operation who did not notice that an oxygen tube became disconnected. As a result, the patient died. The jury convicted him of gross negligence manslaughter. This qualified as a criminal case of manslaughter as it was proven, 'beyond a reasonable doubt', that his actions were unreasonable, a standard higher than that of civil actions proven on the balance of probability.

Yet the question of consensus was never quite convincingly resolved in law, at least in American law. As an American jurist instructed in 1992, in *Jones v. Chidester* ([1992] 531 Pa. 31, 610 A.2d 964), there is an

additional principle of law known as the two schools of thought doctrine. This principle provides that it is improper for a jury to be required to decide which of two schools of thought as to proper procedure should have been followed in this case, when both schools have their respective and respected advocates and followers in the medical profession. In essence, then, a jury of laypersons is not to be put in a position of choosing one respected body of medical opinion over another when each has a reasonable following among the members of the medical community.[192]

Unspoken, this finding draws into question the assumptions about the verities of science, put forward in the idealization of science – 'scientific facts are facts and cannot be questioned and those espousing them are experts and cannot be overruled' – that underpinned the United States Supreme Court's 1993 Daubert opinion (*Daubert v. Merrell Dow Pharmaceuticals, Inc.*, [1993] 590 U.S. 579, 592–6), which introduced a new regime of judicial scrutiny for the admissibility of scientific testimony.[193] The court held that 'an expert may testify about scientific knowledge that assists the jury in understanding the evidence or determining a fact in issue in the case. Factors that a judge should consider include whether the theory or technique in question can be and has been tested, whether it has been subjected to peer review and publication, its known or potential error rate, the existence and maintenance of standards controlling its operation, and whether it is widely accepted in the relevant scientific community.' The court is clear in its definition of scientific evidence *in a medical context* 'since the adjective "scientific" implies a grounding in science's methods and procedures, while the word "knowledge" connotes a body of known facts or of ideas inferred from such facts or accepted as true on good grounds'.[194] The operative word here is 'true'. In other words, EBM before its time PLUS professional consensus.

Fraud, like negligence, at least in the United States, in these terms, is a matter of civil law. Only claims where the action is a form of larceny, as in Medicaid fraud, which would be defined as misrepresenting your qualifications or the illnesses of your patients in order to receive payment, is it a criminal offence. But civil penalties can be used if those accused of fraud 'claimed to have special knowledge of the subject matter' that the listener did not have; or if the representation was made 'not in a casual expression of belief, but in a way that declared the matter to be true'; or if the speaker was in a position of 'trust and confidence' over the listener; or if the listener 'had some other special reason to expect' the speaker to be reliable.[195]

With the rise of scientific medicine and the successful introduction of a wide range of allopathic treatments for a range of diseases from tuberculosis to syphilis to psychosis, the assumption was that the broad audience for non-state-sanctioned interventions was naive at best; and they were culpable, at worst, for their own misfortune. Much like the Victorian notion of the 'deserving poor', the use of state-approved medications proved that not only the practitioner's views but those of the patient were worth consideration. Fraud is thus also the creation of a false belief, and state-sanctioned medicine seems to create a true belief in the function of specific sanctioned interventions. As a recent commentator stated, such claims are defined 'in terms that entrench the medical profession and that exclude all other forms of healing as the "unauthorized" practice of medicine, a crime. The purported justification is to prevent fraud and protect public health.' The problem is that such claims 'reflect the private interest of the medical academy as a professional monopoly, an interest that does not coincide with the prevention of fraud.' And that, 'rather than protecting public health, the current framework limits consumer choice, denigrates patient autonomy, and diminishes patient welfare.'[196] We can add, because it supports an assumption of the fixed nature of belief systems, including heterodox ones.

If we dismiss all alternatives as quackery, we also fall into the belief that only fixed, state-sanctioned modalities of treatment are efficacious. If thus a practitioner is effective by, say, the 'laying on hands – if he is employing a therapeutic technique of potential benefit to future patients, one that implicates a physiological reality', we often see this as being relegated 'to the realm of faith, on one hand, or [we ban] it outright . . . If the touch of [a practitioner] – while it employs no scalpel, dispatches no pharmacological agent, and operates solely on touch – ameliorates . . . disease, then we must reevaluate our foundational assumptions about the way the law defines "medicine".'[197] Karin Knorr Cetina has observed that modern medicine now straddles the line between modernist optimism about finding objective truths and postmodern scepticism about such claims.[198] And I can add, in this tension lies our examination of quackery.

To define medical fraud, the law must resolve the intention of the perpetrator. *Mens rea*, an awareness that what one is undertaking flaunts the law, is necessary for a crime to exist. But *mens rea* has itself been understood on various levels of consciousness and therefore culpability. Actions can have purpose (the same as intentionality), with the individual achieving or attempting to achieve specific aims; it demands in addition the knowledge that these aims are what is intended; it is recklessness if such knowledge leads one to act even if risk is entailed and is only negligent if one is aware that a potential unjustifiable risk is entailed by the action. Thus, there must be a provable causality between the belief and the *actus rea*, the conscious act.

What if, as we shall see in our case studies, those advocating a certain course of action or theory of healing truly believe what they are selling? And that which is being sold has some type of state sanction or traditional value? And perhaps the claim is the opposite in those who purchase such potions or believe such people. Is an unawareness of being the target of the quack or quackery necessary to be deceived? As the American Supreme Court Justice Oliver Wendell Holmes, Jr, the son of the physician-poet, famously argued, the concept of intent seems so evident that 'even a dog knows the difference between being stumbled over and being kicked.'[199] If, I assume, you are a Reasonable Dog or Man, do you as the purveyor or the consumer of quackery really know the difference? Quackery in use and practice thus covers a multitude of options but, according to the state, can thus be shown to be able to be distinguished from 'real' healing by not truth claims but claims about belief and power. Belief is a tricky category, even if Justice Holmes believed it was not.

When we read of such distinctions, we assume that there is always, at each moment, in the ever-altering landscape of medical research and therapy, a clear-cut boundary between allopathic and state-sanctioned, complementary or alternative medicine, on the one hand, and 'quackery' for the sake of purely financial gain, on the other. Scientific publications, recognized and ranked by academic institutions, would be an index for such a distinction. But we have ample evidence that experts who review papers for publication are prejudiced against alternative forms of therapy to the one in use at that moment. In one case, reviewers were shown a wide range of responses to two versions of a certain paper, with a significant bias in favour of the orthodox-conventional version. It was concluded that 'authors of technically good, unconventional, papers may therefore be at a disadvantage in the peer review process.'[200] We will see that in the creation of ever more specialized medical sub-fields. New scientific journals appeared with the creation of new fields in both allopathic and heterodox medicine as they accept the sort of science, for good or ill, that is unable to be placed in the best 'peer-viewed' journals of the day. And each one, in print or online, makes the claim for their use of evidence and efficacy of treatment.

Here we can move on to our case studies and the sciences and the cultures that shaped and continue to shape them. In each we can observe how shifts in scientific understanding and the development of technology shapes, for good or for ill, clinical practice. And how, as each reach towards the establishment of valid and apparently successful therapies, they are replaced or modified or abandoned as new claims for scientific knowledge evolve. The reciprocity of clinic and bench continues to define and redefine the boundaries between doc and quack in that ambiguous space of healing we call 'medicine'.

2
Stomachs

PEPTIC ULCER DISEASE, or PUD, to use its contemporary acronym, was seen in the age of scientific medicine to be a relatively new disease.[1] The acronym, coined in the 1970s, attempted to lump together a range of earlier diseases of the digestive system. In this chapter, I too shall be lumping together a range of ulcerations: those of the oesophagus (gullet or food pipe), the stomach and the duodenum (upper part of the small bowel). In the 2023 World Health Organization's *International Classification of Diseases*, the international gold standard for naming and then coding diseases, these are still seen as quite distinct (to be found at DA25, 'Oesophageal Ulcer'; DA60, 'Gastric Ulcer'; DA63Z, 'Duodenal Ulcer'). These distinctions are the most recent attempt to deal with the complexity of the manifestation of such diseases by focusing on anatomy rather than cause. As we shall see, there have been many such attempts to set these boundaries and definitions, all shifting during the age of scientific medicine. Indeed, the boundaries between PUD and other intense internal discomfort and pain in the digestive tract made differential diagnosis, even well into the age of scientific medicine, difficult.[2] Today PUD as now defined is a significant cause of morbidity and mortality both in the United States and worldwide, with a lifetime prevalence estimated at 5–15 per cent. But it has a complex history.

Early in the age of scientific medicine it was claimed that the ancients did not know of ulcers of the digestive system, though a wide range of symptoms associated with them were recorded.[3] The *morbus niger* (black vomit and stools) of the Hippocratic corpus seemed only to describe haemorrhage, which may be due to diseases of the spleen or gastric cancers, not ulcers per se. Talmudic medicine does not cite stomach ulcers, although perforations of the stomach (open and closed), which rendered animals unkosher, are mentioned.[4] Vesalius, who may well have suffered from PUD, did not register peptic ulcers.[5] The first postmortem demonstration of this disease seems to be that by the physician Marcello Donato in 1586. Donato found that the inner layer of the stomach near the pylorus was eroded ('*exesam*'), and he does 'not doubt that this was the cause of the disease', without commenting on what could have caused the erosion. He also avoids recounting any of the symptoms of a chronic ulcer, without a doubt because the patient was dead.[6] Until the eighteenth century, as we shall see, the ability to distinguish the location and intensity of various ulcers of the digestive system was only possible posthumously.

By the eighteenth century, the symptoms of PUD as narrated by patients appeared more frequently in the medical literature without being linked to either a specific aetiology or a disease process. Were these then new diseases or merely a rearrangement of various symptoms to provide an excuse for innovations in treatment? Names matter. Cardialgia, heartburn, pyrosis, biliousness, dyspepsia and indigestion were terms regularly found in the medical and popular literature and seemed interchangeable in terms of symptoms.[7] Rare terms, such as cardialgia, came 'from *cardia*, the heart, or rather the left orifice of the stomach, and -*algia*, to be pained, the pain of the mouth of the stomach or heart-burn. The ancients called the mouth of the stomach *cardia*.'[8] Pyrosis, first documented in 1776, was defined as different from 'dyspepsia . . . This disease appears to be a peculiar spasmodic affection of the stomach . . . it usually comes on in the morning or forenoon, at those times when the stomach is most empty, with a pain and sense of constriction at the pit of the stomach, as if it was drawn backwards . . . After some continuance, it brings on an eructation of a thin watery fluid, sometimes acrid, but generally insipid, and in considerable quantity.'[9] More common terms, such as dyspepsia, still have their echo in our use of 'dyspeptic' today. Documented in English as early as 1706, it was outlined thus:

> a want of appetite, a squeamishness, sometimes a vomiting, sudden and transient distensions of the stomach, eructations of various kinds, heartburn, pains in the region of the stomach, and a bound belly, are symptoms which frequently concur

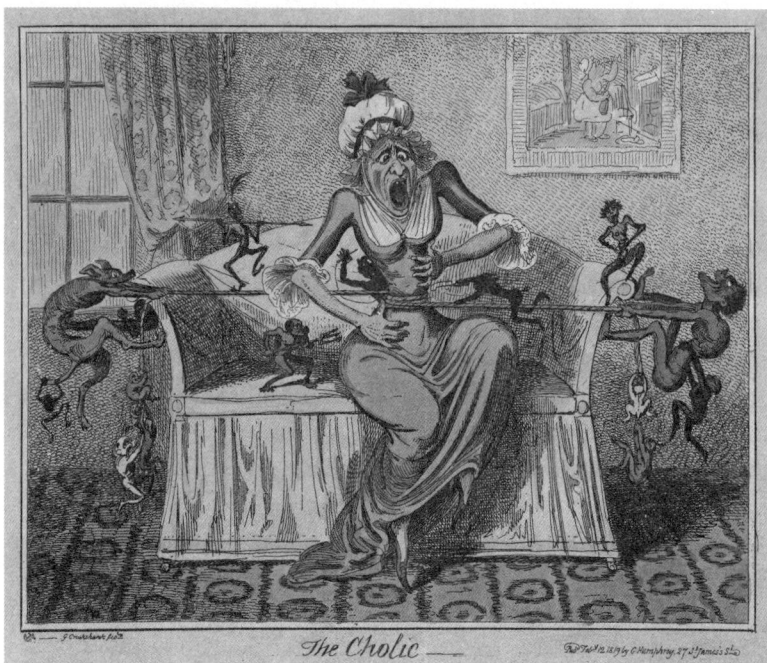

George Cruikshank, *The Cholic*, 1819, etching depicting a woman suffering the pain of stomach cholic. On the wall hangs a picture of an interior with a disreputable-looking woman drinking, implied as the cause of her disorder of the digestive tract as dissolution was often seen as the cause and such maladies were treated by the local docs and quacks.

in the same person . . . But as this disease is also frequently a secondary and sympathetic affection, so the symptoms above mentioned are often joined with many others; and this has given occasion to a very confused and undetermined description of it, under the general title of nervous diseases, or under that of chronic weakness.[10]

Everyone had digestive ills, no matter what they were labelled. 'Headache and dyspepsia are my worst ailments,' complained Charlotte Brontë in 1857.[11]

Popular terms or terms that became popular could not have much cachet in medicine, defined as such by the social status of the physician's use of Latin. The term '*Gastritis inflammatoria*' simply translated the French '*Inflammation de l'estomac*' while others preferred '*Ulcus ventriculi*', or indeed even '*Ulcus ventriculi chronicum*'. '*Ulcus duodeni*' seemed to have some traction with the anatomist, as it was specific to the duodenum. Various and sundry terms are used by noted physicians from Hermann Boerhaave and Gottfried van Swieten to Frederick Hoffmann, Giovanni Baptiste Morgagni and Samuel August Tissot, from the eighteenth century on, for a range of diseases of the stomach that probably ranged from cancerous lesions to ulceration. Peptic ulcer, '*Ulcus pepticum*', appears first in 1795 in a rather complete German translation of Daniel Christian Franzen's Latin medical handbook of 1790–92, where the Latin term is bizarrely not present.[12] By the way, 'peptic ulcer' first appears in English as a recognized medical term only in 1900, in Dorland's *Medical Dictionary*.[13] Names matter.

The relationship between symptoms and post-mortem examinations had been always questionable. Since you cannot ask the cadaver what symptoms they had, and when the narrative of the symptoms may well only be able to be loosely correlated to remembered symptoms much later during an autopsy, it became clear that what was experienced (for example, dyspepsia) might or might not be caused by anomalies of the cadaver's digestive system. What caused the discomfort followed *the* science.

Among the German Vitalists, who believed that the life force was more than mere chemistry, Georg Ernst Stahl (MD, University of Jena, 1683) coined a set of terms – '*vena haemorrhoides interna*', '*vena splenica*', '*vas breve*' – looking at the impairment of circulation in the stomach as the cause of a range of maladies.[14] But again, for what reason? In 1772 John Hunter (no advanced degree; came in 1748 to London to assist in the preparation of dissections for the course of anatomy taught by his brother William, a famed obstetrician) linked his theory of blood circulation to the preservation of the stomach from what he labels auto-digestion, which caused ulcers. For post-mortem, there is 'a dissolution of the stomach at its great extremity; in consequence of which there is frequently a considerable aperture made in the *viscus*. The edges of this opening appear to be half dissolved.'[15] There is acid in the stomach, which the chemists acknowledge, and it can so act to dissolve the organ. But why?

Differential diagnosis was also undertaken to try and distinguish PUD from other diseases of the digestive tract. Matthew Baillie (MD, University of Oxford, 1789) described peptic ulcers in detail using data from autopsies in 1793. Baillie carefully provided a differential diagnosis, in contrast to stomach cancer and 'schirrus' (a cancerous tumour), defining the anatomy of the stomach ulcer in terms of it resembling 'common ulcers in any other part of the body, but frequently they have a peculiar appearance. Many of them are hardly surrounded with any inflammation, have not irregularly eroded edges as ulcers have generally, and are not attended with any diseased alteration in the structure of the stomach in the neighbourhood.'[16] It is seldom seen to warrant detailed description in his morbid anatomy, with clear differential diagnoses to other, more frequently seen diseases.

Even in the nineteenth century duodenal and peptic ulcer disease still seemed rare enough that they were labelled well to the end of the century as 'la maladie de Cruveilhier' (and indeed so still haunts medical dictionaries with that eponym), after the French anatomist and pathologist Jean-Baptiste Cruveilhier (MD, University of Paris, 1816), who again in the 1840s distinguished gastric ulcer from gastric cancer.[17] As Roy Porter noted, the wide range of such digestive disorders 'taxed the medical and moral imaginations of nineteenth century physicians, before another spin of [the] whirligig of maladies a la mode brought the twentieth century fashion: the ulcer.'[18] Yet even then PUD was a disease that seemed so unusual that in the first edition of his standard medical textbook in 1892, Sir William Osler still thought that post-mortem data overestimated the incidence of peptic ulcer.[19] Or did it?

What Causes PUD?

In the age of scientific medicine, Heinrich Irenaeus Quincke (MD, University of Berlin, 1863) used the term 'ulcus digestione' in 1879. He is given the role of the first physician to employ the claims of science concerning the origin of PUD by many later writers, looking for the origin of PUD in the age of scientific medicine.[20] He described three post-mortem cases of lower oesophageal erosions associated with upper gastrointestinal haemorrhage as 'ulcus oesophagi ex digestione', or oesophageal ulcers due to digestive juices.[21] Quincke had been a student of Ernst von Brücke in Vienna, one of Johannes Müller's best students, and then of the pathologist Friedrich Theodor von Frerichs (MD, University of Göttingen, 1841) at the great public hospital, the Charité in Berlin, who had also worked on ulceration of the stomach. By 1879 Quincke was professor of internal medicine at Kiel and is credited with performing the first lumbar puncture. Seeking a scientific explanation, Quincke argued that peptic ulcer is caused by the effect of pepsin breaking down proteins as well as the corrosive effects of gastric acid. No acid, no ulcer.[22]

Yet he was not alone. The great cellular pathologist Rudolf Virchow, in the most exhaustive history of the concept to date, argued in 1853 that such ulceration was the failure of the blood, that he deemed to be alkaline, to neutralize stomach acid. He noted that the popular term '*chronische Unterleibsbeschwerden*' (chronic lower-body complaints) runs from constipation to hypochondria and hysteria. Given its vagueness it has called for a response from the 'doctors, the quacks, and lay people.'[23] He uses '*einfache*' (simple) and '*sogenannte perforirende Magengeschwür*' (so-called perforating stomach ulcer) as his terms of choice, simply using the German terms of the day. No Latin terms for him! But what these lesions were and what had directly caused the failure to neutralize the acid seemed beyond the science of the day. These views of the aetiology of PUD were made concrete by the Croat internist Dragutin (aka Carl) Schwarz (MD, University of Vienna, 1891) in 1910, who hypothesized that it was the hypersecretion of gastric acid that was the cause of peptic ulcer.[24] More acid, more ulcers. But why was there too much acid? What evidence could the physician apply to find cause and, perhaps, cure?

Perhaps one of the problems of PUD was that, like its kissing cousin gout, if there was an ultimate cause imagined in the popular mind, it lies in the agency of the patient, whose dissolute life was seen as the cause of the ailment. So much so that in 1863, the noted advocate of scientific medicine, the pathologist Lionel Smith Beale (MD, King's College, London, 1851), then a young physician who had just been elected to both the Royal Society and the Royal College of Physicians, delivered a series of lectures, entitled *The Stomach Medically and Morally Considered*, to a lay audience. He proclaimed that 'the stomach may justly be considered as the grand antagonist to moral and intellectual improvement.'[25] The Devil incarnate. PUD was claimed to be the result of the rise of a bourgeois society willing to sacrifice abstemiousness for pleasure, the result of soft and corrupting city life. As the noted naval physician Thomas Trotter (MD, Edinburgh, 1788) in his *View of the Nervous Temperament* (1807) observed, recently there has been an 'increase of a class of diseases, but little known in former times, and what had slightly engaged the study of physicians prior to that period. They have been designated in common language, by the terms NERVOUS; SPASMODIC; BILIOUS; INDIGESTION; STOMACH

COMPLAINTS; LOW SPIRITS; VAPOURS, &c.'[26] And names do really matter. And this infiltrated the underlying assumptions of scientific medicine. In *The Lancet* at mid-nineteenth century 'a French writer calls dyspepsia "the remorse of a guilty stomach".'[27]

The aetiology of dyspepsia as a reflex of human action is as varied as the descriptions. The polymath Erasmus Darwin (MB, Cambridge University, 1755) in 1784 writes of '*Dyspepsia a pedibus frigidis*':

> When the feet are long cold, as in riding in cold and wet weather, some people are very liable to indigestion and con- sequent heart-burn. The irritative motions of the stomach become torpid, and do their office of digestion imperfectly in consequence of their association with the torpid motions of the vessels of the extremities. Fear, as it produces paleness and torpidity of the skin, frequently occasions temporary indiges- tion in consequence of this association of the vessels of the skin with those of the stomach as riding in very bad roads will give flatulency and indigestion to timorous people.[28]

In 1881 Sir John Russell Reynolds (MD, University of London, 1852), as of 1878 physician-in-ordinary to the queen's household, sees that 'dys- pepsia, and tight-lacing, and ball-dressing, and all that they involve, are disregarded' by women of fashion when they seek out the care of the specialist.[29] Dyspepia is always caused by the patient's lifestyle.[30]

Who lightly admits to having caused their own discomfort? As we have seen, even a medical diagnosis that linked the wide range of symp- toms presented was murky at best. And the less able the physician was to define the problem, the more scope for quack medicine, as defined by medical science. Indeed, medications and other interventions for dyspepsia and related illness dominated the nineteenth-century patent medicine market in the United States, such as 'Brown's Iron Bitters, a True Tonic, cures Dyspepsia, Indigestion, Malaria, Weakness, etc.,' and which was 'highly recommended for all diseases requiring a certain and efficient TONIC; especially Indigestion, Dyspepsia, Intermittent Fevers, Want of Appetite, Loss of Strength, Lack of Energy, Malaria, etc. Enriches the blood, strengthens the muscles and gives new life to the nerves . . . As Brown's Iron Bitters is specially adapted to diseases incident to the female, we will send in a plain sealed envelope to any lady desiring it, a circular containing testimonials from ladies.'[31]

In the age of the Muckrakers, such medications are often cited as proof of fraud and quackery, as the journalist Samuel Hopkins Adams noted after the beginning of state oversight over quack medicines in the case of

Stuart's Dyspepsia and Catarrh Tablets
Conspicuous in the Rogues' Gallery of Quackery is the F. A. Stuart Co. of Marshall, Mich. To read this firm's advertisements, one would suppose that their pills could repair a disordered stomach with the ease and certainty of a tinker mending a kettle. In the advertising booklet Stuart's Dyspepsia Tablets 'cure dyspepsia in all its varied forms.' That, of course, is a wholesale lie. Knowing it to be such, and appreciating the true meaning of the Food and Drugs Act, the concern made no claims of cure on the label: it offered merely to relieve.[32]

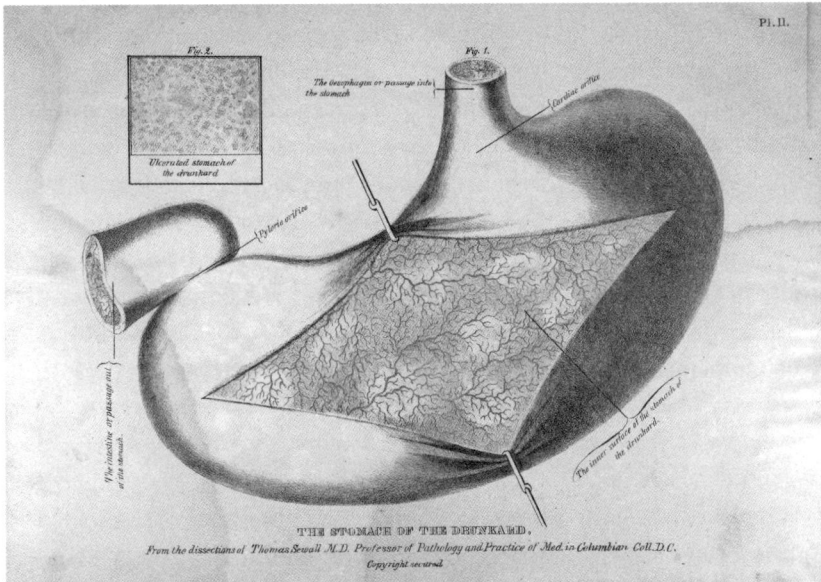

THE STOMACH OF THE DRUNKARD.
From the dissections of Thomas Sewall M.D. Professor of Pathology and Practice of Med. in Columbian Coll. D.C.
Copyright secured

Excess leads inevitably to ulcers and such dissolution can also be read on the drunkard's face, as claimed by Thomas Sewall, MD, professor of pathology and the practice of medicine at the Columbian College (which later became George Washington University), in *The Pathology of Drunkenness; or, The Physical Effects of Alcoholic Drinks, with Drawings of the Drunkard's Stomach* (1841). This illustration of 'the stomach of the habitual drunkard, or hard drinker . . . [shows] the mucous or internal coat, to be in a state of irritation, with its blood vessels, which are invisible while in a healthy state, to be enlarged and distended with blood . . . It bears a strong resemblance in its vascular structure, to what are denominated the rum blossom, seen upon the face of the hard drinker'.

PUD in all its forms, through all of its clinical diagnoses and therapies, was regularly over the centuries the target of quackery, however
defined. As we shall see, each shift in the scientific theories of diagnosis, causation and treatment, each and every abandonment of
established views when thrown into the dustbin as false, old-fashioned,
became, in so many words, mere quackery.

The production of scientific medical specialties soon calved off
the study and treatment of diseases of the digestive system. Gastroenterology as a medical specialty appears first in 1886 in Berlin, where
Ismar Boas (MD, University of Halle, 1881) designated himself as a
specialist for 'stomach and gut diseases' and then as a 'gastroenterologist' to the great consternation of his colleagues, who saw this type
of specialization as anathema to good medical practice, especially
when advocated by a 'pushy' Jew. By 1913 he had created the Society
for Gastroenterology, trailing a bit after the American Society for
Gastroenterology founded in 1897, as a research society, as espoused
by the AMA, rather than a professional one. 'Gastroenterology could
do little better than apply a general label to patients' maladies – that is
"dyspepsia" – and dispense general-purpose medicine for a variety of
conditions, little understood.'[33] The AMA only recognizes gastroenterology as a clinical sub-speciality in 1940, and the American journal by
that name is founded in 1942. The British Society of Gastroenterology
came in 1937 and *Gut*, the premier British journal, arrived on the scene
only in 1960. All well into the world of scientific medicine. Studying
disease processes so intertwined with notions of excess and moral
turpitude made this specialty come very late on the scene.

Seeing Ulcers

To be able to see into the living stomach and observe these biological processes at first hand had been undertaken in 1833 by William
Beaumont (after a two-year apprenticeship, in 1812 the Third Medical
Society of the State of Vermont certified his ability to practise). He
was able to explore the digestive processes of the French-Canadian fur
trader Alexis St Martin, who had been shot in the stomach and whose
open fistula never completely healed, allowing Beaumont to peer
directly into his stomach. Beaumont explored changes in the appearance of his stomach lining and noted that his cantankerous subject,
in 'fear, anger, or whatever depresses or disturbs the nervous system',

developed, among other symptoms, 'irregular circumscribed red patches'.[34] That St Martin had developed ulcers, given his experiences with Beaumont, would surprise no one.

Such direct observation within the stomach was then repeated over and over in the nineteenth and twentieth century. After creating artificial fistulas in dogs, researchers, among other things, undertook to measure the impact of anger and rage on the development of their peptic ulcers. As in the case of one unfortunate fifteen-year-old in 1878 studied by Charles Richet (MD, University of Paris, 1869; Nobel Prize, Physiology or Medicine, 1913, 'in recognition of his work on anaphylaxis'), who had developed an abdominal fistula having been poisoned ingesting potassium hydroxide. Perhaps the most famous researcher who investigated the relationship between gastric activity and external events was Ivan Pavlov (MD, Medical Military Academy, St Petersburg, 1879; Nobel Prize, Physiology or Medicine, 1904, 'in recognition of his work on the physiology of digestion, through which knowledge on vital aspects of the subject has been transformed and enlarged'), a great fan of Beaumont, who, in the 1890s, in a famous series of experiments, was able to generate gastric acids in his dogs through external stimulation, by ringing a bell. We remember the bell and the saliva, but not the reason for the experiment.

If finding patients who had an open fistula was difficult, then the idea of directly examining the digestive system through technology seemed to be an answer. Today, endoscopy of the gastrointestinal tract in modern clinical practice is most often undertaken under moderate sedation using such agents as midazolam, diazepam, pethidine and the ever popular, highly addictive social scourge fentanyl.[35] So, entering the body even to see ulcers posed much discomfort and some risk.

The history of that risk is one that tracks the rise of modern scientific technology in medicine.[36] In 1806 the physician Philipp Bozzini (MD, University of Mainz, 1796) invented a set of specula and mirrors reflecting candlelight by which he could make examinations within the openings in the body.[37] His '*Lichtleiter*' (light conductor) built on older specula but enabled the physician to look deeper within the body's cavities. He demonstrated his device to great acclaim to the members of the Viennese St Joseph's Academy at the end of 1806 and the beginning of 1807; an announcement of this was published in the local Viennese newspapers at the end of January. It was greeted as an 'ingenious invention', to no little degree because such examinations were (he claimed)

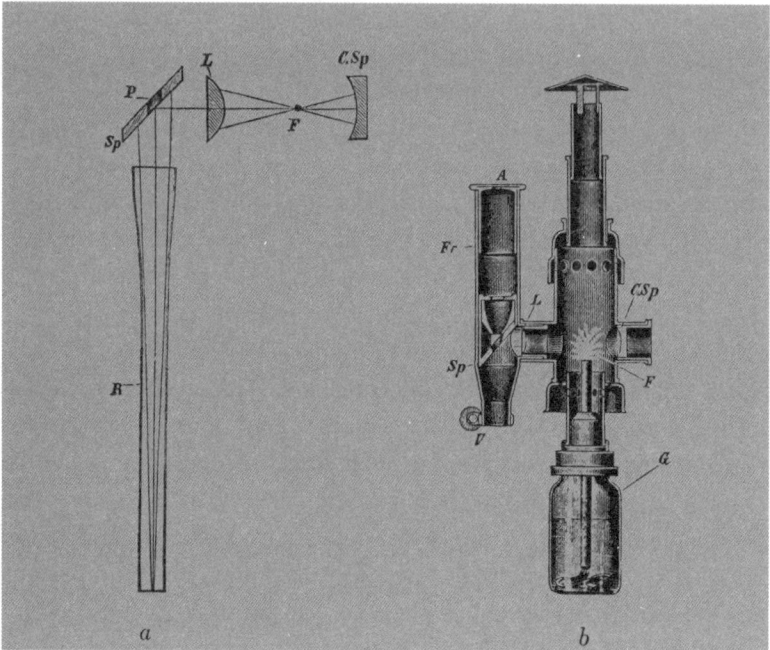

Adolf Kussmaul's rigid oesophagoscope, from Theodore H. Bast,
The Life and Time of Adolf Kussmaul (1926).

painless. The members of the Academy then sent the instrument in February to the Medical Faculty of the Viennese University, headed by the emperor's physician, Andreas Joseph Stifft (MD, University of Vienna, 1784), who was 'on principle an enemy of all new ideas'. They dismissed it, in their 'expert's opinion', as 'a mere toy', and more importantly warned physicians not to buy the instrument.[38] Quack medicine.

It was not until 1853 that the French surgeon Antonin Jean Desormeaux (MD, University of Paris, 1844) used an improved version of the device, with an external light source, a gasogene lamp, to successfully diagnose urethral and bladder diseases in living male patients. It was his use of the device in surgery for the first time that meant modern endoscopy was finally introduced into clinical practice. He too wrote widely about the device and tried to popularize its use. But the deeper you probed into the body through such technology, the poorer your evidence became, as rigid materials and limited illumination made the patient's experience unpleasant and the physician's ability to examine the interior of the body unproductive.

The German army surgeon and later professor of medicine at Heidelberg Adolf Kussmaul (MD, University of Heidelberg, 1848) is generally credited with the first gastroscopy in 1868. He truly was 'shouting in the marketplace', as it was only possible to test his straight rigid metal tube when a cooperative sword-swallower, whose *nom de théâtre* was 'Iron Heinrich', agreed to be the first to be the subject of his 'gastroscope'. Kussmaul had a local musical instrument-maker named Fischer fashion tubes 47 centimetres (18½ in.) long and 13 millimetres (½ in.) in diameter, one being round and the other elliptical in design, the tubes fitted with conical wooden collars (mandarins) to facilitate insertion. For a light source, he used a mirror reflecting light from the Desormeaux device, which he received from Paris, but in the end found it inadequate. He also quickly discovered that gastric secretions were a problem, despite using a flexible tube he had developed earlier to empty the stomach before the procedure.

The value of his efforts was the demonstration that the curves and bends of the oesophagus and oesophago-gastric junction could be traversed with careful manipulation and that the gastric pouch could be visualized, if with great care and potential pain. Kussmaul apparently demonstrated his 'gastroscope' several times in various medical schools, but the illumination was too poor to allow a clinically useful image.[39] And, I suspect, his sword-swallower ran out of patience. With

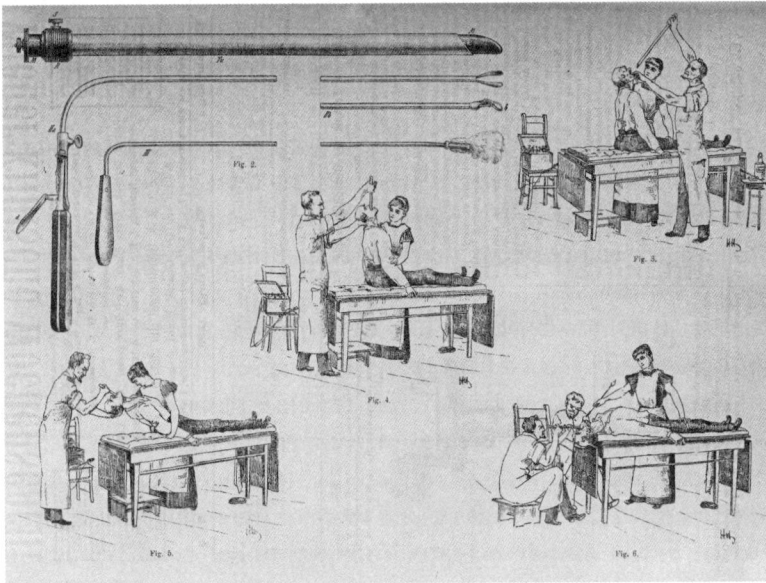

Victor Ritter von Hacker, professor of surgery at the University of Innsbruck, presenting at his teacher Theodor Billroth's Viennese clinic in 1895 the usage of a rigid Mikulicz-Leiter oesophagoscope, with a reflective electric lamp for illumination.

the addition of electric light sources in the 1890s more and more invasive endoscopies were possible, unlike Bozzini's initial one, only now
with the use of anaesthetic. Georg Wolf, a Berlin manufacturer of rigid
endoscopes established in 1906, produced the first 'Sussmann flexible
gastroscope' in 1911, enabling the detailed examination of the upper
digestive tract. From there the improvements followed the improvements in light conduction, with eventually the fibre-optic endoscopes
in the 1950s. Modern endoscopy becomes professionalized shortly
before that when in 1941 the American Society for Gastrointestinal
Endoscopy is founded.

If endoscopy provided one form of technological innovation by
the 1890s, by the close of the nineteenth century there was at least the
possibility to observe the digestive process with X-rays, accidentally
developed by the Würzburg physicist Wilhelm Röntgen in November
1895, and for which he received the Nobel Prize for Physics in 1901 'in
recognition of the extraordinary services he has rendered by the discovery of the remarkable rays subsequently named after him'. In 1897
X-rays were first used during a surgical procedure, trying to locate
a bullet. But it came with the quick realization that they were much
less able to capture images of soft tissue. The simple fact that soft
tissue vanished meant that it was less useful for the examination of
the digestive system and led interpreters of such images to flights of
fancy. By 1920 we had X-rays that depicted the 'hysterical gut', *'coxalgia
hysterica'*, a condition that simply does not exist except in the eye of
the beholder convinced by the new science that all pathologies could
finally be seen.[40] That these flights of fancy were a problem from the
very beginning was clear. In 1896 the hand of a cadaver was X-rayed
with the circulatory system filled with a contrastive, radiopaque substance, which was helpful, at least on cadavers. Seeing via this new
technology, especially a technology which provided perhaps much too
great a latitude for fanciful interpretation, was simply less scientific, or
perhaps less satisfying, than unmediated observation.

Carl Wegele (MD, University of Würzburg, 1882), in 1896, used a
metal wire inserted through an oral gastric tube to provide a loose
sense of where the oesophagus and stomach were on the X-ray plate.
In March 1896 Wolf Becher (MD, University of Berlin, 1888) in Berlin
presented the use of a contrast agent in demonstrating the gastrointestinal tract of a guinea pig. Sadly, the substance used was toxic.
John Hemmeter (MD, University of Maryland, 1884), at his alma mater,

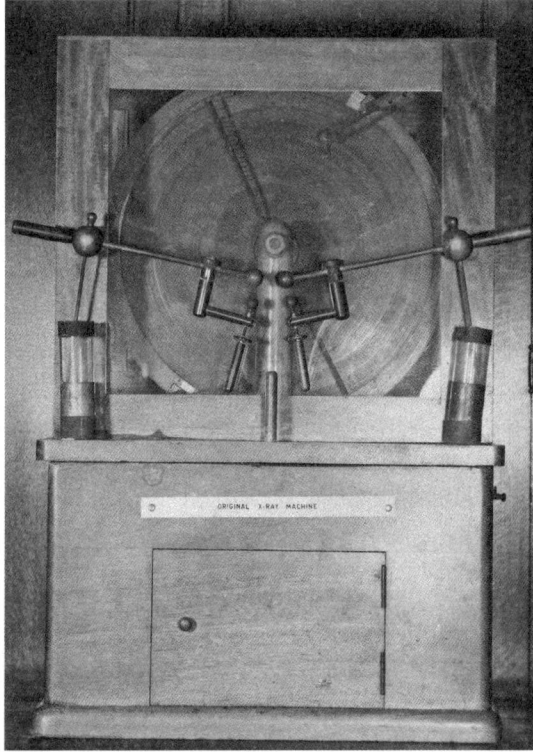

X-ray machine used by the physiologist Walter Bradford Cannon to investigate the mechanical process of digestion, 1896–8.

put lead acetate in a rubber bag in 1897 and had his patients swallow it. It was truly unpleasant and was quickly discontinued.

It was the Harvard medical student Walter Bradford Cannon, who received his degree in 1900, about whom we will read much more later in this chapter, who used fluoroscopes, moving X-ray images, to capture the moment of a liquid mixed with bismuth subnitrate passing through the digestive system of a cat. Now, bismuth was already well known to the physicians and the patients as it was a standard component of both compounded and quack medication for gastric distress.[41] Even as late as 1930, the pitfalls of radiological examination for PUD were clear, as

> inaccurate diagnosis has undoubtedly been a source of much confusion and error in the past. Too often the radiologist alone has had to bear the burden of diagnosis, and under such circumstances, errors of commission and omission are unavoidable . . . Many ulcers on the posterior part of the bulb are visualized only with palpation under the fluoroscopic

screen and may not appear in the films. Furthermore, the obvious visualized defect of the duodenum may be the cicatrix of a healed lesion in a patient whose present symptoms are due to another cause.[42]

It was not only the new technology that could locate lesions but the general introduction of anaesthesia and antisepsis that turned the corner on seeing PUD as the focus of surgical interventions. Surgery becomes not only imaginable but possible with this confluence of factors: you can visualize, identify and then operate. Today upper GI series uses barium for X-ray visualization of the gastrointestinal tract, but the perils of interpretation have led to other forms of visualizations (CAT scan, fMRI) complementing or replacing X-rays. The more complex the technology, the more information could be acquired. The more complex the technology, the more focused and limited the information acquired. The more complex the technology, the more complex the procedures for the patients. Living patients, more detailed images and the ability for the patients to narrate their symptoms should result in easy diagnosis and focused clinical interventions, but the lived reality, as we shall see, is quite different.

Infections Cause PUD

There was a compelling argument in scientific medicine that PUD was one of the modern mass diseases, a disease that came to the fore in the Enlightenment, as part of the Industrial Revolution and the rise to social dominance of the bourgeoisie. Paralleling this was the popular claim that the disease had its origin in the misbehaviour of exactly that class: overeating, excess in all things, indeed even the daily life of the new middle class; the radical social divisions propagated by these shifts were also postulated as a potential cause. But it is just as compelling to see its history as distorted by the plenitude of symptoms, labels and aetiologies which made it impossible to define a specific disease and sought causes within and beyond the body. Indeed, were the Romans, at least in the fantasies of Petronius' *Satyricon*, any less prone to excess, to stress and indeed to ailments of digestion? As in many cases during the rise of scientific medicine in the nineteenth century, the conflicts between aetiologies and therapies play themselves out in the understanding of the origins and meanings ascribed to PUD. Explaining where the disease came from was as important in treating the patient as any intervention would be. For 'knowing' the cause of your malady almost always was assumed to have an impact on compliance with treatment.

By 1857 William Brinton (MD, King's College London, 1848) speculated on its origin and looked for psychogenetic causes:

> There can be no doubt as to the physiological circumstances which predispose to this disease. Old age, privation, fatigue, mental anxiety, and intemperance are such frequent coincidences of its occurrence, that we are fully entitled to regard them as its more or less immediate causes in a large proportion (I think we might say a majority) of cases . . . But that careful clinical study of the malady which my Hospital opportunities have afforded me, leaves me just as little doubt with respect to the remarkable influence of poverty and intemperance . . . in the production of the gastric ulcer.[43]

The popular answer to such claims about the social location of PUD was regularly made also in the public sphere from the 1850s through to the 1870s. For example, by G. H. Lewes, philosopher and amateur physiologist (as well as George Eliot's domestic partner), in a series of bestselling books on digestion and indigestion – studies, which were, by the way, admired by Ivan Pavlov. He saw urban life as the cause of such ailments and felt the treatment should be thus: 'a walking excursion especially in mountain districts and, with resolute avoidance of walking too much, will be of great service to the dyspeptic.' Get out of the city with its 'bad air' and into healing nature.[44]

By the age of Robert Koch and Louis Pasteur, mere evocation of poor lifestyle and the vagaries of life did not suffice. Even though in 1858 Hermann Brehmer, a student of Johannes Müller in Berlin, where he received his MD in 1851, had already opened a tuberculosis sanatorium and exposed his urban patients to fresh air with a remarkable rate of cure. In 1885 this was copied when the Adirondack Cottage Sanatorium for the urban poor was established in Saranac Lake, New York, by Edward Livingston Trudeau (MD, Columbia College of Physicians and Surgeons, 1871) and became the model for getting the chronically ill out of the cities and into G. H. Lewes's healing countryside. Between the two dates, on 24 March 1882, Robert Koch announced the discovery of the tubercle bacillus. Now science demanded clear and direct causation for disease processes, and given that this was the age of bacteriology, it would be nice if those causes could be seen under a microscope. Seeing had indeed to come before believing.

Seeing had to be placed in the service of the new scientific medicine defined by bacteriology. One of Koch's most dedicated opponents, the hygienist and bacteriologist, Max von Pettenkofer (MD, Ludwig Maximilian University, Munich, 1845), felt that seeing was simply not sufficient. He advocated strongly that bacterial infection was possible primarily in a social context, as poor nutrition, bad hygiene and adverse environment factors were necessary to transform the germ into the actual cause of an epidemic (what Pettenkofer called 'epidemic mutation'). To this end he produced a range of studies of human metabolism, examining the function of food and digestion on the potential for infection. To provide evidence for his theories he developed the modern urine test. Even though urine had been examined for colour, scent and taste since the Greeks, standardized tests for specific gravity, sugar and urea promised to turn urinalysis into a scientific tool useful for evaluating a patient's clinical status.[45] Suddenly digestion became accessible through urinalysis, now not merely seen but documented through chemistry. Social norms could be measured in the laboratory.

Such theories, no matter the evidence, demanded that the social and economic location of the patient would be causal for PUD – unlike bacteriology, which argued that the cause was the invasion of the system by those 'foreign' actors, bacteria and viruses, that worked regardless of the status, age or social location of the patients. The Viennese anatomist Carl von Rokitansky, who constantly sought the 'anatomical' seat of illness, had proposed in 1842 a theory of the origin of dyspepsia that postulated that it was caused by high fever, resulting in an overproduction of stomach acid as a response to the innervation of the stomach. The acid resulted in the overstimulation of the vagus nerve (the tenth and longest cranial nerve running from the brain to the intestines) because of the fever having caused a rise of intracranial pressure, which in turn caused hyperacidity and thus ulcers. Most of his cadavers suffered from an 'intracranial disorder', which had accompanied a fatal fever. His diagnostic differential is to a local infection, which he discounts.[46] But some sort of disease process was taking place elsewhere in the body, impacting on the lining of the stomach. This was seemed to be resolved after the aetiology of tuberculosis, syphilis and cholera all turned out to be bacterial infections and seemed thus to promise immediate therapies (which was sadly not to be so in many of these cases). Bacterial inflammations present in the body could therefore impact the stomach and cause ulcers. But where? Certainly, the most common form of intestinal inflammation seen in the clinic was appendicitis, with its clearly defined presentation and the evident risk of infection spilling into the belly.

Remember that in this age of scientific medicine, one of the heroes, and rightly so, is the Glasgow surgeon Joseph Lister, 1st Baron Lister (MB, University College London, 1852), who sprayed carbolic acid (or phenol, a derivative of coal tar, which we discussed in the last chapter), in 1865 to kill bacteria in the surgical theatre. This was an age in which a mere scratch could lead to death. The poet Rainer Maria Rilke died in 1926 of leukaemia, well into the age of antisepsis, but it was claimed that: 'Rilke gathered some roses from his garden. While doing so, he pricked his hand on a thorn. This small wound failed to heal, grew rapidly worse, soon his entire arm was swollen, and his other arm became affected as well.'[47] The avoidance of infection meant that patients' anxiety about surgery was lessened; indeed, it seemed less risky than even a rose's thorn. The acceptance of antisepsis was relatively slow. On 26 November 1877 Robert F. Weir (MD, New York College of Physicians and Surgeons, 1859), the 24th president of the New York Academy of Medicine, said in a talk before the New York Medical Association that the British and German acceptance of this procedure had outpaced that of the United States. He urged that the smallest detail of the cleansing of patient, surgeon, instruments and surgical theatre be carried out so that the patient is not placed at needless risk. Once this was done, the risks attendant on all surgery decreased sharply because of the reduction in the high incidence of infection.[48] No pain, no pus, much gain.

Lister and Weir were following *the* science, for if Pasteur's understanding of bacteria was correct, then the infections resulting from surgery were also the result of bacteria. They knew that the basic science of putrefaction had already been established in the 1830s, but 'Pasteur's work had been ratified', as Lister stressed, 'by the report of the Commission of the French Academy, first in 1862 and then in 1864.'[49] Not science but status mattered. The pH of a typical dilute solution of phenol in water is likely to be around 5–6 (depending on its concentration). If carbolic acid killed bad germs, then certainly the hydrochloric acid in gastric juice, with a pH between 1 and 3, would do the same, his contemporaries assumed. This problem consumed the interest of Ivan Pavlov, who sought an explanation for the secretion of gastric 'juices' and found it not merely in external stimuli that stimulated the flow of hydrochloric acid but in the ability to store the acid in the follicles of the empty stomach's lining before it destroyed the stomach itself.[50]

In 1912 a lively discussion took place at the Medical Society of London about 'the widely spread evils which might arise from a disordered gastro-intestinal tract'. The speaker 'believed the evil was primarily an infection and recurring infection of the gastro-intestinal tract and was in direct proportion to the number and virulence, and also to the varieties of the infecting germs'. Infection causes ulcers, as 'the bacteria were numerous and constantly reinforced from suppurative processes'. But not in the stomach, as *everyone* knows bacteria cannot exist in its acidic environment. Cure seems to be possible, even on that day well before antibiotics, as all people had to do was cleanse 'their mouths, nasopharynges . . . and so the infection [was] removed, and oils and suitable laxatives and diet administered'. We today – he observed – in the age of Koch know that 'the clinical picture of intestinal stasis was becoming fairly generally recognised in its more exaggerated forms, but the early cases, those in which, if properly treated, a perfect and permanent cure could be guaranteed, were still to be found labelled as "indigestion", "neurasthenia", "duodenal ulcer", &c., a misery to themselves and a source of constant worry and continual disappointment to their medical attendant.' For their intransigence regarding being cured not only irritated the patient's gut but exacerbated the physician's toleration for their patients.[51] Koch and Pasteur made a basic claim for the praxis of clinical medicine. Once infection had become microbial, explaining it without referring to the involvement of microorganisms became almost unimaginable: 'To oppose the claims of bacteriology is now not a rival view, nor an alternative view, nor even a dissident view. It is now a lunatic view.'[52] Not merely a consensus but any opposition was quackery.

Researchers quickly focused on a wide range of focal infections, such as that in the appendix, as playing a role in the aetiology of ulcers. Indeed, in a review of 718 operations for gastric and duodenal ulcers in 1923, Berkeley George Andrew Moynihan, 1st Baron Moynihan (MB, University of London, 1887), a noted abdominal surgeon and president of the Royal College of Surgeons, reported that he had also removed the appendix in no fewer than 307 cases of peptic ulcer.[53] His competition in the United States were the Brothers Mayo – William (MD, University of Michigan Medical School, 1883) and Charles (MD, Northwestern University, 1888) – whose practice began early to include surgery for PUD and 'who had done only 54 abdominal operations between 1889 and 1892, recorded 612 in 1900 and 2,157 five years later.'[54]

The sixth edition of the *Merck Manual* (1934) noted that 'focal infection (teeth, tonsils, etc.) is regarded as a very important etiological factor' for ulcers, a theme that was repeated through to the seventh edition (1940).[55] This is a reflex of the thinking behind what comes to be called Koch's postulates: specific pathogens were defined as causing specific, clearly defined infectious diseases. If infective pathogens were found in teeth, the appendix or the tonsils, might not their presence cause other pathologies elsewhere? 'Circumscribed and confined infection, commonly expressed as focal infections, has long been recognized as an important etiologic factor in systemic disease. Yet as a principle it has not received sufficient attention from practitioners. In my opinion, focal infection is very frequently related to local and general disease.' Indeed, among a large number of patients seen with 'infectious myocarditis' caused by streptococci are sufferers from 'exophthalmic goiter, cholecystitis, ulcer (peptic) of stomach, diabetes mellitus, etc.'[56] Therapies quickly built on these claims and in an age where general and local anaesthesia make such interventions less risky, the removal of teeth, appendectomies, colostomies and colectomies were employed to mitigate or cure PUD, as surgeons sought to locate the hidden sources of infection, often far from the site of the ulcers.

Surgery was undertaken for other potential aetiologies, such as cutting the vagus nerve to ameliorate the production of stomach acid. Surgeons, based on earlier animal studies, including those by Pavlov, began to imagine that severing or restructuring the vagus nerve could cure PUD. Modifying the nerve altered the parasympathetic nervous system, those functions beyond conscious control such as digestion and heart rate, since both seemed also to play a role in acid secretion in PUD. The first resectioning of the vagus nerve in humans, however, by the neurosurgeon Mathieu Jaboulay (MD, Lyon, 1885) at the turn of the twentieth century, was undertaken to palliate the chronic pain of tabes dorsalis, tertiary syphilis, the disease that obsessed allopathic medicine at the time. This became an intervention of choice for PUD after the First World War advocated by George Washington Crile (MD, Wooster

Medical College, 1887), the first surgeon to successfully undertake a blood transfusion in 1906 and, in 1921, the co-founder of the Cleveland Clinic. But such interventions were being phased out by the late 1930s. Such surgery for ulcers was no longer fashionable, as even physicians of the time writing in the American provincial press observed that 'there is one ailment . . . in which surgery is not used as much as formerly because it has been found that medical treatment faithfully carried out brings more satisfactory results . . . Peptic ulcer is the name given to it . . . It is now realized that certain types of individuals – nervous, slender, emotional – are most likely to "grow" ulcers. By teaching them how and what to eat, to rest, how to acquire poise or calmness, the formation of peptic ulcers can often be prevented.'[57] By this moment, the reality was that PUD in its radical explosion in the clinical experience of the twentieth century could not be as easily reduced to the existence of infections to be cured by surgery and that seemed to be a constant across time and geography, if perhaps defined more and more by the character of the patient. Yet, spurred on by the work of the neurosurgeon Lester R. Dragstedt (PhD, Physiology, University of Chicago, 1920; MD, University of Chicago, 1921), vagal surgery never really vanished. Dragstedt, who died in 1975, was one of the pioneers of the 'vagotomy' in the 1940s for PUD, authoring numerous articles on the topic through the 1950s stressing the PUD was the result of 'nervous' rather than 'hormonal' dysfunction and, as Rokitansky proposed a century earlier, was usually caused by trauma. Surgery remained for him the intervention of choice. Well after interest in surgery had waned, his students continued the procedure into the 1990s, calling on the authority of older studies of vagus nerve interventions to validate their continued use.[58] They had to be right, as they were 'standing on the shoulders of giants'.

Correlation, as the old saw has it, is not causality. That the patients seen had infectious pathogens, excess acidification and ulceration did not suffice for a scientific explanation. 'One idea which has been prevalent should be discarded: that peptic ulcer is invariably due to focal infections from the tonsils or teeth. There is little scientific evidence supporting such a theory,' observed Arthur Dean Bevan (MD, Rush Hospital Medical College, Chicago, 1883), president of the AMA in 1918, in 1930. He concluded that 'the theory of focal infections has been made to cover too many sins.'[59] So much for 'following *the* science', this was not science at all, it seems. Perhaps now a bit too much like the promises made by the innumerable quacks shouting their cures for dyspepsia in the marketplace. This dismissal continued to haunt scientific medicine through the 1950s, with widely cited papers still arguing against theories of bacterial infection in the stomach or elsewhere as the cause of PUD.[60] Neat transitions simply don't exist in scientific medicine.

Stress Causes PUD

If infections had played themselves out by the 1930s as a rationale for the origin of PUD, a replacement was already on hand. By the 1930s psychogenetic theories of somatic diseases had become commonplace. Sigmund Freud became one of the major figures in this transition. A trained neurologist with both laboratory and clinical experiences in Vienna and in Paris, two of the centres of the new scientific medicine, he began in the 1890s to answer the claims of biological psychiatry. He remained steadfast to his model of scientific medicine, believing that at some point brain localization would merge the psychology of human beings with their *Seele* (soul/psyche) into brain anatomy. But celebrity neurologists of the day, such as Alois Alzheimer (MD, University of Würzburg, 1888), were only able to examine the brains of cadavers and then hope to associate what they observed with the actions and changes they or others had seen in the living patient. Rather than seeing mental illness as a product of a diseased brain, in analogy to the notion of focal infections as the core of PUD, he argued that physical symptoms could often be the product of a disordered *Seele*.

Freud developed a theory of mind and a theory of society as well as a therapeutic process. This provided him, and the new approach that he called 'psychoanalysis', with the sort of dense model of interpretation and action that Robert Koch and Louis Pasteur had provided for bacterial infection, with the added bonus of being able to locate all in a sociological and historical context. This was highly controversial and was both condemned as well as employed, often without much public acknowledgement, by a wide number of medical specialists. Freud's claim was that the symptoms, as well as perhaps the underlying manifestation of many of the diseases seen by the specialists, such as the peptic ulcers that appeared in the clinics of internal medicine, were psychogenetic, and best dealt with by the psychoanalyst, even if they were a lay person. And best of all, in the 1890s, just as Wilhelm

Röntgen came on the horizon with his X-rays, which needed to be read by medical specialists – radiologists, who did not provide therapy – patients now, by narrating their symptoms to another new specialist, the psychoanalyst, could free themselves of them. What researchers of PUD needed in the twentieth century was something that provided a reading of the peptic ulcer in the popular and medical world of the day.

Sigmund Freud provided this in spades, arguing that disordered mental states rooted in early childhood experiences or fantasies could create physiological symptoms such as ulcers. Richard Wollheim in 2003 outlined the key to understanding, asking

> Why did he think that . . . hysterical symptoms . . . could be psychologically explained? And the answer lies with a discovery that Freud originally learned of from [Jean-Martin] Charcot [the Parisian neurologist], and then repeated for himself, concerning . . . surely the most unpromising of [psychic] phenomena, that is, hysterical symptoms. For it was a trick of Charcot's, a master of theatre, to demonstrate to his students that, in their demarcation, or how much of the body they invade, the symptoms of hysterics observed conceptual boundaries rather than any neurophysiological grouping. When, say, a patient had a hysterical paralysis of the arm, 'arm' meant the area of the body that protruded from a sleeveless dress, though this had no anatomical backing. 'Hysteria', Freud wrote, 'behaves as though anatomy does not exist', and from this he concluded that its symptoms were 'ideogenic', or caused by psychological phenomena.[61]

Could then the ulcer too be 'ideogenic', serving to represent something well beyond the stomach in the psychic body map of the patient?

Before 1914 the core truth of psychoanalysis was that the central psychic force was sexuality. This was very much in line with Freud's absorption of Charles Darwin's mechanism of sexual selection as well as his understanding of models of inheritance. With the horrors of the First World War, Freud suddenly saw the need for an alternative model. The neurologist Ernst Simmel (MD, University of Rostock, 1908, with a dissertation on dementia praecox) had empirically shown the efficacy of psychotherapy over other interventions for the treatment of 'shell shock'. The nightmares that the soldiers recounted as one of their salient symptoms were not explicable in terms of Freud's psychosexual view that all dreams were repressed (and thus disguised) desire. No dream of terror on the battlefield, repeated endlessly, masked any desire. To resolve this Freud returned to the psychophysics of his youth and the work of Gustav Fechner (MD, Carus School of Medicine, Dresden, 1822; PhD, physics, University of Leipzig, 1823), who argued that what the psychic mechanism demanded was stability, homeostasis. With this acknowledgement Freud, in his 1920 paper 'A Supplement to the Theory of Dreams', argued against psycho-sexuality as the sole motivating force for psychic activity. He saw that such terror-stricken dreams were an attempt to deal with the inher-ent instability of one's life in war. Not very psychosexual at all. By the mid-1920s, Ernest Simmel had reworked the concept of '*Organsprache*' developed by one of Freud's original followers, Wilhelm Stekel (MD, University of Vienna, 1893) in 1922. Stekel held that specific somatic symptoms reflected specific forms of trauma. *Organsprache* was trans-lated into English as 'somatization' and became an intrinsic part of the vocabulary of psychogenetic illnesses, focusing on somatic diseases, including those of the digestive tract.[62] Psychic trauma was converted into specific diseases of specific organs.

Seele – soul or psyche – defines the body; psyche is always a component of the physical, either causal or as a direct result, as Freud's views shifted concerning hysterical symptoms of what he calls trau-matic neuroses; today we would say PTSD (post-traumatic stress disorder). He was confronted by his colleagues serving at the front who reported the vivid dreams of those in battle, those labelled as 'the repetitive intrusion of nightmares and relivings of battlefield events . . . whose symptoms seem to reflect, in startling directness and simplicity, nothing but the unmediated occurrence of violent events'.[63] In *Beyond the Pleasure Principle* (1920), he wrote that

> dreams occurring in traumatic neuroses have the characteristic of repeatedly bringing the patient back into the situation of his accident, a situation from which he wakes up in another fright. This astonishes people far too little. They think the fact that the traumatic experience is constantly forcing itself upon the patient even in his sleep is proof of the strength of that experi-ence: the patient is, as one might say, fixated on his trauma . . . In the war neuroses, too, observers like Sandor Ferenczi and

Ernst Simmel have been able to explain certain motor symptoms by fixation to the moment at which the trauma occurred. I am not aware, however, that patients suffering from traumatic neurosis are much occupied in their waking lives with memories of their accident. Perhaps they are more concerned with *not* thinking of it.[64]

Freud elaborated this in *Beyond the Pleasure Principle*, adding to his theories of repression the ultimate state of psychic stability: the death drive.

Physical experiences can shape the unconscious, which in turn can be expressed in symptoms from paralysis to ulcers by the body. By the Second World War these were labelled as 'military dyspepsia' or 'war ulcers' in Britain and it was claimed that, in contrast to the First World War, 'in this war it is the stomach that shakes not the hand.'[65] Psychosomatic illness created or exacerbated by repression; not purely psychogenic, as it has been triggered by some external reality. That such an awareness was not new can be seen in the claims by a veteran of the American Civil War, writing in the 1890s, very much at the beginning of the age of Freud, that war cures, rather than causes, dyspepsia: 'Well, who ever heard of a soldier having dyspepsia? Of all the ailments that came along to make the soldier's life miserable, indigestion was one of the things he never complained of. Ye dyspeptics, who swallow nostrums and patent medicines by the barrel, consider the ways of the soldiers and be wise. Go to the war and be shot, and you'll have no more dyspepsia. Nor will you have any more even if you are not shot.'[66] Fear cures as well as causes? Or merely an ironic comment of a Civil War veteran on the horrors survived.

The notion of 'diseases of civilization' became commonplace by the end of the nineteenth century. Everything moved too fast, trains were at fault, electricity blinded rather than illuminated, and the world in general whirled by in confusion; people were forced into situations beyond their ability to function. The ease and simplicity of the American frontier, at least its reflection in prose and poetry, had been lost as the frontier closed in the 1890s. Certainly, the best example of this 'American' problem before the Civil War is to be found in Walt Whitman's pseudonymous series of newspaper essays in 1858 on 'Manly Health and Training' which 'is part guest editorial, part self-help column, published in the *New York Atlas*. At first, it reads as a straightforward diet-and-exercise guide for *men*, yet, over its course, the series accretes additional genres. In the end, one might call it lots of things: an essay on male beauty, a chauvinistic screed, a sports memoir, a eugenics manifesto, a description of New York daily life, an anecdotal history of longevity, or a pseudoscientific tract.'[67] And that is particularly the case in his discussion of indigestion as 'THE GREAT AMERICAN EVIL'.[68] In the main, all of Whitman's ruminations about health and disease have their roots in dyspepsia, its causes and alleviation: 'the subject of digestion is, in effect, treated and affected by the whole tenor of our paragraphs, under almost every one of the different headings of our subject – and partly because the main thing is to impress upon him who really wishes to acquire perfect health, that equal and thorough digestion is indispensable.' But it is self-help, not medicines, that is vital: 'Do not depend on medicines to place your stomach in order; that is but casting out devils through Beelzebub, the prince of devils.' For the problem of the 'American' disease is the increased speed of modern life, which defines their experience of quotidian existence for Whitman (and his contemporaries) at the dawn of the age of scientific medicine:

> In America, a great deal of the indigestion that prevails, is the result (we cannot too often recur to this, [*sic*]) of a cause we have elsewhere alluded to, *excessive mental action*. Those who think much, or whose business cares return upon the mind, and are brooded over and over, are often, perhaps generally, the very men whose habit it is to eat copiously of rich viands, perhaps at the hotel table, and to deluge the stomach with liquids. How can anyone bear up under such inflictions, when the same person is probably the one who, week and week, and year after year, takes no systematic exercise, and does not know even what the training for health means?

Civilization is at fault with its rich food and stress resulting from our desire to afford it. 'Simple and hearty food, and no condiments, must be his motto. This too is the continual lesson of nature. By reason of it, we see that fine state of health which characterizes hunters, lumbermen, raftsmen, and sailors on shipboard.' Rural and working-class America is the apotheosis of health and masculinity. Not the excesses of 'frightfully injurious dinners and dinner habits of most people who, as they would call it, "live well." Look over the bill of fare of any hotel or restaurant, or even the dinner-table of an ordinary boarding-house – see the incongruous dishes that, on the bills, stand in long lists, and that men devour, often three or four different kinds – soups, pastry, fat, fish, flesh, gravy, pickles, pie, pudding, coffee, water, ale, brandy – and heaven knows what else!' But a return to an idealized menu unfazed by the stresses of modern life would cure all forms of dyspepsia.

By the appearance of the neurologist George Miller Beard's *American Nervousness* (1881), which codified the immensely popular view of the stress that accompanied modernity, this had become a truism. In a passage that betrayed a multitude of anxieties about rapid technological and cultural change, Beard argued that nervousness could be traced to the principal features of 'modern civilization', namely 'the moderns differ from the ancient civilizations in these five elements – steam-power, the periodical press, the telegraph, the sciences and the mental activity of women. When civilization plus these five factors, invades any nation, it must carry nervousness and nervous disease along with it.'[69] Now, when this quote is cited, and it is the most common passage from Beard to appear in the historical literature over the past decades, it is because of its misogyny. But note that it is also 'science' that is, for him, a radical force undermining health. Beard was a renowned neurologist, having obtained his MD degree from the College of Physicians and Surgeons of New York in 1866. By the 1880s he had an active clinical practice that he mines over and over for cases showing this 'nervousness'. He is (and they are) confronted with the new world of scientific medicine and he does not like it because science itself has become a social disrupter. His patients' central nervous systems are exhausted, their energy reserves depleted by the world that they inhabit. And its impact manifests itself, among other diseases his patients present with, in 'dyspepsia, with its accompaniments, constipation, insomnia, nervousness, and emaciation'.[70] All of which are missing 'among savages everywhere'.[71]

In fact, Beard notes that 'twenty-five years ago nervous dyspepsia was diagnosed in Germany as the "American disease"'.[72] Indeed after Beard this was a touchstone, as 'in the distribution of diseases among nations the English got gout, the French syphilis, and the Americans dyspepsia . . . For practical purposes we may divide dyspepsia, or gastric indigestion, into chronic catarrhal gastritis, nervous dyspepsia, and gastric ulcer'.[73] Why does a physician in Belleaire, Ohio, ask then 'is dyspepsia so common in America? I believe it is due to too much hurry in eating, too great mental strain, worry, too high tension in living, which breaks down the nervous and digestive systems.' And notes that Sir William Osler 'condemns ice-cream and the soda fountain.'[74] What Sigmund Freud did with his reading of Beard was to redefine this as repression in the service of maintaining societal order and move away from Beard's litany of the symptoms of civilization, including peptic ulcer or at least its primary symptoms.[75] Leaving, I might add, the local problems of the dangers of soda fountains, by this point found in virtually every pharmacy in America, with Coca-Cola, ice cream sundaes and the social danger of young men and women fraternizing over an egg cream, which contained neither egg nor cream.

What Sigmund Freud also added to the mix was a psychological reading of 'civilization' (in his 1930 *Civilization and Its Discontents*) as the force that, through repression, generated that vocabulary of symptoms, including peptic ulcers. Freud echoes Darwin, seeing human beings as aggressive and the rules which are instituted to control that aggression, which he calls civilization, as necessary but also causing repression.[76] He is in this sense a follower of the seventeenth-century philosopher Thomas Hobbes, who sees the state as necessary for human existence, if not flourishing. Freud thinks that what society needs to control is human sexuality, the root of all aggression for him. But the competitive world can provide some false promises, which are the core of the notion of happiness and success in the rules established by society. What results is 'a flight into neurotic illness – a flight which he usually accomplishes when he is still young. The man who sees his pursuit of happiness come to nothing in later years can still find consolation in the yield of pleasure of chronic intoxication; or he can embark on the desperate attempt at rebellion seen in a psychosis.'[77] For Freud, therefore, it is neither the train nor the telegraph that deforms psychic life in civilization, as

> civilization is built up upon a renunciation of instinct, how much it presupposes precisely the non-satisfaction (by suppression, repression or some other means?) of powerful instincts. This 'cultural frustration' dominates the large field of social relationships between human beings. As we already know, it is the cause of the hostility against which all civilizations have to struggle. It will also make severe demands on

our scientific work, and we shall have much to explain here. It is not easy to understand how it can become possible to deprive an instinct of satisfaction. Nor is doing so without danger. If the loss is not compensated for economically, one can be certain that serious disorders will ensue.[78]

Peptic ulcers as a symptom of much deeper-lying repressed desires.

The brother of one of Freud's earliest patients, whom he had diagnosed with hysteria, presented with a 'typical neurasthenia of early manhood, and this ruined his career . . . Starting originally with a good constitution, the patient is haunted by the usual sexual difficulties at puberty; there follow years of overwork as a student, preparation for examinations, and an attack of gonorrhoea, followed by a sudden onset of dyspepsia accompanied by obstinate and inexplicable constipation. After some months the constipation is replaced by intracranial pressure, depression and incapacity for work.'[79] A disease of civilization in an individual presenting with a range of illnesses, including PUD. Here, in 1892, Freud still asks whether this is hereditary or not, leaving open its cause. But soon PUD comes for him to be potentially a risk for all human beings, especially after his son Ernst and his sister-in-law Minna develop them, since he sees the repressive structures of civilization concerning sexuality exist not only in modernity and the Global North but in the 'civilization' of colonial expansion.

Gastric and duodenal (peptic) ulcers captured the attention of both the medical and the public sphere engaged with the new science of 'psychoanalysis' in the new century. The idea that dyspepsia and attendant ills were 'frequently attendant upon persons of a nervous or irritable temperament, and hence common to the hysteric, dyspeptic, and choleric', as J. Mason Good in 1823 had claimed, was long a commonplace.[80] But the notion that anyone and everyone might be at risk given the circumstances was quite revolutionary.

Psychosomatic models for the widest range of symptoms proliferated within and then beyond psychoanalysis to explain and outline treatment not so much of the symptoms but of the repressed causes. All centred on theories of specific forms of repression and their expression in specific diseases. The Hungarian psychoanalyst Franz Alexander (MD, University of Budapest, 1913; trained at Berlin Institute of Psychoanalysis under Hanns Sachs, then teaching at the University of Chicago after 1930) came to be fascinated by peptic ulcers, for him one of the paradigmatic psychosomatic diseases, which also came to have a heavy symbolic value in the post-First World War context.[81] He sees them as the somatic manifestation of crying for mother's milk, as a compensatory oral mechanism. But Alexander picks up right where Freud left off in the 1920s, seeing the development of a peptic ulcer in the light of a reimagined set of causations about shell shock during the war:

> It is difficult to hold a man responsible for his gastric ulcer; it is much easier, as the experience in the war showed us, to hold him responsible for his hysterical symptom; and still easier to blame a man for his irresponsibility, his gambling, and his incapacity to engage in serious work. To have the right to consider such people as pathological, we should have to extend and re-define considerably our concept of disease. One might regret that in doing this one places the organically sick in rather bad company.[82]

But ulcers thus could be the unconscious symbolic incarnation resulting from 'dependent, help-seeking, and love-demanding desires' which, ungratified, yield emotional stimulation that exerts a specific effect upon the functions of the stomach because of their link with orality.[83] However, his model also reflects the conflicts seen in the economic as well as cultural situation of males in this moment, as 'the inhibition of the desire to receive after the receptive urge has taken the aggressive form of wishing to take. The underlying emotional syllogisms can be formulated as follows: "I cannot accept anything from a person whom I really want to rob" ... This same emotional syllogism is of primary importance also in gastric neuroses and in peptic ulcer formation; it explains the inhibition of oral receptive tendencies as a reaction to an extreme aggressive demanding attitude.'[84] This reflects what he labels his 'Specificity Theory', that tied together specific patterns of physiological arousal that resulted from and were concomitant with specific, chronic emotional states that in turn lead to specific somatic disturbances.

Alexander developed a list of diseases, known as the Chicago Seven, which were considered paradigmatic psychosomatic diseases: peptic ulcer, ulcerative colitis, bronchial asthma, neurodermatitis, rheumatoid arthritis, essential hypertension and thyrotoxicosis. (No, not the other 'Chicago Seven', those tried in 1970 for disrupting the 1968 Democratic Convention in Chicago because of their opposition to the Vietnam war, about whom we shall hear more later.) Now, there was in the 1920s and 1930s strong interest in psychogenic factors in organic disease within the now dominant field of 'internal medicine', perhaps the medical specialty, arising imperial Germany, that best exemplified the claims and impact of scientific medicine – and yet still could not explain and thus treat all of the pathologies of the digestive system. Alexander's psychoanalytically based ideas were published, among other places, in the mainstream and venerable *Journal of the American Medical Association*.[85] There he stated to this medical audience, who seemed attuned to having an explanation that matched the idea of changing roles and definitions of success and masculinity at the psychogenic roots of peptic ulcers:

> I have had occasion in several cases to establish the psychic origin of functional stomach troubles that preceded clinically diagnosed peptic ulcers . . . I was able to distinguish certain specific psychic tendencies that seem to have a very near affinity to the functions of the stomach. If certain wishes and claims of a receptive nature, the wish to be loved, to be helped, to be taken care of by others, longing for the maintenance or revival of the infantile relation of the child to the mother, are repressed in the unconscious, they have a definite tendency to influence the functions of the stomach. Such tendencies, if present in adults, have to be repressed because they are incompatible with the dominating ambitions of the conscious personality: with the strife for independence, masculinity or activity. Repressed and thus excluded from gratification, they maintain a permanent tension which can be considered as a chronic unconscious psychic stimulus . . . Every hysterical organ disturbance is the dynamic substitute for omitted actions. The emotions and wishes to which the individual cannot give expression and relief in actions concerning the environment find expression in the unintelligible tacit language of inner organic processes.[86]

Such psychosomatic views dominated the understanding of the aetiology of PUD through the 1940s.

Helen Flanders Dunbar (MD, Yale School of Medicine, 1930), a pioneering figure in psychosomatic medicine and the pastoral care movement, attempted to establish a 'specificity theory' of psychosomatic illness, where certain kinds of personalities could be associated with specific diseases. She found patients with peptic ulcers are 'nasty to anyone who helps them . . . If they can make their doctor so impatient that they have to go to another one, or if they can get the doctor sick or bored, they feel that they have scored a real triumph. The reason for this is that they themselves are sick and bored, and they want the doctor to feel what they feel. This is an attitude which is found with special frequency among sufferers from ulcer and colitis.' They present with what she labels 'the jellyfish personality', which 'does not mean that they are always perfectly flaccid and harmless, for they are not. The jellyfish that stings is still a jellyfish. And the sting can be mighty painful.'[87] In the countertransference with the patient with PUD, thus, the analyst too is at risk of emotional harm. For Dunbar, the range of such views seemed always linked to an understanding of both patients' character, as an abstraction, and their situation, such as the 'struggle for life'. But people with PUD are different in their psychological as well as their physiological make-up, at least when we follow *the* science of the time. There too, where and when such people exist seems to play a major role despite the science.

Social Pressure Causes PUD

Some writers and thinkers in mid-twentieth century America do see that lived experiences can drive the development of PUD. But what experiences and for whom? What is vital in understanding the relevance of these approaches is that it answered one of the central moral questions of the day, one that F. Scott Fitzgerald, who according to his diaries also suffered from stomach ulcers, postulated in his last, unfinished novel *The Last Tycoon* (1941).[88] The novel reflects on his central concern in the Jazz Age: how do the institutions of modern capitalism impact the internal lives of those striving to exist within a destructive system? For Fitzgerald, in this novel, the film studios epitomize the relentless pressures of the illusion of reality sold by Hollywood and the studio system that rests on the instability of the lives of those who inhabit a system built on stress. Typical is the scriptwriter Jane Meloney, as described by one of the other characters in terms quite familiar from the image of the 'blue stocking', the woman defeminized in seeking masculine roles in Victorian culture, and suffering the social and physical consequences:

> a dried-up little blonde of fifty about whom one could hear the fifty assorted opinions of Hollywood – 'a sentimental dope', 'the best writer on construction in Hollywood', 'a veteran', 'that old hack', 'the smartest woman on the lot', 'the cleverest plagiarist in the biz'; and, of course, in addition she was variously described as a nymphomaniac, a virgin, a pushover, a Lesbian, and a faithful wife. Without being an old maid, she was, like most self-made women, rather old maidish. She had ulcers of the stomach, and her salary was over a hundred thousand a year. A complicated treatise could be written on whether she was 'worth it' or more than that or nothing at all.[89]

Franz Alexander notes that those with peptic ulcers were also compensating 'for their strong unconscious receptive-dependent attitude by assuming responsibilities and by concentrated efforts in work'.[90] Work makes you sick; being sick makes you work. Thereafter, so it was that, for specific 'diseases of civilization' such as gastric and duodenal ulcers (peptic), this obtained: 'not unnaturally, in those post-Freudian days, psychosomatic influences were for long thought to be the cause of peptic ulcers, stress being the major culprit. The complications of peptic ulcer were an important cause of death, severe haemorrhage being common and perforation, particularly of duodenal ulcers, being a frequent surgical emergency.'[91] Modernity generates stress; stress kills but not everyone.[92]

Out of Franz Alexander's theories there had developed the assumption, as we have seen in the comments of Helen Flanders Durbar, that specific personalities, 'ulcer types', reacted to anxiety by developing gastric complaints.[93] This merged with the notion of body types reflecting psychological states pioneered by the German psychiatrist Ernst Kretschmer (MD, University of Tübingen, 1913). This belief in a constitutional psychology became wildly popular through the work in the 1940s of W. H. Sheldon (PhD in psychology, University of Chicago, 1925; MD, University of Chicago, 1933), whose three somatotypes – slim ectomorphs, muscular mesomorphs and soft endomorphs – had clearly distinctive personality types connected to each body form, echoing seventeenth-century discussion about the humours and character. Sheldon also defines his types in the light of race, with racial types presenting as exaggerations of his somatotypes. 'Ulcer types' were usually male, had a long thin face, slim build, and boundless energy, combined with restlessness and a tendency to suffer fear or anxiety. They could cope with most of the day-to-day stress of life, unless they experienced a stressor so severe (as in war time) that the resultant tension would be discharged through the channels of their autonomic nervous system and manifest in the organs of the digestive tract.

The character type most impacted by psychological stress was named quickly as 'Type A'. 'Type A' was one of the personality dimensions sketched by British psychologist Hans Eysenck (PhD, Psychology, University College London, 1940), who focused on hostility, state and trait anxiety, that is, the difference between having specific emotional responses to specific circumstances ('state') and being 'pre-programmed' for such responses ('trait'), and depression. By comparison with cardiac patients, who by the 1940s had come to be the cohort that defined 'Type A' behaviour ('coronary-prone behaviour pattern'), the peptic ulcer groups were similar on most of his other variables, involving a constellation of time-urgent, hard-driving, competitive and hostile behaviours. But 'Type As' are simultaneously aggressive and often accomplished workers.[94] What makes them successful makes them ill.

Ironically, earlier work on ulcers in lower animals had proved inconclusive, for the claim was that 'the animal kingdom does not develop "peptic" ulcer.'[95] As we earlier noted, the claims were that ulcers could not be the result of infection, as 'infection and thrombosis should occur in domestic and wild animals – ulcer does not.'[96] It is a sign of the human condition. In the light of Eysenck's work, which was widely publicized, the American behavioural psychologist Joseph V. Brady (PhD in psychology, University of Chicago, 1951) showed that the 'executive' ('Type A') monkeys subjected to his electric-shock test were more likely to develop ulcers than their passive counterparts, even when both were treated identically.[97] Brady's designation of his dominant monkeys as 'executives' in 1958 says everything that needs saying about the image of the elite worker in modern capitalism and the post-Second World War world.

That level of assumptions about the psychogenic origins of peptic ulcers permeated not only the psychological but the sociological literature of the day. In their extensive and detailed study of *The Authoritarian Personality* (1950), in the light of the rise of fascism and post-Second World War racism, the philosopher Theodor W. Adorno, the psychoanalyst Else Frenkel-Brunswik and the psychologists Daniel Levinson and Nevitt Sanford understood the ulcer to be an index of that personality type. They too invented a set of criteria by which to define personality traits, and ranked these traits and their intensity in any given person on what is called the 'F-scale' (F for fascist). These traits can be measured by means of the F-scale with good correlations between F scores and measures of antisemitism and 'anti-Negro' prejudice. They saw many of their male informants as presenting 'counter-cathective defenses [that is, rigorous denial of emotional responses] . . . producing compulsive features of psychosomatic manifestations such as stomach ulcers (men)'.[98]

These informants arrived with somatic complaints, 'some of them psychosomatic symptoms which could be understood as expressions of suppressed affects such as fear or rage', and 'the most frequent physical complaints of the high-scoring men in our group were stomach ulcers and physical expressions, such as tremors, sweating, etc., of tension and anxiety.' One of the most extensive cases, in which 'the special importance of illness, as a condition under which dependence can be admitted and gratified', was defined by PUD: 'Mack's stomach ulcer was very probably psychogenic and . . . in this case it could be regarded, in accordance with generally accepted theory, as an expression *par excellence* of unconscious dependence.' Anti-social psychopathology is loudly expressed by the body of the racist as ulcers through which he can declare his own feared weakness. Here is the counter case to the businessman (and they were always men) with an ulcer seeing it as a badge of success; yet the racist, after the fall of the Third Reich, closeted and fearful of exposure, suffered from identical manifestations of stress.

Sloan Wilson's 1955 novel *The Man in the Gray Flannel Suit* (and subsequent film of 1956 with Gregory Peck as Tom Rath, the protagonist working as a public relations executive at a television network) reflected a fantasy of the combative world of American middle-class life in Eisenhower's America. Its immediate popularity reflected a post-Second World War world that gave rise to assumptions about the body/mind dichotomy that lead both to important innovations in diagnosis as well as to their overturning, and that acknowledged the moral penalties of the striving for success that blinded middle-class males (at least) to the impact of such striving on their psyches. This became a set critique of the moral vacuity of the immediate post-war world echoed by social critics of post-world-war materialism such as the sociologist C. Wright Mills, who wrote of the 'new ulcered entrepreneur [who] operates on the guileful edges of several bureaucracies. With his lavish expense account, the new entrepreneur sometimes gets into the public eye as a fixer – along with the respectable businessman whose work he does – or even as an upstart and a crook: for the same public that idolizes initiative becomes incensed when it finds a grand model of success based simply and purely upon it.'[99] He also argues that seeing them as inherently unhappy in a culture that defines itself by accumulated wealth may be naive.

Sloan Wilson stressed the loss of any moral orientation of overly ambitious businessmen, especially those in the world of advertising, in the 1950s; the radical sociologist Paul Goodman put a finer spin on this in his 1960 *Growing Up Absurd: Problems of Youth in the Organized Society*:

> the committed Organization Man also *really* belongs, he has status and salary and must protect them. Therefore, the junior executive is in a terrible contradiction. He is cynical about the aims of the firm, yet he fears that his own ineptitude will be found out. He has no recourse to concrete performance, for there is little contact with unambiguous material and there are no objective standards. How to meet a purely subjective demand? In pain (even ulcers) he has to get by by role playing, interpersonal relations abstracted from both animal desire or tangible achievement. He meets expectations, he conforms, he one-ups, he proves he must know how by attaining a higher status.[100]

The relationship between masculine success and peptic ulcers seemed clear, especially in retrospect. The numbers of those defined with PUD peaked at mid-century, impacting about 10 per cent of employed men, and reflected, it was claimed, their economic setting.

The peptic ulcer came to symbolize the oppressive power of capitalism; indeed, it signified the very nature of the system. In 1968 mass demonstrations took place in Chicago during the Democratic National

Convention that eventually nominated Hubert Humphrey for president after Lyndon Johnson refused a second nomination because of the extraordinary opposition to the war in Vietnam. Abbie Hoffman, the leader of the Youth International Party, the Yippies, addressed the crowd on 27 August 1968 on tactics and the police:

> Cops are like Yippies – you can never find the leaders. So if you're good at guerrilla theatre, you can look a pig right in the eye and say that to him, you know, and he'll do it. You know, that's the thing, to get him to do it. You just let 'em know that you're stronger psychically than they are. And you are, because you came here for nothin' and they're holdin' on to their fuckin' pig jobs 'cause of that little fuckin' paycheck and workin' themselves up, you know. Up to what? To a fuckin' ulcer. Sergeant. We got them by the balls.[101]

Hoffman became one of the 'Chicago Seven' (not Franz Alexander's psychosomatic diseases but here the leaders of the Yippies and the SDS [Students for a Democratic Society], reacting to those forces that they believed caused them), who were convicted in 1970 for 'crossing state lines with the intent to incite a riot'. Eventually their convictions were vacated. They represented the 1960s on the street – they didn't have ulcers because they were representing a valid cause. They fought those to whom the system had given merely a facsimile of power. This illusionary power gave those representatives of authority ulcers. Adorno proved to be right: the authoritarian personality was represented by the ulcers of those suffering under the system, even though they had the illusion of power, at least in the USA.

Post-Second World War West German Society Confronts PUD

The social chaos of 1968 was a global phenomenon. Yet capitalism takes on different implications across the world in the immediate post-Second World War generation. The Federal Republic of Germany, created in 1949 out of the three zones occupied by the United States, Great Britain and France, focused exclusively on rebuilding for an economically secure future. The passage of time and the ageing of the youngest generation born at the very end of the war or in its immediate aftermath, those who had no conscious awareness of the Nazi period and were shaped largely by the Cold War and the gradual Americanization, for good or ill, of West Germany (BRD), suddenly became aware of their parents' own potential culpability. This generational distancing from the Nazi past formed the generation of 1968. In 1967 two German psychoanalysts, Margarete (MD, University of Tübingen, 1950) and Alexander Mitscherlich (MD, University of Heidelberg, 1941), asked how one could selectively forget the past while focusing only on an economic future in their study entitled *The Inability to Mourn*.[102] An immediate bestseller in Germany, the text seemed to focus all of the anxiety about the past felt by the youngest generation on the to-that-point-unspoken question: what did you do in the war, Daddy? (And it really was 'Daddy' who was asked.) In 1967, when the West Germans were at the peak of the German *Wirtschaftswunder* (economic miracle), the extraordinary economic resurgence after the Second World War, what the Mitscherlichs saw in West Germany was the total refusal to come to terms with history, marked by what they defined as the refusal to mourn the past and to understand the deep emotional bond that the Germans had had to Hitler and fascism. That denial was present did not surprise the Mitscherlichs, but what did was the fact that this was not repression but the absence of any moral awareness.

Alexander Mitscherlich was a serious student of psychogenic illnesses, quite aware of the very different work of Franz Alexander, Walter Cannon and the ego theorist Heinz Hartmann. Yet following *the* science seems to have had very different meanings in Frankfurt in the 1960s than those it had in Chicago at the same time. What the Mitscherlichs found was odd. Based on their readings, 'the researcher in the field of psychoneurotic and psychosomatic illness might reasonably have predicted that after the collapse of the Third Reich there would be a large number of such cases.' They note that the confluence of 'various psychological processes might have been expected to interact'. Having been as children formed 'to make them loyal and obedient tools of aggression and megalomania . . . such insoluble internal and external conflicts were to be expected, leading to psychologically determined illness.' But they simply did not appear. Looking at 4,000 patients 'who attended the psychosomatic clinic of Heidelberg University [a clinic founded by him in 1949] because of neurotic or physical illness in recent years', they seemed to 'show very little to connect their symptoms with experiences during the Nazi period'. They simply did not manifest physical or psychological symptoms relating to guilt or even moral awareness. The recalcitrant Nazis felt no guilt and were happy to join right-wing parties that still shared their ideology; the others felt that the acts of the regime were not criminal. Indeed, they felt that they were the victims of 'foreign' occupiers.[103] And it was specifically these foreigners, as George Miller Beard observed, that had imported the 'American disease', dyspepsia, PUD, into imperial Germany.[104] After the Holocaust: no guilt; no neurosis; no neurosis; no symptoms. Most important for us, West Germans in the Mitscherlich clinic did not come to them because of PUD. On Adorno's 'F scale', they were not repressed fascists at all, at least in terms of their psychogenic illnesses.

Yet at the peak of the *Wirtschaftswunder*, Alexander Mitscherlich turned to a, for him, new manifestation of the *Wirtschaftswunder*: the appearance in the elite of the Federal Republic of PUD. The world that he and his spouse had examined in 1967 subordinated the politics of the past to the economics of the present. And that world suffered from PUD. Trained as a psychoanalyst in a world where German psychoanalysis had been transported to Great Britain and the United States by exiles, he turned, not to a reading of the aetiology in the competition inherent in late capitalism, but to universals of depth psychology, looking to explore both the unconscious as well as the experiential basis of the human psyche. He mapped the infant's dependence on the mother for sustenance, the anger generated when this dependence is not immediately fulfilled and the overcompensation, the aggression and fear that accompanied it on to the adult's 'pride and guilt' at being sustained by the competitive world in which he finds himself. Not evident because of repression, it presents as symptoms. The resulting hypersecretion of stomach acid, the vasoconstriction of the stomach and the impact of the endocrine systems result in peptic ulcers.

Alexander Mitscherlich highlighted the fact that psychogenic illnesses may well have their roots in such early childhood experiences but those other contributing factors, such as adult social experience and its stressors, also played a role, perhaps a dominant one. Now, this was also the explanation for the absence of psychosomatic diseases among the same population. The child, they had argued in their book, responds to childhood conflict by projecting it on to a 'persecutor ostensibly equipped with mysterious powers'.[105] When this delusion collapses, as after 1945, one can either accept what had happened or, as the child does, protect the ego against punishment by denying guilt. But memory in this restructured form does not lead to the stress that manifests itself in ulcers. In the period of the early Federal Republic, in the time of economic expansion and brutal competition, Germans with ulcers reflect universal childhood trauma, not past actions and beliefs. Evoking psychosomatic work on the nature of those with ulcers, he notes that most have a predisposition to the disease because they already have higher rates of stomach acid because of childhood experiences. And this was not specific to time or place. That ulcers result in adults from overcompensation and competitive aggression was furthered in the workplace by a 'rigid model for work'. We today might read this as a variant of his view of the 'culture-specific childhood neurosis that had helped make them loyal and obedient tools of aggression and megalomania', but this specificity is now missing. For Mitscherlich there are therapeutic interventions. Some patients can be treated with talk therapy if their chronicity is only the result of unresolved and for the patient unresolvable conflicts. Other patients may suffer a chronic form of ulcer that is only amenable to surgical treatment, as the pain resulting from the lesion is part of the self-punishment of the patient.[106]

Gastric ulcers had a particularly bad reputation in post-war German medicine, as virtually any ingestion of food was known to produce hydrochloric acid, which exacerbated the ulcers, which in turn caused bleeding and further erosion of the stomach. At that moment Germany had redefined itself, not as a conquered nation responsible for unimaginable horrors, but as the perfect, modern capitalist society, defined by its work ethic and its productivity, against all odds. In this the subjectivity of patients is key to Mitscherlich's concept of psychosomatic disease. This informs his continuous criticism of the use of statistical methods of a science-based medicine to validate individual diagnoses and hypotheses. But he shapes this to fit his sense of how his patients too shift over time.[107] Germany became the instantiation of the United States' self-image, not only in the 1950s: it had also done so in the post-First World War Weimar Republic, with its obsessive importation of the victors' culture and values. Indeed, this was one of the charges that the far right lodged against the new Republic. As Dagmar Herzog has noted, Mitscherlich integrated 'elements of Heinz Hartmannesque American ego psychology (Hartmann was the dominant figure in the U.S. – the 50s in America are referred to in psychoanalytic circles as "the Hartmann Era") with frankly left-liberal political commentary on current events with (what in hindsight may seem rather un-analytic and conceptually clunky) persistent enjoinders to West Germans to develop what he variously referred to as "ego-strength" (*Ichstärke*), "self-control", "capacity for critical thinking", or "the critical thinking-capacity of the ego".[108] The Austrian psychiatrist and psychoanalyst Heinz Hartmann (MD, University of Vienna, 1920) created ego psychology, examining the complexity of how we defend who we believe we are in a world of psychic conflict and contradictions. Fleeing the Nazis in 1938 for New York, he became in 1950 the long-time president of the International Psychoanalytic Society and thus a pivotal figure in post-war German psychoanalysis. For Mitscherlich, he represented a theoretical model of dealing with the past, both in terms of his life story as well as his approach to ego defence. And thus, perhaps, provided a model as how to avoid PUD.

The *Wirtschaftswunder* was not solely the result of post-war Germans repressing their guilt into work. Between 1955 and 1973 the Federal Republic had developed a system to import workers from a wide range of nations from Italy to Turkey to Yugoslavia. After the erection of the Berlin Wall in 1961, when the labour flow from the German Democratic Republic was stopped, the numbers increased. While the assumption was that these workers would return to their homelands after one or two years, most remained, altering not only the workplace but the overall culture. By the 1970s the image of the ulcerated male took on a new and complex form when cultural conflict in post-war Germany, dealing with 4 million *Gastarbeiter* (guest workers) by 1973, came to be at the core of the aetiology of PUD.

Case in point is the Turkish-German Güney Dal's first novel *İş Sürgünleri* (Exiles of Labour, 1976; published in German translation by Brigitte Schreiber-Grabitz as *Wenn Ali die Glocken läuten hört*, When Ali Hears the Bells Toll, 1979).[109] Documenting the 1973 Ford strikes in Cologne, the author focuses on the story of one of the 'guest workers', Kadir Derya, a Kurdish worker at a pharmaceutical company in Berlin, who, as readers learn at the end of the novel, has been given oestrogen pills by his boss at the laboratory to alleviate the pain he suffers from a peptic ulcer. As his breasts develop – a side-effect of the medication – he grows more and more depressed, and at the end, he mutilates himself while trying to excise his breasts. This is not that unusual a therapy, as a 1953 paper noted: 'Estrogens have been used extensively in the treatment of peptic ulcer during the last fifteen years, especially in Europe . . . A surprisingly large number of favorable reports have emphasized the increased sense of well-being and prompt relief of ulcer distress, especially in patients with gastric ulcer, in males, and in women during the menopause.' But the paper concludes that the results 'are not impressive for several reasons: the relatively brief periods of observation, the concomitant use of other therapeutic measures, and the lack of adequate controls. The favorable results have been observed chiefly in early uncomplicated cases, likely to respond to any therapy, including the injection of inert materials.'[110] In other words, it is 'merely' a placebo, a phenomenon within scientific medicine we shall examine in detail in our discussion of acupuncture.

Ulcers were such a common problem among labour migrants in the 1960s and 1970s that PUD was referred to as 'Guestworker Ulcer' (*Gastarbeiter Ulcus*), very specifically as the 'Turkish ailment' (*Türkenkrankheit*).[111] They became a theme in the popular culture of the time. When in 1974 Rainer Werner Fassbinder presents his film *Angst essen Seele auf/Ali: Fear Eats the Soul*, reflecting the complexity of the integration of the Turkish 'guest workers' into the post-war *Wirtschaftswunder*, he creates a love story between a Moroccan man known only as Ali and a German woman, Emmi Kurowski. Ali momentarily seems to abandon Emmi and she has a nervous breakdown; when finally reconciled this leads too to his physical collapse, but with a gastric ulcer, that forces him into the hospital. Perhaps the exemplary film of the 'New German Cinema', Fassbinder's account of the medicalization of both the Germans and the guest workers reflects Mitschlerlich's notion of a post-war world that is unstable in very different ways for its players.

The presumed aetiology for PUD in West Germany in the 1970s was that seventeenth-century Swiss disease 'nostalgia', suffered by soldiers sent abroad to fight during the Thirty Years War. It is what Svetlana Boym has called the 'hypochondria of the heart'.[112] Nostalgia is understood in the 1970s by the factory physicians as caused by the 'uprootedness' (*Entwurzelungsreaktion*) of the guest workers, which mirrored the 'inauthenticity' (*Uneigentlichkeit*) of everyday existence in modern capitalism, as Peter Sloterdijk described it in the 1980s.[113] These were 'artificial diseases', a term that originated in the social medicine of the nineteenth century and referred to the role of social and environmental conditions in the onset of the illness. At least one epidemiologist of the time noted (writing in 1984) that as PUD begins to reduce in the Global North, it is substantially increasing among *Gastarbeiter* in Western Europe and 'Blacks' in South Africa. Do we need to note that the uprising in Soweto, one of the 'townships' in apartheid Johannesburg, had occurred in 1976 and that this was one of the highpoints of state repression, with over 700 of the 20,000 students marching murdered? He relativizes the psychogenetic view that ulceration was the result of an imbalance between aggressive and defensive factors, as, and here he throws up his hands, other factors probably need to be considered.[114]

While it is clear that Alexander Mitscherlich's image of the ulcer patient was a reflection of his understanding of psychogenetic illness in West Germany and the compensatory function of economic success as an answer to the failures of the Third Reich, Güney Dal's view sees West German capitalism as exploitative and therefore deadly. This was something he knew at first hand, as he had arrived in Berlin in 1972. The medicalization of the labour migrant's body during the strike parallels the author's critique on economic exploitation but also the impact of medical theory on the lived experience of his character. Alienation, in this view, causes ulcers, but medical practice does not focus on the worker's life in Germany, only on the distance felt from their land of origin.[115] Now, Güney Dal's novel appears well after the end of the world that saw local infections as causing PUD. He sees ulcers having a psychogenic cause, not because of alienation, as did Mitscherlich, but because of their physiological aetiology, stress, and thus they came to be treated with pharmacological or indeed surgical interventions rather than psychotherapy, which could never change the society in which these workers functioned. Ignoring the psychological effects would not have improved the worker's health, as it would have substituted one pharmaceutical for another, ignoring, as the author stresses, the social location of the patient. Capitalism is at the very core of PUD. Its exploitation results in stress, whether you feel yourself at the bottom or the top of the system. In 1985 the investigative journalist Günter Wallraff, following the model of John Howard Griffin's 1961 *Black Like Me*, in which Griffin disguised himself as an African American to write about the experience of American racism at first hand, 'became' a Turkish worker in the pharmaceutical industry. There, as he described it, he became a human guinea pig, first testing barbiturates and then quitting when he refused to take Mesperinon due to its side-effect of gynaecomastia, male breasts. There is no mention of ulcers, but the roles played by the various actors seemed to be interchangeable.[116] Capitalist exploitation gives you symptoms, whether because of work or of therapy.

Race Science and PUD: African Americans

As early as the Enlightenment, race was considered a precipitating factor in defining the aetiology of a wide range of illness, but almost exclusively in the 'inferior races': African Americans in the United States, the Irish in the British Isles and Jews in Western and Central Europe. The development of the scientific perspective on 'race' emerged alongside the epistemological shift within Western European society from religious doctrine to scientific doctrine, whereby authority was relocated from the Church to the laboratory, with the scientist as an independent and unbiased observer true-to-nature. The debates about outlawing slavery in Great Britain and the civil emancipation of European Jews beginning in the late eighteenth century were paralleled by the growth in the rhetoric of scientific racism throughout Western Europe. The movement towards civic and legal emancipation collided with the claims of the new scientific medicine and the role of civilization. What was race and what role did it play in disease?

Under slavery, dyspepsia, according to the plantation physician Samuel Cartwright, 'is, par excellence, a disease of the Anglo-Saxon race. I have never seen a well-marked case of dyspepsia among the blacks. It is a disease that selects its victims from the most intellectual of mankind, passing by the ignorant and unreflecting.'[117] The *Southern Medical Journal* noted in 1913 that 'digestive discomforts' afflicted 'those higher in the social and financial scale'. 'Very sparing doses of . . . aids to digestion have generally sufficed for the gastric infirmities of our negro patients, – in fact, I have many times earnestly wished that some of the prompt and satisfactory responses shown by these humble invalids could be duplicated among those higher in the social and financial scale – those to whom surcease from digestive discomforts would mean bountiful emoluments to the medical attendant.'[118]

For George Miller Beard in 1881 the African Americans he observed in the age of Jim Crow were moving from not evidencing 'dyspepsia' to beginning to show the strains of 'modern life'. The African American surgeon based in Cleveland Charles H. Garvin (MD,

Howard University, 1915) predicted (again) in 1924 that the rising social status of African Americans would make them more vulnerable to various diseases: 'It is not a direct race question but a question of civilization and its "hustle and bustle" and "burning the candle at both ends".'[119] The increase of perceived social pressure in the past decades, the 'ever-increasing rapidity of progress, exacts a toll in the health of those who choose to run in its race', specifically 'the syndrome of peptic ulcer', observed Andrew B. Rivers (MD, Creighton University, 1917) at the Mayo Clinic in 1934, referring to those he characterized as 'the better educated, more ambitious and more intensive members of society. Their abilities and their willingness to accept responsibility naturally increase the complexity of their lives far beyond that of those who follow along unperturbedly so long as others guarantee a more or less comfortable existence.' But he also found fundamental differences among African Americans who did not present with this disorder. His image shadows that of Beard quite closely as he sees them as 'slow-moving' and 'easy-going . . . untouched by aspiration for culture'. Despite 'unbalanced diets, abuse of alcohol and tobacco, irregular sleeping habits, reckless behavior, and unhygienic living conditions, peptic ulcer was absent among them.'[120] We need to note that tobacco abuse was claimed already in the 1820s to be 'employed very often to such excess, whether in smoking or chewing, as to become a very alarming cause of dyspepsy'.[121] Excess in all things harms, especially those most at risk.

Documenting peptic ulcers in 79 patients, the Chicago specialist in internal medicine Samuel C. Robinson advanced in the 1930s a similar modification of the overall psychogenic theory. Ulcers, he noted, were found largely among susceptible individuals of the white race – 'usually the long thin type who are given to worry and nervous instability'. These views paralleled theories of constitutional psychology such as W. H. Sheldon's somatotypes, which also made claims in the 1940s about inherent racial predisposition reflected in body types. For Robinson the peptic ulcer is the ultimate disease of modernity as 'the Negro and lesser pigmented races seldom if ever do and the Caucasian race rarely does [suffer from them even] under primitive conditions.' On the other hand:

> The pure blooded negro is practically immune to the disease although he eats the same food and is subjected to the same

'focal infection' as the white man. Why does this disease skip an entire race? The answer is an anthropological one based on hereditary differences of psychological structure and function. The negro race in its evolutionary ascent has not, as yet, acquired the habit of worry so peculiar to the white race under pressure of routine civilized living. The negro meets life's frustration with greater calm and equanimity – sometimes even with laughter.[122]

The danger for poor, working-class whites, however, was just as evident. In her 1900 temperance novel, *The Daughter of a Republican*, Julia Babcock (writing under the nom de plume Bernie Babcock) presents her image of the 'drunk' suffering from 'the disease caused by the legalized drink traffic [consumption of alcohol] [that] was eating his life away little by little, and as the fire burned it called for more fuel. One night when every little gland and fiber in his whole being and all the great ulcers in his diseased stomach seemed like fierce flames cutting and licking and torturing him, half-drunk, he staggered from one grog shop to another, begging for something to drink.'[123] 'The white race alone is susceptible' to the curse of alcoholism, a weakness that revealed why members of the newest immigrant communities (read: the Irish) also developed ulcers. Certainly not all of them, only those who in addition show signs of degeneration. 'Most ulcer patients show some nervous instability, especially undue anxiety, fear and worry.' Such patients present as a form of decayed masculinity since 'the male sex is predominantly susceptible, 6 to 1 . . . The few females that develop ulcers often show some masculine traits.'[124] Shades of F. Scott Fitzgerald's 'blue stocking', the woman defeminized. A eugenic weakness of moral fibre lies at the heart of white predisposition to PUD; Black 'indolence' at the core of African American immunity from the disease.

The counterargument about 'type' against the sense of Sheldon's somatotypes was made in 1944 by the African American surgeon Ulysses Grant Daley (MD, Northwestern University, 1906), who also argued for 'an ulcer habitus, or, more modernly, an ulcer constitution. The ulcer patient is apt to be a lean but dynamic individual. He is usually quite well nourished, but it would be rare to discover a stomach ulcer in a stodgy, obese person. The ulcer patient would usually be a male.' Thus, his African American patients are not predisposed by *race* but by *type*, as 'peptic ulcers occur in all occupations, all social strata, and in all parts of the world. The ulcer patient might therefore be farmer, bank clerk, stevedore, playboy, senator. He could be black or white, Jew or gentile. Although the literature of a quarter of a century ago contains many statements concerning the infrequency of ulcer in the Negro, racial predisposition as such is no longer alleged, all races being about equally susceptible, depending upon personality, environment and habits of diet.'[125] By then the debate about innate race differences had heightened, a debate that Sigmund Freud had dismissed in the 1890s when he transformed what had been ascribed to racial characteristics in the lectures and medical textbooks of his own schooling into qualities ascribed to all human beings, appearing in different circumstances and forms based on the historical location and the 'civilization' in which these differences were manifested.[126]

Otto Klineberg (MD, McGill University, Montreal, 1925; PhD, psychology, Columbia University, 1927) was a Canadian psychologist (and colleague of Franz Boas at Columbia University), whose popular book *Race Differences* (1935) answered theories of innate racial differences, placing primary emphasis on environmental factors. Fredrick Steigmann, a Chicago physician, agreed in principle with Klineberg, as 'environmentally conditioned psychic factors play an equally important role in the genesis of peptic in White and Negro patients.' Thus, the physician had to deal with 'the problem of peptic ulcer in the Negro with the same attitude as he does in the White patient.'[127] It took until 1950 for this view to appear in the *Journal of the National Medical Association*, published by the Black medical association that paralleled the then segregated American Medical Association. In a letter to the editor, Henry Arthur Callis (MD, Rush Hospital School of Medicine, 1921) described what he had labelled 'discriminatory neurosis'.

> Since hypertension has been found absent in the African Negro when undisturbed by the white man, it may be assumed that the great toll of hypertensive heart disease among American Negroes is related to his struggle at a disadvantage, in his American social and economic environment. In such a disease as cancer which is no respecter of wealth, class, or race, there is no significant difference in total incidence between white and Negro. Among Negroes many emotional disturbances arise chiefly from job discriminations. Many of the

reactions are accommodative and often over-compensatory. Others are anti-social. In the wake of the disturbed psyche the following physical syndromes are frequent: migraine, peptic ulcer, cardiospasm, simple angina, cardiac irregularities, neurodermatitis, spastic colon, colitis, urinary dysfunction, glaucoma, and in adolescents, even acute appendicitis.[128]

After the Second World War the aetiology of peptic ulcer disease is tied to the legacy of Jim Crow.

African American physicians, a decade earlier, were less certain. In the *Journal of the National Medical Association*, two physicians noted in 1934 that 'Peptic ulcer is not a very common disease in the Negro race' and that 'Upper abdominal disease is not well borne by the Negro.'[129] What they did establish was to counter the claims that syphilis was at the root of these rare cases. The idea that African Americans had a higher toleration for syphilis was also at the core of the notorious 1932 Tuskegee experiment, which left subjects untreated even after specific treatments for the disease were available after the Second World War. Syphilis was (and is) a disease with moral opprobrium, so showing that it did not cause ulcers freed their patients from the charge of immorality. Race really did matter, then and now, as anyone who was diagnosed had to be able to see a physician, and that was difficult for many African Americans in the 1930s. This counterview has a very long life, indeed seems to reappear regularly in the colonial medical literature, as can be seen in a letter from 1960 to the BMJ from a physician station in Aden, stating

that the incidence of duodenal ulcer is very much lower among the general population than among those holding posts of responsibility. 'Stress' was an obvious factor in the latter group, and several volunteered the information that their symptoms were exacerbated during periods of overwork and mental strain. It may well be that as Africans take over the burdens and responsibilities of administration and management in business and politics, so the frequency of peptic ulcer will rise in this group, while it will remain a comparative rarity in the non-civilized areas where the African continues to live his happy-go-lucky, day-to-day existence, letting to-morrow take care for [sic] itself.[130]

Race matters in scientific medicine then and now; race matters in access and therapy then and now.

Stress because of racism is a topic that surfaces repeatedly. In 2023 Arline T. Geronimus (ScD [Doctor of Science], Harvard School of Public Health, 1985; Professor of Health Behavior and Health Education, University of Michigan) published the result of decades of work on the impact of stress on health.[131] In her *Weathering: The Extraordinary Stress of Ordinary Life in an Unjust Society* she attributes the decay of the health of minorities to the impact of stress on the organism, seeing ulcers, hypertension and a range of other infirmities not as the result of any genetic predisposition but of life circumstances.[132] She, and we shall see this repeatedly, is monocausal in reading stress as a purely mechanical phenomenon, arguing that the constant, unmitigated stress of living in racist societies produces an endocrine rush, the fight-or-flight response, which should, she argues, need to be activated only rarely and for very short periods of time. This is an uncited variation on the work of Hans Seyle (MD, German University of Prague, 1929), who, beginning in the 1930s, defined stress responses as an answer to psychoanalytic theories, as we shall discuss later in this chapter.

Geronimus calls the constant repetitive occurrence 'weathering' and sees all deviations in health outcomes because of this process. Higher rates of cardiovascular disease and cancer are to be found in communities as diverse as white inhabitants of rural Kentucky and Black inhabitants of the South Side of Chicago. Both groups, as she notes, are viewed with 'contempt, fear or resentment' by those around them. Women in both groups suffer higher rates of morbidity and mortality in pregnancy or childbirth, according to her views, as they are doubly stigmatized. The lack of social capital in these contexts adds to the burden of those defined by their social location. So compelling was this argument that the playwright Harrison David Rivers wrote a drama, *Weathering* (2023), about the crisis of childbirth in the Black community. That this could be one of the aetiologies of somatic diseases and their negative outcomes is without a doubt but there are others, some somatic, along with purely social ones, such as the lack of access to healthcare, that certainly play major roles. Thus a mechanical notion of stress is evoked to explain all somatic ills without any 'magic bullet' that would resolve such pathologies. Much like 'trauma' – undefined and thus unlimited in its scope – 'weathering' describes but does not propose specific ameliorations except to change the world.

Race Science and PUD: The Jews

If the stereotype of the African is a 'race' without the diseases of civilization, the image of the Jew in the literature of the nineteenth and twentieth century is quite the opposite. The nineteenth century was for Western European Jews the best of times and the worst of times. Civil emancipation, increased economic and social mobility and access to secular education were all slowly acquired by European Jews, yet counterbalanced by the rise of a political antisemitism that sought to reverse civil emancipation and the reappearance in altered form of older forms of antisemitism such as the medieval 'blood libel', now cast in political rather than theological terms. Meanwhile, political realities within the Russian Empire led to massive pogroms and the flight of millions of Eastern and mainly unacculturated Jews to the cities of Western Europe and beyond following the 1881 assassination of Tsar Alexander II. Consequently, there was a range of Jewish responses to these political realities, including assimilation and conversion, the rise of political and cultural Zionism and the establishment of secular Jewish political parties (at least in the Austro-Hungarian Empire). This snapshot is reductive as well as accurate.

Throughout Western Europe the gradual integration of Jews into the body politic was seen as the cause of Jewish psychopathology as well as a source of danger to the nation state. Various theories were put forth to explain the nature of Jewish predisposition to various diseases. All these explanations functioned to produce a uniform biological category, labelled 'the Jews'. Even the liberal pathologist Rudolf Virchow was persuaded to undertake a massive statistical study in 1886 of the hair, skin and eye colour of 6,758,827 German schoolchildren to see whether there were any uniform standards that would define race. He was surprised that there weren't but acknowledged that this undermined 'race' as a biological category. Few of his contemporaries agreed. The Munich psychiatrist Georg Burgl (MD, University of Munich, 1876) observed in his handbook of forensic medicine of 1912 that the degenerative nature of the Jew can be easily observed in the 'physical signs of degeneration such as asymmetry and malocclusion of the skull, malocclusion of the teeth, etc.'[133] Wilhelm Erb (MD,

University of Heidelberg, 1864) commented that the 'Semites . . . are a neurotically predisposed race. Their untamed desire for profit and their nervousness, caused by centuries of imposed lifestyle (*auferlegte Lebensweise*), as well as their inbreeding (*Inzucht*) and marriage within families (*Familienheiraten*), predisposes them to nervousness.'[134]

Yet the emancipation of the Jews was also read as one of the explanations of their predisposition for madness. The dean of *fin-de-siècle* German psychiatrists, Emil Kraepelin (MD, University of Leipzig, 1878), professor of psychiatry at Munich, spoke with authority about the 'domestication' of the Jews, their isolation from 'nature and their exposure to the stresses of modern life'.[135] Even acculturated Jewish doctors had to accept this type of predisposition, as had their African American counterparts, as it was part of what defined clinical medicine at the time. Jewish academic physicians were forced to deal with the potential of Jewish illness in their own research and the claims of such potential impairment reflected on their own stability.

If the African American was a 'primitive' and thus shielded from diseases of civilization, then the Jew was a 'degenerate', unable to respond to the pressures of civilization. In 1857 Benedict-Augustin Morel (MD, University of Paris, 1839) defined the degenerate as 'a morbid deviation from a primitive type'.[136] The Paris-based physician Max Nordau (MD, University of Pest, 1872), one of the founders of modern Zionism, in one of the most widely read (and translated) books of the 1890s, *Degeneration* (1898), continued this line of argument and defined degeneracy as 'a morbid deviation from an original type. This deviation, even if, at the outset, it was ever so slight, contained transmissible elements of such a nature that anyone bearing in him the germs becomes more and more incapable of fulfilling his functions in the world; and mental progress . . . finds itself menaced also in his descendants.'[137] Health and disease are virtually interchangeable, depending on their location: 'As a matter of fact there exists no activity and no state of the living organism which can in itself be designated as "health" or "disease." But they become these in respect of the circumstances and purposes of the organism. According to the time of its appearance, one and the same state may very well be at one time disease and at another health.'[138] For the Jews, the context of health and illness is everything. He sketches the history of the Jews, distinguishing between the so-called 'master-race' and Jews as 'slaves'. He argues that, in antiquity, 'the Jewish race' generated a 'slave revolt in morality' against the 'master-race which had long oppressed the Jews'.[139] In regard to his own time, the age of scientific medicine in which he was trained at the medical school in Pest, civilized life is considered bad for everyone's health as 'many observers assert that the present generation ages much more rapidly than the preceding one' and especially for the Jews.[140] The 'struggle for life', even if successful, has its medical consequences.

Now, we need to note here that Nordau was 'shouting in the marketplace'. He wanted attention paid to his claim that modernity was degenerate in all its forms, from opera to philosophy to politics. William James called *Degeneration* 'a pathological book on a pathological subject', and William Dean Howells, in a review, blasted it as 'a senseless and worthless book' whose 'insufferable pages' show Nordau to be 'a bad-tempered, ill-mannered man' and 'a clever quack advertising himself'.[141] Just another Jewish quack misusing medicine for his own ends.

The 'Jews', now as a racial category, displaced from their place of origin, both in time and geography, cannot adapt to civilization (in the Global North) or can adapt so well that they become invisible: 'It is pretty well known that the Semitic peoples possess a power of acclimatization, or adaptability to climate, superior to that enjoyed by the Aryan races.'[142] Their adaptability, however, does not preclude presenting with diseases of modern life. 'Everywhere Jewish men and women are peculiarly liable to diseases of indigestion or dyspepsia, to diabetes, cataract, etc., which would seem often to arise from eating too much and digesting too little, frequently aggravated by want or deficiency of regular exercise in the open-air,' noted the Brighton surgeon J. Lawrence-Hamilton in 1893.[143] Indeed, this is a reflection not only of lifestyle but of race: 'Easterns, of whom there are many in Manchester, are markedly more susceptible to neurotic troubles than the English – I speak of the males. Greeks, Syrians, Armenians and Eastern Jews are very much inclined to hysteria, "visceral neuralgias", as you would call them, and so forth.' And they suffer from 'a series [of ailments] which would contain kinds of dyspepsia, of arthritis, of phlebitis, of arteritis, of nephritis, of angina pectoris, of migraine, of hypochondriasis, of insanity, of eczema, of glycosuria, of neuritis, of bronchitis, of tonsillitis, of haemorrhoids, and so forth'.[144] All diseases where 'Jews' seem to proliferate as patients.

Jewish physicians acknowledge this but limit how they define those 'Jews' at risk. 'Nervous dyspepsia is a very common disease among Jews, and acid dyspepsia (hyperchlorhydria) is also more frequently met with among them. Physicians who have experience among them find that acute indigestion is particularly met with among orthodox Jews on Sundays.' This from Maurice Fishburg (MD, New York University, 1897), the leading Jewish public health specialist in New York City in the first half of the twentieth century. Not a problem of the hustle and bustle of city life, but of antiquated traditions imported with the new Eastern European migrants flooding the Lower East Side. As he continues, 'A prominent clinician, a specialist in diseases of the stomach in Berlin, states that three-fourths of the Russian Jewish patients who consult him belong to the class of neuropaths and hypochondriacs. This is seen mostly in Russia and Poland, but rarely among the Jews in Western Europe and America, because here, as a rule, they do not prepare their Sabbath food on Friday to be kept in the oven till Saturday.'

Yet even here in New York City, among Jews now well integrated into American social norms, 'chronic dyspepsia is very common. It is due to the fact that Jews generally, owing to deep absorption in their business, rarely have regular hours for meals, and can hardly spare time to masticate their food properly.'[145] The debate rages well into the twentieth century, with counterclaims in the 1950s that in the newly founded State of Israel 'immigrants from Europe had a significantly higher rate of ... peptic ulcer, while Oriental Jewish immigrants suffered from a very high rate of intestinal infections.'[146] The sabras, the native-born Israelis, are unmentioned as they, as the unspoken baseline, seem to suffer from neither.

The claim that the Jews suffered from gastrointestinal diseases was answered by an extensive literature praising Jewish dietary laws, the Laws of Moses, with their restriction on what could and could not be consumed, as the source for Jewish vitality in the light of persecution.[147] Referring back to Fishburg's comment about Jewish dyspepsia on the Sabbath, there is the argument that the status of food in religious practice provides healthier food (paraphrasing a contemporary view that Moses was the first hygienist): 'The food of the Russian Jews is considered to be above reproach. The meat consumed, as is well known, has, before being placed on sale, undergone a thorough inspection as to the health of the animal killed. The meat is therefore more wholesome and more fit for human consumption than that in the average non-Jewish butcher shop.' Also, the Eastern European Jew's diet is rich in fish. Yet the amount of 'healthy' food consumed is relatively small as 'another important fact is that the Jews do not eat much: – a pound of meat per diem is sufficient for a poor family of a husband, wife and a few children.' If there is dyspepsia and peptic ulcers it is

> primarily, the deleterious effects of poverty and over-crowding, and also the insufficient use of green vegetables and whole-some food in general, and probably the early maturing of the sexes. Diseases of the stomach are extremely common among the Jews, particularly among the Jewish poor – more common than they are in other races of this dyspeptic country. The cause of this is not intemperance in eating, which plays such an important part in producing stomach trouble among the general American population, for the Russian Jews are quanti-tatively frugal. Hasty eating, however, poor food – or, rather food unsuited to this climate, tea drinking, and perhaps undue indulgence in soda water and kindred beverages, all these serve to produce gastric disorders.[148]

Acculturation, not tradition, causes stress and stress causes illness.

We can return for the moment to Arline T. Geronimus and her concept of 'weathering' as the explanation for the higher rates of minorities, such as African Americans, living under constant racial strain having a wide range of chronic illnesses such as ulcers. In 2011 she and a colleague looked at Jewish self-perception of health by analysing the National Jewish Population Survey and found that the self-rated health of Jews seemed to converge with that of African Americans and was significantly worse than that of other whites, even though educa-tion levels and income were substantially higher. If, and that was the assumption of this study, a 'white ethnic group with a favorable socio-economic profile reported significantly worse health than did other Whites' then it was assumed that the result was 'the complex inter-play of cultural, psychosocial, and socioeconomic resources in shaping population health'. For they assumed that 'Jewish Americans as Whites have frequent interactions with mainstream American social institu-tions in their daily encounters . . . they may as "outsiders" experience othering and exposure to stigmatizing messages. These experiences could adversely affect their health.'[149]

Now, we need to examine this set of assumptions in 2011 when the present rate of antisemitic incidents had not yet become a social factor in American life, indeed at the moment when Jews, however defined, had become the 'model minority'.[150] That 'self-reporting' itself might be at fault rather than any statistical presentation (with its own set of complex contradictions) seems to not be understood. Social position is indeed frangible, as we have seen, but its reading is always contextual. Is 'class' one of the variables here, echoing the debates about 'Type A' characteristics and stress which we have discussed? Not stigma per se but attempting to fulfil the social expectations of the 'model minority'. And what could be understood as an index of poor health could also be read as an openness to speaking about such matters in a scientific location such as a social science survey. The meaning of stress, as, of course, of 'race', shifts over time, as does its presentation and perception.

Physiological Explanations for PUD

While psychosomatic explanations dominated the discussion about the aetiology of peptic ulcers, this was simultaneously the age in which biological explanations competed for public attention with Freudian ones. As we have seen, anatomists such as the Viennese Carl von Rokitansky in 1842 proposed a neurogenic theory of the origin of dyspepsia in cases of acute perforating ulcers, seeing it as caused by an overstimulation of the vagus nerve. And Jean-Baptiste Cruveilhier fifty years later had intimated that such alterations in gastric function and the appearance of peptic ulcers were attributable to external factors, such as emotional states.[151]

In the 1880s William James (MD, Harvard Medical School, 1869) and Carl Lange (MD, University of Copenhagen, 1859), quite independently, had argued that physiological stimuli automatically induce bodily changes, and that the feedback of these bodily changes to the brain is constitutive of the feeling of the emotion. Then Walter Cannon (MD, Harvard University, 1900), by then the George Higginson Professor of Physiology at Harvard Medical School, argued that the emotions were generated in subcortical brain regions, especially the hypothalamus, linking the realms of endocrinology and neurology.[152] This was the same William Cannon who figured out how to X-ray a cat's digestive system while a medical student at Harvard.

Cannon's focus became the aetiology of gastric disorders in psychic states, but he rejected the Freudian model of repression as the underlying cause for symptoms. He sees the relationship between the expression of such emotions as 'fear, horror, and deep disgust' and the digestive process. For him the expression of such emotions on the musculature of the face mirrors the state of the gut. Cannon uses the term 'emotions', which he defines as 'not restricted to violent affective states but includes "feeling" and other affective experiences. The term is also used in the popular manner, as if the "feeling" preceded the bodily change.' Cannon stresses that the emotions he is evoking are not of the unconscious, as his model is behavioural in the extreme, citing Ivan Pavlov and his dogs' flow of saliva when exposed to stimulation, but also augmenting it with a case of a young boy whose gastric secretion appeared only when he was chewing something 'agreeable'. It was erroneous, he wrote, 'to assume a predominant importance of the psychic state in the causation of digestive disease', countering the Freudians. Nevertheless, he concluded, the patient's mental state had to be considered, 'for just as feelings of comfort and peace of mind are fundamental to normal digestion, so discomfort and mental discord may be fundamental to disturbed digestion.' And it was vital for therapy, as 'the mental state of a person complaining of digestive difficulty may have marked effects on both the motility and the secretion of the alimentary tract. The mental state of the patient, therefore, must be considered before passing judgment on the nature of his trouble, for just as feelings of comfort and peace of mind are fundamental to normal digestion, so discomfort and mental discord may be fundamental to disturbed digestions.'[153] Cannon follows this initial argument in 1909 with dozens of articles and books reclaiming space for a psychogenetic component for the aetiology of PUD from the psychoanalysts.

In 1920 the British neurologist Sir Arthur Hurst (BM [Bachelor of Medicine], Guy's Hospital [London], 1904) had described the effect of mental and physical fatigue on the appearance of symptoms of duodenal ulcer; his position linked quickly with that evolved by Cannon.[154] The causative role of the nervous system in PUD came to be an answer to Freudian arguments about repression, still seeing the aetiology in affect but not in the unconscious. The internist Thomas R. Brown noted that perhaps peptic ulcer was 'not a local but a constitutional disease, and that in its origin and in the recurrence of symptoms psychic factors are important'.[155] This view appeared in his section on peptic ulcers in the first edition of what will come be to known as the 'best known medical textbook in the world,' — by 2024 in its 27th edition – *The Text-Book of Medicine* (1927), edited by Russell LaFayette Cecil (MD, The Medical College of Virginia, 1906, with further study in Vienna and the Johns Hopkins University School of Medicine). The Brooklyn gastroenterologist Emanuel W. Lipschutz claimed the next year that virtually every physician conceded that the 'neurotic, worrisome, emotional and hard working person' was at highest risk to develop peptic ulcer.[156] This was a theme that resonated across the medical literature. Studies that focused on the physiology of acid secretion assumed that where there was a 'high secretion of hydrochloric acid', this 'may be caused by increased nervous tension'. The answer to excess stomach acid is that 'the increased nervous tension must be relaxed and its causes removed, whether they be in the external environment or are the effect of toxins upon the nervous system.'[157] If this were the case for all people under stress, then the claims that race formed a major predisposition for PUD was answered by the claim that it was racism that caused stress, not race per se.

That same year, 1930, saw the appearance of the Stanford-trained (MD, 1910) gastroenterologist Walter C. Alvarez's *Nervous Indigestion*, which emphasized listening to the patient's emotional as well as physical history to rule out organic causes as well as to understand the psychic roots of the individual's distress. This reinforced the affective relationship between physician and patient, what the Freudians call 'transference' and 'countertransference'. Alvarez quietly but authoritatively brought the psychoanalysts back into the medical discussion: 'If she does not immediately give me a frank, convincing answer I say, "Come on now, let us have the whole story; it will do you good to tell someone about it" and it often does. Freud has pointed out that nausea in nervous women may be a sign of disgust over a disappointing love affair, and I have seen some cases which would support this view.'[158] That behavioural and psychoanalytic models competed was clear; but all insisted that the patient's account of their distress was itself an interpretable moment that moved the diagnosis and thus the therapy forward.

Looking at a specific subset of patients under clearly demonstrable physical stress, earlier in the century Thomas Blizard Curling (no degree, but Assistant Surgeon at the London Hospital as of 1833 and President of the College of Surgeons in 1873) found non-chronic peptic ulcers ('Curling's ulcers') in his patients with extensive burns.[159] Harvey Cushing (MD, Harvard School of Medicine, 1895) provided an explanation of ulcers that focused on causation as well as physiological mechanism. He suggested that the 'interbrain' (the endocrine structure of the brain, epithalamus, the thalamus, the hypothalamus and the subthalamus), which was newly recognized as an important but hitherto overlooked station for vegetative impulses, was 'easily affected by psychic influences', including 'emotion or repressed emotion, incidental to continued worry and anxiety and heavy responsibility . . . [and] other factors such as irregular meals and excessive use of tobacco'. This neurogenic claim was that underlying character, such as being 'highly strung', made people particularly susceptible to ulcers. Even though it echoed psychological categories such as 'repression', in this view ulcers could only be cured if the patient was put on mental and physical rest. Symptoms were bound to recur when they returned to normal tasks and responsibilities because of the patient's inherent character.[160]

Cushing in the 1930s postulated a direct relationship between brain dysfunction, in the case of his three patients who died after successful cranial surgery, intracranial tumours of the cerebellum and peptic ulcers, as 'intracranial injuries and diseases affecting these same basilar regions of the brain are known to be accompanied by ulcerative lesions of the upper alimentary canal. It is reasonable to believe, therefore, that the perforations following the cerebellar operations forming the base of this study were produced in like fashion by an irritative disturbance either of fiber tracts or vagal centers in the brainstem'.[161] That the brain and gut were anatomically linked in such patients was clear but was there also a psychological theory that linked them in terms of the patients' experiences in the world?

A complex behavioural theory rooted in a biological explanation was subsequently offered by the Canadian endocrinologist Hans Selye (MD, Prague University, 1929), who described the general stress reaction from stimulation of the adrenal gland.[162] Selye, in a note to *Nature* in 1936, began the field of biological stress research by showing that rats exposed to noxious stimuli responded by way of a 'general adaptation syndrome'. One of the main features of Selye's theory was the 'formation of acute erosions in the digestive tract, particularly in the stomach, small intestine and appendix'.[163] What was most powerful about Seyle's claim is that it co-opted the psychoanalytic model that claimed that repression could manifest itself in any number of seemingly unrelated symptoms. 'Koch's postulates', the concept that specific causal factors generated specific sets of symptoms, seemed not to hold for Seyle's rats. Rather it looked a great deal like Claude Bernard's view of a *'milieu intérieur'*, that the body demanded a stable interior balance, and that this homeostasis was achieved by a negative feedback system. This paralleled on the physiological level Freud's psychological theories of the homeostatic psyche, that the *Seele's* job was to ameliorate the excitation of stimulus. Seyle was able to link his endocrinological work on the hypothalamic-pituitary-adrenal axis to the way the body coped with stress and thus provided experimental evidence that peptic ulcers could be caused by stress.

The consensus in the world of post-Second World War society – whether one accepted a psychosomatic or a biological explanation – was that stress was intrinsic in the formation of peptic ulcers. All therapies were linked to this set of assumptions. Ranging from long-term talk therapy to pharmaceutics such as the tranquillizer Miltown, the most widely prescribed pill of the 1950s, or radical surgery such as severance of the vagus nerve (vagotomies) and removal of most of the stomach (gastrectomies), all sought to ameliorate either psychic stress or the biological response to stress. If the psychoanalysts were obsessive about finding a patient's ultimate repression, the 'surgeons went mad to do something to prevent all recurrent ulcers, instead of using the simplest treatment and waiting to see how the patient fared'.[164] But even the simplest treatments, such as anti-reflux and antacid medications, saw exceptionally high rates of recurrence. Peptic ulcer and duodenal ulcer were understood as highly relapsing diseases, unless continuous acid suppression was used (and indeed to a lesser extent even when it was). By the 1920s such medical interventions had become so commonplace that the home and 'quack' remedies were replaced by the first American over-the-counter antacid, created in 1928 by pharmacist James Howe and marketed in 1930 as TUMS, a pill composed of sucrose (sugar) and calcium carbonate ($CaCO_3$). No longer concerned with bacterial infection, popular medicine sought only to ameliorate acid production, which provided some temporary relief. It thus created life-long customers for their medications.

Yet therapeutics for peptic ulcers continued to rely on such home remedies: 'the standard then for any stomach upset in a Scottish household was baking soda. A teaspoon of baking soda stirred into water and as you know the side effect was CO_2 and a big belch and, "That's me, I'm off to work", that was the standard remedy for upsets.' 'Roter tablets', which first appeared on the market in 1948, were popularly linked to milk as a remedy for dyspepsia: 'Oh aye Willie, it was all fish and these milk puddings (before starting Roter tablets). He's got these Roter tablets and now it's all fish suppers, curries and stews.'[165] Milk became one of the medicinal interventions in this modern age of cows' milk as a universal food: post-pasteurization, with its elimination of the risk of bovine tuberculosis and the marketing of milk as the health drink, milk came to be seen not only as prophylactic but therapeutic for peptic ulcers. Reducing stomach acid levels became the goal and Carl Schwarz's dictum 'No acid, no ulcer' (1910) became an unspoken rule. Physicians such as Bertram Welton Sippy (MD, Rush Medical College, Chicago, 1890; postgraduate study in Berlin and Vienna) created full regimens of health food and his 'Sippy diet', with its reliance on milk, to which eggs and other bland foodstuffs were added after the lapse of several days, became the go-to therapy for ameliorating gastric distress.[166]

In Britain over-the-counter medications such as Rennies, Alka-Seltzer, Milk of Magnesia, Bisma-Rex, Bismag's 'Bisurated' Magnesia, Moorland tablets and Queens Health & Liver Salt, as well as Roter tablets, claimed to be effective in acid suppression. Many of them contained bismuth. By the 1980s much more sophisticated drugs to control stomach acid production, known as h2 blockers, were employed to control peptic ulcers. The bestselling of these was Smith, Kline & French's Tagamet (cimetidine), which blocked production of gastric acid and became the first drug ever to reach $1 billion annual sales by 1986. Soon thereafter came Zantac (ranitidine), which only increased the market for such drugs. h2 blockers treated ulcers as a chronic condition, which meant, like the antidepressants, you were yoked to them forever. If working in advertising agencies gave you peptic ulcers, then perhaps their hawking of such cures might (or might not) help. Zantac certainly did not, as in 2020 ranitidine was declared by the FDA to be carcinogenic. Stomach cancer was definitely not ulcer relief.

Now, this concatenation of aetiologies and cures based upon them may well have seemed confusing, as Sarah Murray Jordan (MD, Tufts University School of Medicine, 1921), who in 1942 became the first woman president of the American Gastroenterological Association, had already noted about peptic ulcer disease in 1930: 'the laity . . . is frequently offered that there is a shifting of thought from one vogue to another, and that what was considered good therapeutics five years ago is discarded today, only to be resuscitated and justified in another five years. While to a certain extent such criticism may be justified when superficially considered, the underlying truth is usually that one or another factor, in a complicated group of factors, assumes greater or less significance as investigative work progresses.'[167] And that comes to be the case even more with PUD, but as each shift occurs the boundary between 'real' and 'quack' approaches gets reinscribed.

A Nobel Prize-Winning Cure

Now let us move across to a rather distant world, that of Australia in the 1940s. About as far from stress, one could imagine, as one could have gone at the time. Yet in the 1940s Australian medicine began to see a spectacular increase in cases of peptic ulcers in men. In a survey of over a thousand cases from 1939 to 1944 in Adelaide, hardly the stress-centre of Australia at the time, it was clear that men outnumbered women 7 to 1 and that their morbidity rate hovered at about 8 per cent, a rate double what was to be expected. Why more male than female patients and why such a high death rate was deemed unanswerable: 'It is intimately bound up with the cause of the condition, which is unsolved at the present moment.'[168] But what it mirrored was a major shift in the Global North as to who developed peptic ulcers. The earliest recorded hospital admissions for gastric ulcer were in the 1840s in London and New York. The numbers increased to about 1910 and then declined. However, the increase in admissions in London was far greater than that even in New York, with four times the number of admissions by 1920. Although the rates increased in similar decades in the two cities, far higher rates were reached in London and Berlin and even higher further north in Edinburgh. Over the same period, ever so slowly, admission rates for duodenal ulcer exceeded those for gastric ulcer. It was only in London in 1938 at the Royal Free Hospital and 1948 at St Bartholomew's that the number of duodenal ulcers surpassed that of gastric ulcers; in New York this dominance had already been reached in 1925 at Bellevue.[169] Location, location, location – not aetiology. Still, as we noted, they were understood to be relatively rare occurrences.

In the early nineteenth century, the typical patients in Australia had been young women of the 'servant class' who developed acute gastric ulcers; by the end of the century, they appeared more and more in young and middle-aged men and later in older men.[170] What also shifted among men was the type of ulcer: gastric ulcer was highest in men born around 1885, while the risk of duodenal ulcer was highest in those born about ten to thirty years later. That was true across modernizing societies including colonial Australia.[171] (We must remember that while Australia became a 'commonwealth' in 1901, it became independent only in 1986.) That is what the figures in Adelaide also showed in the 1940s. But the question remained about causation. What caused the lesions and were there any corollaries to the psychosomatic or the physiological generation of stomach acid? For the baseline remained that it was increased acid production that underlay the problem. Maybe the answer did not lie in the age or the gender or the class or the race or the location of the patient but in something that transcended all of these?

The view from Melbourne at the time was little different. Not location, but then what? The surgeon Leo Doyle (MB, Melbourne University, 1913) at St Vincent's Hospital stated in 1947 that 'in peptic ulcer we have a disease for which we have as yet no completely satisfactory explanation' and then gave us one: food allergies.[172] Allergies too are a discovery of the first age of scientific medicine; the Viennese paediatrician Clemens von Pirquet (MD, University of Graz, 1900) noticed in 1906 that when his patients were given a second smallpox vaccination they developed a hypersensitivity, which he called 'allergy'. (He will reappear later in this case study.) Physiological interventions appeared first around the First World War, with the development of immunotherapy, and pharmaceutical treatments, in the form of the newly discovered antihistamines, were widely available in the 1930s. Of course, ulcers of all locations could be just one more allergic reaction. But, even in Australia, they weren't. So, the Australian medical establishment imported whole hog all the psychogenic and physiological theories about acid production, from inflammation to functional causes, as well as potential underlying psychic traumas that might well explain shifts in patient populations with the rise of modernity.

But there were other things in Australia that attracted the public's attention to medicine in the late 1940s, such as a cure for cancer. At about the time that PUD was beginning to spike, in 1948 the New South Wales government instituted an inquiry into the claims of John Braund – a 78-year-old self-described 'quack' – that his secret treatment had cured 317 cancer sufferers. The 'Braund controversy', as it became known, was one of Australia's most prominent cases of medical fraud and coloured much of the discussion about mainstream and alternative approaches not only to treatment but to alternative conceptualizations of medical intervention.[173] The question was not so much whether he was a quack but how to deal with his claims. The committee appointed to examine him examined his method: 'Mr Braund . . . proceeded to massage the toes by his special method . . . He rubbed and squeezed each side of the toes, particularly the great toe, emphasizing that the blood was forced through the gland alleged to be at the side of and near the tip of the great toe. It may be mentioned in parenthesis that no such gland exists.'[174] Needless to say, the committee's findings were clear. They concluded that 'his methods are based upon unsound physiological and grossly incorrect anatomical bases . . . If any apparent benefit has resulted in certain patients, it can be attributed, without any doubt, to its psychical effects which are seen in certain patients upon varying therapeutic procedures.'[175] Now, Australian law was as much a jumble as elsewhere in this regard, perhaps because there had been many fewer claims about quackery or perhaps simply because there was a greater tolerance for such claims. After the Second World War

> the medical profession in Australia had achieved profession-alisation milestones of legislated restrictions on entry to the profession, an autonomous medical board, and control of work conditions through industrial action leading to the collapse of medical friendly societies. The subsequent events of the Braund case in the late 1940s shows that both the medical profession and the scientific approach to health had achieved sufficient status and regard to move the government to protect the monopoly of the profession and the dominance of scientific medicine without medical organisations having to expend much (or, rather, any) effort.[176]

Braund had been fined earlier for advertising himself as a 'doctor' and 'manipulative surgeon'. When he no longer claimed this 'the Braund controversy raised the question in the press and in parliament of whether legal measures were needed to curb mistakenly enthusiastic or downright fraudulent claims for cancer cures by non-medical people.'[177] Braund was a quack by the medical definition of his day but his sole punishment was to have the premier of New South Wales politely ask that he stop treating cancer patients, a request that he ignored, continuing to practise until his death in 1955.

The Braund case illustrated that the medical profession in Australia after the Second World War was highly attuned to quackery, as 'Braund was . . . cited as the arch quack who had shown that cancer treatment needed regulating.'[178] This accusation was an especially touchy area in Australia at the time as Australian medicine's sole worldwide medical celebrity was a self-anointed nurse without any formal medical training, 'Sister' Elizabeth Kenny, 'sister' being a grade below 'matron' in the hospital system. During the ever-greater global panic about polio earlier in the twentieth century, standards of post-infection treatment had been codified, including the fixing of weakened limbs with splints and plaster casts to alleviate cramping and to provide support to weakened muscles. Kenny introduced warm wool compresses that worked much more efficiently to treat the leg cramps and thus enable patients to begin early rehabilitation. And in a world where there was no prophylaxis for polio, such innovative treatment was immediately questioned. Between 1936 and 1938 a commission was set up to examine her claims, rejecting them in 1938: 'The abandonment of immobilization is a grievous error and fraught with grave danger, especially in very young patients who cannot co-operate in re-education.'[179] She noted in a magazine article in 1944, not too long before the Braund affair: 'At first, I was called a quack, a charlatan, and worse, year after year, in Australia, England and the United States, by men who simply refused to believe that a nurse from "the bush" could devise a treatment which succeeded where they had failed.'[180] Indeed, as one member of a commission examining the fallout from the Braund affair twenty years later noted, 'if an investigating committee had the powers in relation to the after-care of polio [that was to be given to a new cancer oversight committee in 1967] . . . Sister Kenny would have been for a long time a guest of Her Majesty in one of our State Penitentiaries.'[181]

But despite her being labelled a quack by the medical profession in Australia, Kenny's approach was accepted first in the USA and then worldwide, to the point that in 1946 Rosalind Russell portrayed Sister Kenny in an Academy Award nominated film. In 1951 she topped Eleanor Roosevelt as the most admired woman in the world. Kenny?

Braund? While the legislatures in Australia wrestled with this, the professional organizations were hyper-aware of both the risk and the profit of confronting established medical practice. How could the state and the medical professional organizations 'stamp out the John Braunds of the world but still allow for the Sister Kennys'?[182] As with all institutions, the tendency is always centripetal, to stress continuities not ruptures.

And now we return to ulcers, to stress and to quackery. But whose? To try and answer this we need to go to Perth, a city as far out of mainstream Australian medicine as possible. There Robin Warren (MB, University of Adelaide, 1961), a pathologist, had observed spiral-shaped bacteria in stomach biopsy samples taken with endoscopes in association with gastritis. He understood that the pH of stomach acid did not preclude their presence, counter to the prevailing view that the stomach did not tolerate bacteria that could cause ulcers.[183] This was the academic science that had to be followed, but Warren demurred. These bacteria became ever more easily visible when he stained them with a silver stain. Thus, two innovations, the modern flexible endoscope that made observing within the digestive tract easier (certainly easier than in the world of Alexis St Martin and Iron Heinrich) and the insight that a silver stain would make whatever bacteria was present easier to see, made it possible for Warren, considered to be 'a bit eccentric' by his colleagues, to become interested in what exactly their impact on the patients would have been.[184]

Into this world came a young gastroenterologist, Barry Marshall (MB, University of Western Australia, 1974), looking for an offbeat research topic. The result was a meeting of two physicians who were simply unwilling to follow the common wisdom of the day. The bacteria they found were first labelled *Campylobacter*-like organisms and then in 1988 were reclassified as *Helicobacter pylori*. The notion that peptic ulcers were caused by a rather simple bacterium seemed reactionary, even though both British and German researchers in the 1930s and even earlier, well known to both Marshall and Warren, and easily found in the research literature, had claimed much the same thing. The focal theory of PUD, abandoned under the growing influence of psychogenetic theories in the 1930s, had seen infection as the primary cause. Where that infection was localized was consistently revised. But given the emotional and financial investments in both drug therapy and the psychosomatic approaches, what would have been seen as a rather mechanical observation, certainly in the age before antibiotics, was dismissed out of hand once a convergent theory of peptic ulcers was available. Now, after the Second World War and the beginning of the mass employment of antibiotics, even where inappropriate (as we now know), the notion that not the unconscious but a bug could be the cause of PUD seemed outlandish, but grew to be more and more imaginable, as the investment of older theories seemed to be a thing of a more complicated model with little immediate relief. And antibiotics were Occam's razor, simplifying treatment and potentially signifying the end of infectious diseases. As the citation for the Nobel Prize for Physiology or Medicine for 1945 – awarded to Sir Alexander Fleming (MBBS [Bachelor of Medicine, Bachelor of Surgery], St Mary's Hospital Medical School, London, 1906), the discoverer of penicillin, as well as Sir Ernst B. Chain and Sir Howard Florey, both of whom oversaw its mass production – stated: 'for the discovery of penicillin and its curative effect in various infectious diseases'. Pfizer began to mass produce penicillin in March 1944; by the 1980s it was every physician's first drug of choice for virtually every infectious disease, whether bacteriological or not. 'Various' could cover PUD, couldn't it? Only if it were an infectious disease, and that claim had been dismissed decades earlier.

Alternative theories of the aetiology of PUD in Australia were appearing by the 1960s. The explosion of easily available NSAIDS (nonsteroidal anti-inflammatory drugs) such as the brand-new ibuprofen, developed in 1961, and naproxen, developed in 1967, as well as our ubiquitously available old friend aspirin were seen as a major cause. The post-Second World War global pharmaceutical industry reached into every nook and cranny even of rural Australia. A higher rate of aspirin consumption was documented in female gastric ulcer patients, even though most patients were men – with or without consuming aspirin. So this really could not be a variable. But what caused the ulcers, then?[185] Infection? Not really.

Medicine, certainly in Perth, had already determined what was good practice, as Barry Marshall observed: 'When I was in medical school, I was given the impression that everything had already been discovered in medicine. It must have been the way it was taught. So I never thought that medical research would be interesting, but as I did my internship . . . I realised there were a lot of people who had things wrong with them that you couldn't do anything about particularly.' When it was suggested that he check out Warren, who 'was always

'Penicillin Chewing Gum', a British blotter issued by Allen & Hanburys in 1949
advertising the new super drug as a painkiller and active against oral infections.

carrying on about seeing bacteria in [stomach] biopsies', Marshall was
hesitant but followed up the suggestion.[186] After all, *everyone* knew
that the stomach was bacteria-free, stomach acid making it impossible for colonies of bacteria to thrive. After working for months, they
cultured the organism from all 13 patients with duodenal ulcers and
from 24 of 28 patients with gastric ulcers, out of their sample of 100
patients.[187] Both then wrote separate letters (not articles) to *The Lancet*
describing their findings in 1982.[188]

The letters appeared the following year. Yet the Australian
Gastroenterological Society, in 1983, heard them present a paper on
their findings. They never finished their paper because they were
laughed off the stage. They were called quacks 'by colleagues' both
in Australia and, after the letters appeared in *The Lancet*, globally.
The investment in older, established therapies was underscored by
their prestige, physicians' and pharmacists' continuous income from
dealing with chronic illness and by explanatory models that seemed,
both from the psychological and psysiological perspectives, coherent: whatever the reason, increased stress causes increased acidity
(and gastritis) that eventually may lead to peptic ulcers and indeed

cancer.[189] Therapies were at hand and yokels from rural Australia were no match for accepted wisdom, especially when they aimed to overturn the basic premise of the pathology. Yet of course they were right in the light of their model. Stress seems to play little or no role. A well-regarded psychoanalytical approach to peptic ulcers in the immediate post-Second World War moment saw in their ulcer patients a 'conflict situation' associated with a marked dependency.[190] Perhaps also an explanation of the medical establishment's response to the radical new theory. And the fact that every other infectious disease had been treated with antibiotics, with the abandoned model of focal infection omnipresent in the background, meant there was both anxiety about returning to something that looked 'old-fashioned' and the temptation to use something that seemed 'cutting edge'.

But how could Marshall prove what he and Warren had found, as the clinical evidence seemed not to persuade his peers? They had, Marshall claimed, fulfilled all of Koch's hypotheses in the laboratory. 'My attempt to fulfil Koch's postulates started in January 1984 with experiments on four piglets.'[191] But we need to be reminded of the simple fact that 'Unfortunately, Koch's postulates have frequently been applied to issues of causation with a mathematical zeal that is not warranted in the biological world . . . The power of Koch's postulates comes not from their rigid application, but from the spirit of scientific rigour that they foster.'[192] Such claims on science were not sufficient; publicity needed to follow. Their mass of data was not convincing and the slow but steady stream of studies that supported their theory did not put a dent in the official explanation. So, in 1984, Barry Marshall undertook a self-experiment. This has a long but chequered history in medicine: in the eighteenth century John Hunter self-experimented with the penile discharge of a patient and developed gonorrhoea; in 1900 Jesse Lazar allowed himself to be bitten by a yellow-fever-carrying mosquito and died; Max von Pettenkofer avoided that end after ingesting cholera vibrio in 1892, in order, one can add, to show that Robert Koch was wrong in claiming that it solely caused cholera. He developed diarrhoea but not cholera: Koch, of course, was right and Pettenkofer lucky. Self-experiment seemed to be as much public relations as medicine.[193]

After Marshall performed an endoscopy and gastric biopsy on himself to rule out any pre-existing pathology, he swallowed a vial of the bacteria taken from a patient who had stomach ulcers. Two weeks after drinking the bacterial soup, Marshall developed acute gastritis, documented by another endoscopic examination. He was self-treated by a stew of the newest antibiotics – amoxicillin, tetracycline, erythromycin and tinidazole – with the addition of bismuth, in the form of the proprietary medication De-Nol, as Marshall had read about its apparent bactericidal effects in an old textbook of medicine by Sir William Osler.[194] It was bismuth that had proved the British over-the-counter treatments for peptic ulcers to be much more effective than TUMS. And bismuth, of course, that had enabled the first examinations of the peptic ulcer by X-ray fluoroscopy. Even with empirical and clinical evidence Australian medical practice remained sceptical, even though British researchers quite independently began to track bacteria in cases of peptic ulcer.[195] As one witness to Marshall's self-experiment stated: 'Marshall could show that Helicobacter pylori could cause gastritis, but so could a contaminated burger eaten at the weekend. It was a very long step from gastritis, which no-one understood anyway, to ulcer and even further to gastric cancer, as suggested by Marshall.'[196] Even though their work showed that a majority (58 per cent to 100 per cent, depending on the sample across a series of studies) of his patients presenting with peptic ulcer also presented with the bacterium.

Here the Braund/Sister Kenny problem resurfaces. Practitioners in Australia were entrenched in seeing peptic ulcers, as elsewhere in the world, through specific models that made Marshall's claims seem radical. Yet he did use what was the newest and most widely accepted form of intervention, with seemingly good results for the patients he treated, including himself. Was he 'Braund', a quack, or 'Sister Kenny', a home-grown saviour? This was a particularly Australian set of problems that made even those who would have been positive towards Marshall's empirical and clinical evidence refuse to take a position. What if we were wrong?

Marshall left Australia in 1986 and moved to the medical school of the University of Virginia, hoping that American medicine would be more receptive to his views. 'I was disappointed. It was to be another eight years before the bacteria was finally accepted there, following the consensus conference held by the National Institutes of Health in February 1994.'[197] Indeed after Marshall published a detailed double-blind study of the efficacy of the treatment in 1988, 'more research' was demanded before such interventions would be accepted. Marshall responded to this claim by noting that large therapeutic trials would certainly not be supported by the pharmaceutical industry, since the drugs he used were all cheaply available as generic, and that it would take many more years for such a study to appear.[198]

Not enough proof was the standard claim at the time by those opposing the causal relationship between smoking and lung cancer. Never enough proof. The parallel rates of increase in cigarette sales and lung cancer during the twentieth century did not seem to be a compelling enough argument against the charge that the danger was 'unproven'. More science was always needed; statistical proof was not 'real' proof. There was a gold standard set by the bench scientists, who did the 'real' science that had to be answered before 'proof' was present. In his brilliant history of the tobacco industry in the United Allan Brandt subtly shows how all these claims were constructed by the tobacco industry itself. The claims for what was, and was not, 'real' science in the age of statistical reasoning and bacteriology was an artefact of tobacco's interest in making every possible argument seem 'unproven' and, therefore, impossible to take seriously before more work was undertaken. As Brandt notes, it was as if one should have asked John Snow to leave the handle on the Broad Street pump in 1854 until we really knew what caused the cholera, since one could not rely on mere statistics.[199] Luckily, Snow simply took the handle with him, since it was only in 1883 that the agent that caused cholera was identified and even longer before the biochemical processes of infection were adequately described. Science was not followed but limped slowly behind.

The Microbiome

By the mid-1990s the newly reinvigorated bacterial thesis moved from quackery to accepted practice. Ulcers were the product of an infectious disease. The head of the u.s. National Institutes of Health wrote in 1994 an article virtually dismissing psychological factors and emphasizing that *Helicobacter pylori* is directly causally responsible for ulcers.[200] *Helicobacter pylori* tripled or quadrupled the risk of PUD.[201] This led to the near universal adoption of antibiotic therapy for ulcers as the essential treatment for peptic ulcer: 'Kill the bug, cure the disease!' And by century's end 'the rôle of *H. pylori* in the pathogenesis of duodenal ulcer disease is no longer disputed and eradication of this infection is now regarded as the first-line treatment for this common disorder.'[202] Barry J. Marshall and J. Robin

Warren were awarded the Nobel Prize for Medicine or Physiology in 2005 'for their discovery of the bacterium *Helicobacter pylori* and its role in gastritis and peptic ulcer disease. Thanks to this pioneering discovery, peptic ulcer disease is no longer a chronic, frequently disabling condition, but a disease that can be permanently cured.' But, of course, stress and modern life did not vanish as a result. Nor did PUD. Yet the new understanding permeated popular culture of the twenty-first century in real time.

Mad Men, the prize-winning American TV series about the New York advertising industry in the 1960s and '70s, which ran from 2007 to 2015, seemed ironically to capture a world still in thrall to what by the twenty-first century was thought an antiquated and indeed false notion of causality. By that date patients with peptic ulcers were being treated by internists with antibiotics, not by analysts with couches. In the first season of *Mad Men* in 2007, in episode seven, we find the protagonist Roger Sterling, senior partner of the Sterling Cooper advertising agency, on the phone with his wife. 'I *am* drinking my milk,' he reassures her. And sure enough, he's got a half-full glass of milk in front of him, which he tops up with vodka and drinks down. The milk was a prophylaxis, which we (wink, wink) in our twenty-first-century popular medical knowledge 'know' will cause high cholesterol levels and lead to cardiovascular disease. In the TV fantasy of the 1960s 'the milk, on the other hand, was supposed to treat ulcers. Turns out, ulcers were considered a badge of success on Madison Avenue [epicentre of New York's 1960s ad. industry], because all the high-ranking executives like Roger had them. In fact, around the middle of the twentieth century, Madison Avenue was popularly known as "Ulcer Gulch".'[203] The therapy was, of course, the renowned 'Sippy diet'.

When Roger subsequently has a heart attack, it is implied to be as a result of his overconsumption precisely of this prophylaxis for ulcers; he complains: 'All these years I thought it would be the ulcer. I did everything they told me. I drank the cream, ate the butter. Then I get hit with a coronary.'[204] In the mind's eye of the viewer, it was the overconsumption of his therapeutic milk for his incipient ulcers, with or without vodka, that created the cardiovascular disease through high levels of cholesterols (or not)! For the viewer in 2007, dairy products were closely associated with cardiovascular disease because of saturated fatty acids, which were then believed to increase low-density lipoprotein cholesterol levels.[205] As with much of the popular reception of medical knowledge in the twenty-first century it was a belief that unravelled quickly over the next few decades; indeed fermented dairy products, such as yogurt, *kefir* and cheese, came to be seen as having a positive effect on heart health, in fact could be seen as anti-inflammatories.[206]

So, we have cycled through biological theories in the age of bacteriology, through psychogenetic theories in the age of psychoanalysis, through a new age of bacteriology in an age of evidence-based medicine. Many side alleys have been unexplored, such as the Freiburg pathologist Ludwig Aschoff's 1918 claim that friction of food through the narrow pyloric part of the stomach resulted in peptic ulcers.[207] Ghosts of the early twentieth-century American food faddist Horace Fletcher's axiom, widely popular at the same time, who claimed that 'nature will castigate those who don't masticate.' At least forty times for each mouthful. A method Fletcher evolved to cure his own dyspepsia, without Aschoff's urging. And which the AMA's Morris Fishbein, then the editor of its distinguished journal, quickly dismissed as quackery: 'The result of such a pronouncement was a thorough disturbance of the entire body and the development of intoxication and general disability. Professor William James, the great psychologist, is quoted by John H. Kellogg as saying, "I tried Fletcherism for three months. I had to give it up – it nearly killed me."'[208] Fletcher was a quack to no little degree because although, as Fishbein admits, he advocated for 're-establishing a simple fact that had been known for centuries', he was a lay practitioner in the age of scientific medicine.[209]

By the time of writing, we have returned to what may well be the most obvious problem in 'following *the* science': that looking for single causes may well obfuscate complex disease entities, even though researchers in all cases wish that they exist. With *Helicobacter pylori* we suddenly had it: case closed. Yet the claim that *H. pylori* is the cause of all stomach ulcers is a correlation without absolute causality. If we return to Robert Koch's postulates we are stymied. Barry Marshall's 1984 self-experiment proved, to his and eventually the press's satisfaction, that the contents of the stomach of a patient with PUD will create, if not an ulcer, the symptoms of a pre-ulcerous condition. But was that the only factor in his developing 'dyspepsia', to apply our older term? Were there other conditions, such as the stress he was evidently under to prove his theory and create a professional identity for himself, playing a role? Can we now state that *H. pylori* cause peptic ulcers, or do we need to be much more careful and state that people with peptic ulcers have *H. pylori* present in their stomachs?

What we need to be able to find is a reservoir of *H. pylori* in a wide population that does not have PUD and monitor the percentage of individuals who do develop ulcers. And we want to be able to eliminate those factors in individuals who did *not* develop the disease which served to protect them. This indeed was one of the extraordinary questions raised not when Koch announced his discovery of the tuberculosis bacillus in 1882 but when there were cheap, universal tests for exposure to the bacillus. The test was an offshoot of a failed attempt by Robert Koch, who in 1890 claimed to have developed a vaccine against tuberculosis which he called 'tuberculin', an attenuated mix of dead bacteria and antigens from the fluid in which the bacteria had been grown. When administered as a vaccine a hypersensitivity manifested itself in a flagrant skin rash. Sadly, with all that, the vaccine did not prevent the disease. The Viennese paediatrician and creator of the study of allergies Clemens von Pirquet, mentioned above, recognized that this inflammation had diagnostic properties with his patients who had been given smallpox vaccine for a second time. He was able to rethink tuberculin's function, not as a vaccine, but administered in a highly titrated form, as a diagnostic tool. Clean the forearm, two quick scratches with a needle, a drop of tuberculin on each scratch, wait 48 hours. If an inflamed area of at least 5 millimetres (less than ¼ in.) appeared, then the individual had been exposed. Moreover, he found that of 1,400 clinically disease-free children under the age of fourteen he examined, more than 80 per cent tested positive.

Over time it turned out that less than 10 per cent of people who tested positive developed the disease. Massively more people had been exposed than had developed the disease.[210] By 1921 a vaccine, BCG (Bacillus Calmette-Guérin), was available, and the test became universal. But the result was that by the 1920s attenuated tuberculin was being administered as a test for exposure to millions of schoolchildren across the world. Why, physicians suddenly asked, were they immune? Or were they? Since, once they were exposed, they tested positive, if an individual did not develop tuberculosis after the vaccine was administered, was that a success or was it merely the case that the individual belonged to a majority of people who would not have responded in any case? Likewise with peptic ulcers?

In an epidemiological study in 1995 of the general population of San Marino, about 50 per cent of the population showed the presence of *H. pylori* infection (based on the diagnostic examination of blood serum, documenting the response of the immune system to pathogens). It found that, retrospectively, the probability of bacterial infection and ulceration occurring simultaneously was 0.7 out of one. But the *prospective* probabilities suggested a rather different picture: the conditional probability of ulcer given *H. pylori* infection was only 0.18 out of one while the conditional probability of ulcer given no infection was lower at 0.08 out of one, but not insignificant. Nearly a third of the people with ulcers did not or never had harboured the bacteria. But the most striking datum is that the conditional probability of being ulcer-free even if they had *H. pylori* present was 0.82 out of one. While it was clear that infected persons were more than twice as likely to have an ulcer as uninfected persons, infected persons were more than four times as likely to *not* have an ulcer despite being infected.[211] Were there other variables? A study from 2012/13 argued 'that psychological factors play a significant role as predisposing to vulnerability, modulating of precipitation, and sustaining of gastric ulceration'.[212] And we can add to this the growing problems attendant on the therapies employed for treating *H. pylori*.

Is this the next phase in understanding PUD in an age that is beginning to discount the power of evidence-based medicine to provide uniform, consistent and unwavering answers to what are complex and evolving human situations? Certainly, the bacteria 'think' so. There are also other players in this world of scientific medicine, ones without whom such experiments could not even be conceived. Yes, we have experimenters and subjects; there is also the agent, which has been often ignored in the studies of PUD, except as the target of therapy. Microbes have a sort of blind agency. They are visible in their effects globally but not in their essence, which appears only in the laboratory, as Bruno Latour illustrated in his account of Louis Pasteur, for 'you do not need to muckrake or look for distorted ideologies to realize that a group of people, equipped with a laboratory – the only place where the invisible agent is made visible – will easily be situated everywhere in all these relations, wherever the microbe can be seen to intervene. If you reveal microbes as essential actors in all social relations, then you need to make room for them, and for the people who show them and can eliminate them.'[213]

That *H. pylori* was inherently different from anthrax or diphtheria was lost on the clinicians who espoused its eradication. But Latour also missed the boat in his description, for Pasteur began his career not seeking after the causes of rabies but the cause for fermentation. Not 'bad' microbes at all, that may well shape the social as well as physical environment where scientific medicine functions, but 'good' microbes that were necessary for food production. Beginning with figuring out what spoiled milk, he quickly began to grasp the essence of the positive role played by bacteria. Necessary in his world for the making of wine but also the agent of its spoiling. His answer was heating the milk and the wine to stop or prevent spoilage. Pasteur considered that the normal biota (flora) was essential to life. Ilya Ilyich Mechnikov, one of the founders of immunology and winner of the 1908 Nobel Prize in Physiology or Medicine with Paul Ehrlich, 'in recognition of their work on immunity', believed that normal flora was antagonistic and competed with the host.[214] Antagonistic but necessary for life. In 1907 Mechnikov set out to find scientific evidence supporting his theory that not all germs were disease-causing. Such contrary thinking was a hard sell to make during the age of scientific medicine, when it seemed that new discoveries about 'infectious diseases and their relation to microorganisms were being announced like corn popping in a pan'.[215] The irony was that the researchers dealing with *H. pylori* saw it as equivalent to the cause of anthrax, not equivalent to the lactic acid bacteria that play a major role in the production of wine. That they could be both seemed impossible to imagine in 1994, when the bacteria were declared public enemy number one as the cause of ulcers.

Long after the Nobel Prize ceremony was a faint memory, Martin Blaser (MD, NYU School of Medicine, 1973), who by 2014 had run the Epidemic Intelligence Service of the Centers for Disease Control and Prevention and did seminal work on *H. pylori*, noted that he accepted the trajectory of Warren and Marshall's work already in 1983. 'Everyone "knew" that ulcers were caused by stress and excess stomach acid. I, too, was skeptical. I could see that he had discovered a new bacterium, but to me, he didn't have much evidence then at all about ulcers.' For him Marshall was a 'mad man'. But he was quickly converted to the new aetiology for PUD and eventually established the role of *H. pylori* in the causal link to gastric cancer, as 'people without ulcers had it about 60 per cent of the time. So, while it seemed necessary for ulcers it was not sufficient.' Over and over, he found that their arguments about the bacterium held but there were niggling questions. 'Even though *H. pylori* is carried from early childhood to old age, why does ulcer disease start to appear in the third decade of life, peak in the third decade and over the next twenty years or so, and then decline? Why does an ulcer form and then heal after a few days or weeks and then recur weeks, months or years later?'[216] And then suddenly another set of even more basic problems occurred.

By the early twenty-first century Blaser used *Helicobacter pylori*, a bacterium he had been studying for about three decades, to illustrate his 'missing microbiota' hypothesis. Given the success of antibiotic therapy it was 'no wonder doctors around the world began to believe that "the only good *Helicobacter pylori* is a dead one." From ulcers to cancer, everything indicated that *H. pylori* is costly to humans.' Physicians prescribed and then over-prescribed antibiotics to eliminate *H. pylori* in patients with gastrointestinal symptoms. However, he now argued, the bacterium had co-evolved with humans over millennia and is found virtually nowhere except the human stomach – to some purpose, he reasoned. He did epidemiological research on the associations between *H. pylori* and several diseases, the incidence of which has risen in the past few decades – including gastro-oesophageal reflux disease, oesophageal cancers, asthma and allergic rhinitis – and found that the presence of *H. pylori* was inversely associated with these diseases.[217] For Blaser, these findings, which have been replicated by other research groups, underscore the notion of 'amphibiosis' (a term coined by the microbial ecologist Theodore Rosebury [DDS (Doctor of Dental Surgery), University of Pennsylvania, 1928] in 1962) – where 'two life forms create relationships that are either symbiotic or parasitic, depending on context.' Blaser, as a convert to the bacterial thesis, had suddenly discovered the microbiome:

> I believe that the bacteria we carry are not random, but rather have coevolved along with us, passed down from generation to generation in a state of dynamic equilibrium between microbes and host . . . [One study] analyzed the DNA from fecal samples from different hominid species (including *Homo sapiens*) and found that the phylogenic relationships among the bacteria mirrored those among the apes. Interacting with each other and with us in complex ways, our bacteria are a diverse community to which we can apply the term *microbiome*. They

are acquired in a standard, choreographed process, and their composition comes to resemble that of adults by the age of 3.[218]

However, in the age of hygiene as well as antibiotics, Blaser observed, things had changed radically:

Before modern times, microbes were transferred from mother to child during vaginal birth, from the mother's breast during nursing, through skin-to-skin contact and from the mother's mouth by kissing. Now, widespread caesarean delivery, bottle-feeding, extensive bathing (especially with antibacterial soaps), and especially the use of antibiotics has changed the human ecology and altered transmission and maintenance of ancestral microbes, which affects the composition of the microbiota. The microbes, both good and bad, that are usually acquired early in life are especially important, since they affect a developmentally critical stage.[219]

Thus we have new 'diseases of civilization', caused now by all the things that we assumed were prophylactic, as we were told that dirt was bad, that antibiotics cured, that medical interventions such as Caesarean births made deliveries safer. All true yet all with unintended consequences. We had moved from the science of '*anti*-biotics' to that of '*pro*-biotics'.

Overuse of antibiotics, with more than 73 billion antibiotic doses prescribed worldwide annually, had begun to eliminate *H. pylori* as well as 'many microbes from our ancestral bacterial heritage', and 'an ecological shift of this magnitude . . . must have many consequences, good and bad.' Lower rates of PUD, higher rates of a string of other diseases resulting from antibiotic exposure before the age of two and the development of multiple conditions in later childhood, including asthma, eczema, excess weight and obesity, ADHD and learning disabilities.[220] Suddenly every increase in morbidity was the result of antibiotics, in Blaser's view because even good practices may well have their downside.

Initially, the bacteria were found to differentiate into two groups of *Helicobacter*s, *cag* positive and *cag* negative, and Blaser showed that the former increased the risk of gastric cancer by 50–300 per cent.[221] But over the opening decades of the twenty-first century, the actual frequency of both began to wane. Indeed, children whose parents manifested 'normal' amounts of *H. pylori* seemed to have ever lesser counts of the bacterium. Cleaner water, fewer siblings and less exposure to dirt ('matter out of place') in the environment could be precipitating factors. But it was clear that the overuse of antibiotics in each generation destroyed ever more bacteria, given the fact that a course of amoxicillin may eliminate *H. pylori* 10–20 per cent of the time.[222] Yet at the same time gastroenterologists had seemed oblivious to antibiotic overuse, as they assumed that they were dealing with a specific negative bacterium and its total annihilation had positive, immediate outcomes in curing PUD, ignoring the overall risk not only to the patient but to the total ecology. Prescription rates for clarithromycin, the most prescribed antibiotic for *H. pylori* treatment in the twenty-first century, skyrocketed after the beginning of the twenty-first century, as did the rates for quinolones, such as levofloxacin (Levaquin) and ciprofloxacin (Cipro), for the treatment of ulcers. Yet it was also clear that while antibiotics were effective in most patients diagnosed with PUD, they were not effective in all patients, and ulcers also recurred over time.

When the medical profession globally began to become focused on antibiotic overuse, it was not so much because of the soaring rates of prescriptions, analogous to the over-prescription of opioids at the same time, but because of the antibiotics' loss of efficacy.[223] The U.S. National Committee for Quality Assurance listed 'antibiotics of concern' that were overused and clarithromycin, regularly prescribed for PUD, was eventually added to this list. Recent investigations of patients with *H. pylori* infection have reported an increase in clarithromycin resistance from 13 per cent in 2004 to 18 per cent in 2015 as well as a concomitant drop in pan-susceptible strains from 66 per cent to 51 per cent.[224]

But overuse was combined with other clinical problems. Rather than the possibility of indirect *H. pylori* testing (for example breath tests or serology), invasive endoscopy was recommended as the only appropriate tool for clinical investigation and then only those with verified PUD were treated, maximizing the risk of antibiotic overuse. An expensive and invasive diagnostic procedure leads to an expensive and perhaps now less effective therapy. Other new pharmaceuticals, such as the widespread use of potent drugs such as h2 blockers, used to treat duodenal ulcers, and proton-pump inhibitors, which reduce the amount of stomach acid made by glands in the lining of the stomach, also entered the mix, reducing the use of antibiotics. Even with an ageing population, using anti-inflammatory analgesics and anti-thrombotic agents, suddenly there was a rapidly declining prevalence of *H. pylori* infection. PUD disease became substantially less prevalent in the twenty-first century than it had been two decades before. But, as Blaser noted, a wide range of other illnesses, including those of the digestive tract, increased exponentially, including 'globesity', the global pandemic of obesity, and concomitant diseases such as Type 2 Diabetes, which have been laid at the door of antibiotic overuse.[225] Here he gives in to the temptation to have a single answer (his 'hammer') to a wide range of perceived medical problems of the day, just as did all of the earlier theorists about PUD. The simple reality was that, in dealing with ulcers in a world with increasing worldwide antimicrobial resistance, suddenly PUD appeared to be caused solely neither by *H. pylori* infection nor the wide use of anti-inflammatory drugs, such as aspirin, ibuprofen and naproxen. Those without any indication of *H. pylori* made up about a fifth of cases worldwide.[226]

Early on, in the opening chapter of this book, I noted that older models of disease, the diagnoses that resulted and the therapies that were in many cases efficacious never really vanish. Even in a world obsessed by antibiotics and then the radical rejection of them as harmful, the fascination with surgery of the vagus nerve never abated, though the vagotomy became less and less seen as the intervention of choice for PUD. Beginning in 2006 the FDA authorized the use of implants to stimulate the vagus nerve to treat depression and responses to stress. Their efficacy was limited and rarely if ever was PUD the goal of such interventions. Rather, depression and PTSD, seen more and more as having somatic causes in the age of biological psychiatry, were its target. But the notion that the vagus nerve was the key to understanding the widest range of diseases and that its amelioration would cure them extended well beyond allopathic medicine. By 2024 mass culture rediscovered the vagus nerve. With over 70,000 posts on social media with the hashtag 'vagus nerve' and TikTok videos on the topic having been viewed over 70 million times, the vagus nerve became part of heterodox medicine. 'Wellness companies have capitalized on the trend, offering products like "vagus massage oil," vibrating bracelets and pillow mists, that claim to stimulate the nerve, but that have not been endorsed by the scientific community.'[227] This appeared at the same moment that there was a growing conviction by allopathic and heterodox medicine that the 'gut is a second brain', and renewed interest in the enteric nervous system.

This following the claims that the use of antibiotics was destroying our gut biome. Stimulating the vagus nerve is now claimed to treat various forms of mental illness, diabetes, perhaps even long COVID. And PUD remains in the mix, with stress relief as its cure.[228]

Earthquakes, Trauma and PUD

The evident cause for the increase in those cases, as the risk of antibiotic treatment became more and more apparent, was stress. Sigmund Freud had examined the results of being exposed to the horrors of war and the resultant trauma evidenced by soldiers in the 1920s. At 14:46 on 11 March 2011, a 9.1-magnitude earthquake shook the northeastern coast of Japan. Within an hour, a tsunami reached as high as 40 metres (130 ft) in some areas; the Fukushima Daiichi nuclear plant, located on the coast of Tōhoku, the province closest to the epicentre of the quake, was devastated. More than 450,000 people became homeless because of the tsunami. More than 15,500 people died. The response was a national trauma, as the novelist Haruki Murakami reflected:

> 'Why is that?' you might ask. 'Why do so many people think it so natural to live in such a terrifying place? How can they keep from going out of their minds with fear?' . . . From such a perspective, even if humans struggle against the natural flow, that effort will be in vain in the end. The recent earthquake came as a tremendous shock for almost all Japanese . . . Even we Japanese who are so accustomed to earthquakes were completely overwhelmed by the sheer scale of the damage. Gripped by a sense of powerlessness, we feel uncertainty about the future of our country.[229]

Murakami says that the essence of a Japanese aesthetic does offer some cultural solace for such trauma. Yet one thing was quickly noticed. After the 'Great East Japan Earthquake' of 2011 there was an unusual spike in cases of people coming into at least one regional hospital suffering from acute, bleeding ulcers who were *H. pylori* negative.[230] Up to a month after the disaster, as many women as men were diagnosed as having acute haemorrhagic gastric/duodenal ulcers; in the chronic phase the numbers of men substantially increased. Yet none presented with serum *H. pylori* antibodies, and that was significantly different from the previous year's positive rate of 75 per cent with *H. pylori*. Accommodation in a refugee shelter had been seen as a strong risk factor for peptic ulcer bleeding after a large-scale disaster and this turned out to be the case in Japan.[231] A Danish study had showed that psychological stress was associated with an increased incidence of PUD in individuals not testing positive for the bacterium, in part by influencing health-risk behaviours, and that 'stress, socioeconomic status, smoking, *H. pylori* infection, and use of nonsteroidal anti-inflammatory drugs were independent predictors of ulcer.'[232] To which we can add earthquakes, tsunamis and perhaps, if Murakami is right, national aesthetics. A psychogenic, if not a psychoanalytic, reading of PUD.

Murakami had noted that already in his greatest novel, *The Wind-Up Bird Chronicle* (1994–5), where the narrator, Toru Okada, a low-key and unemployed lawyer's assistant, explains that he first met his wife, Kumiko, when he had to 'be in the hospital almost every day back then, to see a wealthy client concerning the inheritance of his property. She was coming to the hospital every day between classes to tend to her mother, who was there for a duodenal ulcer.'[233] The ulcer takes on significance when we eventually learn that Kumiko's childhood was oppressive because her mother had wanted her to take the place of an older sister who had committed suicide at a very young age. Trauma creates PUD and foreshadows the central moment in the novel when Kumiko simply vanishes.

So, are we back to complexity from simple answers? And that in diagnosis and therapy there should be a team approach, often called the Mayo Clinic model, where specialists from a wide range of fields consult, including social workers and psychologists, with each case seen as unique? At that point, it is hoped, clinical medicine will see 'ulcer disease [as] truly curable' only under the following conditions: '[only] when we together fully reject a simplistic Dualism can both psychology and medicine – as cooperative health professions – flourish and find effective and efficient cures for peptic ulcer, as well as other disorders labelled as psychosomatic disease. Let us – psychologists and physicians – now move on and dance together in a celebration of advancing human health and well-being.'[234] Perhaps dancing together is not the perfect image for the complications and boundary drawing that occur when different models, different assumptions and different historical locations all compete for an understanding of aetiology and cure, but it is not a bad goal to aim for in 'following *the* science'.

3

Eyes

AMONG THOSE WHO DEFINED the boundaries of medical practice at the rise of scientific medicine are the eye doctors, the
oculists. Oculists during the Enlightenment had a very
bad rap as 'peripatetic oculists . . . gave specialization a bad name
among physicians. The medical profession viewed specialization as
the province of charlatans and quacks, not respectable physicians.
Physicians too quick to call themselves specialists risked being ostra-
cized by their professional brethren.'[1] Unlike 'gastroenterologists',
who appear as specialists the end of the nineteenth century, 'oculists'
come to be transformed into 'ophthalmologists' at the beginnings of
scientific medicine. Indeed, the modern term for eye doctor appears
first in *The Lancet* in 1825, simply anglicizing the new German scientific term *Ophthalmologie*. In German, *Ophthalmologie* competes
with *Augenheilkunde* (Optical Healing) throughout the age of scientific medicine (in the mid-nineteenth century there were specialist
journals using both terms in their titles). The debate was whether to
use a Latinate term, with its scientific-sounding ring, or its German
equivalent, universally understood but clearly a bit déclassé. Both were
preferable to the quack 'oculist' even though, in the 1890s, 'oculist'
reappears to label those who manufacture and sell glass prosthetic
eyes – not docs at all.

As with patent medicines for PUD, quack oculists certainly had
not vanished by the age of scientific medicine, as in 1893 'a patient suffering from cataract was persuaded that "the skin" had been removed
from her eye, then even signed a testimonial to that effect, but when
she sought skilled advice, the cataract remained. In other cases, the

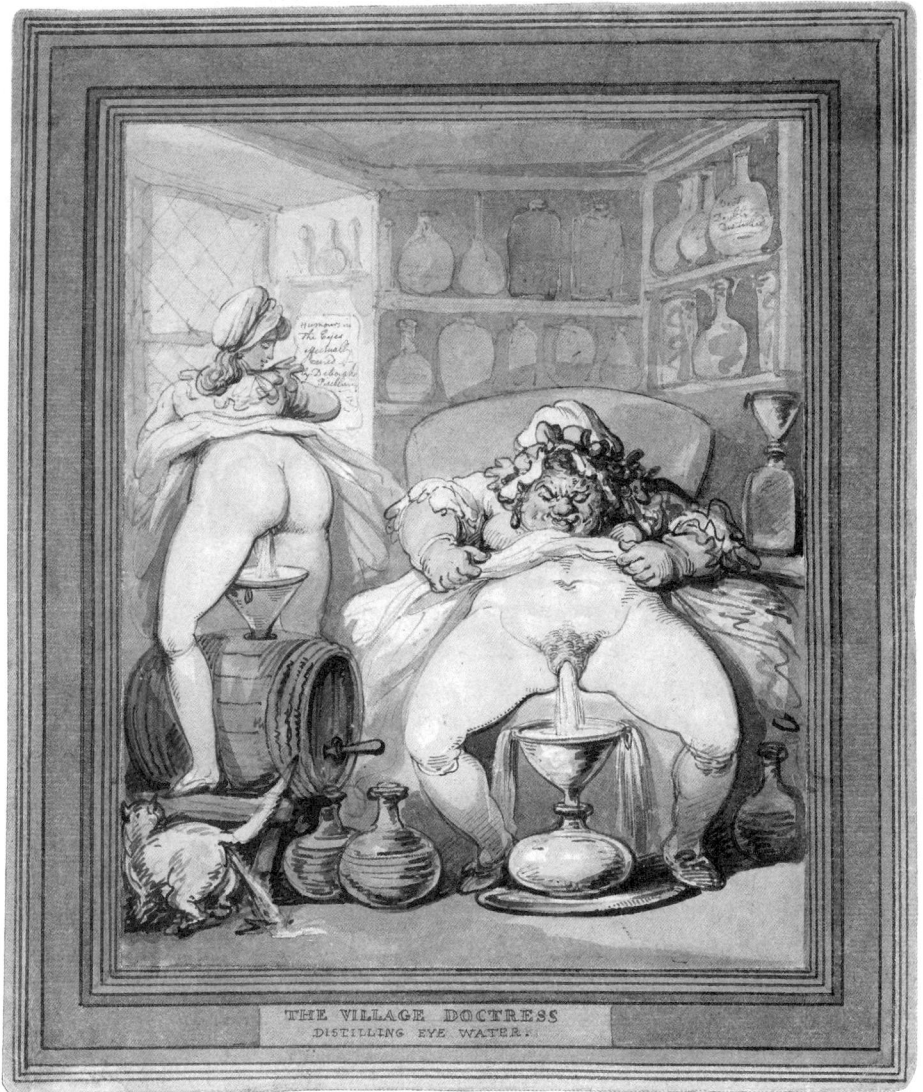

Thomas Rowlandson, *The Village Doctress Distilling Eye Water*, c. 1800. This watercolour shows a rural medical practitioner, a woman, not young, using her own urine to create a medicine which she offers for sale for rubbing on the eyes to dispel bad humours of the eye. She urinates in the right foreground into a funnel over a chemical vessel; another, younger woman urinates in the left background into a funnel placed in a barrel, and a cat urinates in the left foreground on to the ground. 'Humours in the eyes' which are mentioned on the signboard seem to have been a kind of disease, possibly cataract. In the recipe book of Deborah Bragge (also called Deborah Branch), 1725, there is a recipe 'For a homour in the eyes Take a popey head break it into half a pint of watter Lett it be ready to boil then take it off and dape the eyes with it it curred Dr Trotters childs eyes for a homour that fell in them after the small pox' (Wellcome Library, MS 1343, fol. 79r).

quack does some operation, a crude form of couching [piercing the eye near the limbus and pushing the clouded lens back into the eye], and many eyes are lost.'[2] How the former is done is an old ruse of quackery, practised in the twentieth century by 'psychic surgeons' who reach into an invisible wound with their bare hands and painlessly remove tumours. Here the 'stock in trade is some irritating powder, a pair of small forceps and a piece of leather about one-fourth of an inch in diameter. After getting his fee he pinches the patient's lids or conjunctiva enough to make a sharp impression; he then flicks the powder into the eye, exhibits the 'cataract' to the family, and disappears.'[3] Indeed, even into the 1920s a specialist complains that 'scarcely any branch of medicine has been more invaded by advertising charlatans than has ophthalmology.' By that point the problem turns out to be the non-medical specialist, as 'the public continue to think that defective sight is not a matter about which they need consult the family doctor, and so many of them go instead to the chemist or the optician.'[4] With the rise of scientific medicine, the notion of being a specialist came to be not only a positive claim but a necessary one, often contested by those institutions, such as the AMA, that certified the new specialists.

Surgeon or Quack?

In the eighteenth century, the Edinburgh 'quack' John Taylor, a surgeon trained at St Thomas's Hospital in London, undertook a wide range of surgical interventions, from removing scar tissue from the lower lid of a burn victim's eye to removing part of the upper eyelid in a patient who suffered from a drooping eyelid (ptosis), using a procedure which would become commonplace a hundred years later. His reputation rested on his work and innovations as an ophthalmological surgeon, and these were in some manner associated, if only just by him, with his medical training. Despite his evident skill, Taylor was a 'quack', at least according to the Edinburgh Royal College of Physicians, which excoriated him in print.[5]

John Taylor seemed to define the essential 'quack oculist' in his day. Taylor seemed to be as adept in calling out his wares in the public marketplace as he claimed to be in his surgical procedures. He authored a pamphlet advertising his wares entitled *A Parallel between the Late Celebrated Mr Pope and Dr Taylor, Oculist to the King of Great Britain, etc., by a Physician*, in which he praised his skills in treating diseases of vision:

> Hail, curious Oculist! to thee belongs
> To know what secret Springs of Vision move
> The Ball of Sight; what inward cause retards
> Their Native Force; what Operation clears A cloudy Speck,
> > or bids the total Frame Resume the lustre of the lucid
> > Ray . . .
> Fair Vision shines, thither the streaming Rays Converge
> > their Force; and in due Order Range Their coloured
> Forms. Anon the Patient sees
> A new Creation rising to the View In Living Light![6]

Taylor was the son of a surgeon in Norwich and eventually trained as a surgeon in 1727 at St Thomas's Hospital with William Cheselden (London Company of Barber-Surgeons, 1711), an innovator in eye surgery, having developed the procedure of optical iridotomy (described as creating an 'artificial pupil'). But Cheselden had also authored a widely read essay explaining that fear of Blackness (and thus of the 'Black' person) was an inherent rather than a learned quality, when he described how a person, blind from birth, having their sight restored 'was struck with great Horror at the Sight' of a 'Negroe Woman'.[7] What you see matters as well as how you see! Roy Porter noted that Taylor 'received the finest surgical education available', but he also shared in the collapse of the distinction between vision and perception, between looking and seeing.[8] Taylor established himself as an oculist, a profession littered with itinerant practitioners. He also founded a dynasty of oculists, as his son and then grandsons were prominent and respected English oculists in their time.

But was Taylor a quack or a doc? 'Historians want doctors to fit tidily into today's categories. Was a particular practitioner skilful, or a bungling quack? A pillar of the faculty or a coxcomb adventurer? A philanthropist or an opportunist? Taylor, however, resists being exclusively pigeonholed in such ways. In serving thus as a "monster", he can illuminate the wider question of the authorization of the careers of quacks.'[9] Taylor knew his anatomy, as was attested to by his contemporaries, but he was also willing to risk surgery where little or no good could come of it. Indeed, he was accused of having precipitated the

William Hogarth, *A Consultation of Physicians; or, The Company of Undertakers*, 1736. This engraving satirizes the medical profession, depicting a coat of arms with three notorious quacks of the time – John Taylor, Sarah Mapp and Joshua Ward – seated at the top of the shield and twelve physicians below, implying that the quacks and the physicians are one and the same. Taylor, seated at the top left, is winking and holds a cane bearing an open eye, a reference to his dubious ocular surgeries. The motto translates to 'And many are the faces of death' or 'Everywhere the image of death'.

deaths of both Johann Sebastian Bach and George Frideric Handel through his eye surgery.[10] His surgery was conservative: he was still 'couching for cataracts', much as Isaac Newton's bitter rival, the polymath Richard Hooke, had described it in 1681, as 'nothing but thrusting in a fine Needle through the Cornea, and with the Point of it breaking and crushing down to the bottom of the Eye this Mothery Substance'.[11]

Taylor's contemporaries, first Charles Saint Yves (apprenticed at the pharmacy of the Congregation of the Mission in 1686, where he learned medicine and surgery) in 1722 and then in 1747 Jacques Daviel (MD, Medical School of Rouen, 1720), were pioneering a new technique for treating cataracts not by couching, or depression and displacement, as was traditional, but by extraction of the lens. But Taylor, no matter what his actual practice, described the (extra-capsular) cataract extraction before Daviel, although it is again questionable if he ever personally performed this type of cataract operation.[12] The Swiss polymath and physician Albrecht von Haller (MD, University of Leyden, 1727) called him 'a skilful man, but too liberal of promises'.[13] Burchard David Mauchart (MD, University of Tübingen, 1722; Professor of Anatomy and Surgery, University of Tübingen), one of the outstanding eye surgeons of his time, was also quite suspicious of Taylor's claims; however, he testified to his candour, erudition and operative dexterity, confirming that in Amsterdam he had failed to cure only 15 out of 225 cases, even if he did not actually trust his knowledge of the subject.[14] Yet his contemporary the Dutch surgeon Gerhard Ten Haaff (trained as an army surgeon; received his MD in 1747 from the Academy of St Andrews in Scotland) wrote of '*de Beruchte* [the infamous] TAYLOR', and of his incompetence at dealing with cataracts and the many patients operated on for cataracts who after the operation became 'completely [*geheel*] blind'.[15] Taylor, however, also claimed in his autobiography that such surgery 'occasions little or no pain, requires no alternation of diet and admits not even the possibility of a relapse'.[16] Good science of the day: a bridge to the age of scientific medicine, or pure luck on the part of a quack?

That Taylor cried his wares in the marketplace defined him as a 'quack', much more than his skills and knowledge. Indeed, 'Dr' Samuel Johnson (Honorary Doctorates, Trinity College, Dublin, 1765, and Oxford, 1775) famously commented that 'Taylor was an instance

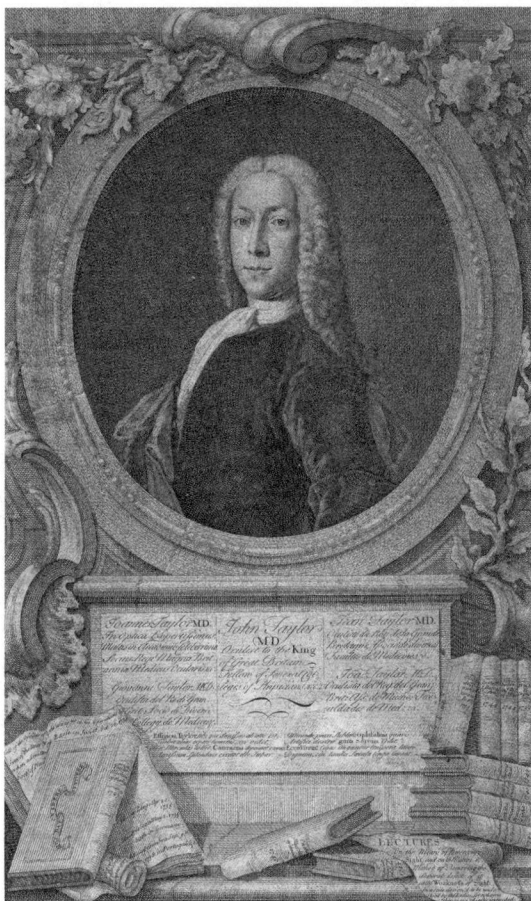

Richard Cooper the Elder, after William Denune, *John Taylor, MD, Oculist to the King, c.* 1745, engraving. This is a very different depiction than the one where he is shown among Hogarth's quacks.

[of] how far impudence could carry ignorance.' Johnson, however, judges him not on his skills as an oculist but 'Talking of celebrated and successful irregular practisers in physick; he said, "Taylor was the most ignorant man I ever knew; but sprightly. . . . Taylor challenged me once to talk Latin with him; (laughing). I quoted some of Horace, which he took to be a part of my own speech. He said a few words well enough."'[17] Good enough perhaps as a surgeon; but a quack because he was a poor Latinist?

Anaesthesia

Pain and fear of infection altered the patient's experience of eye surgery. If there is a subtext to the history of scientific medicine, it is that of all the promises that it fulfilled, the amelioration of pain, however

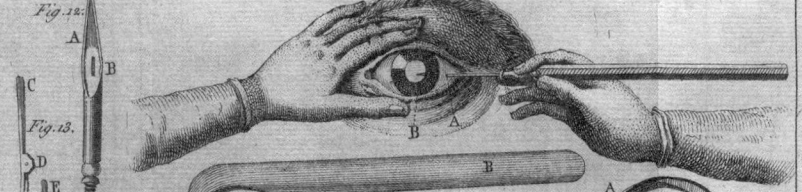

Table XXXVIII.

Fig.12.

Fig.13.

Fig.14.

Fig.1.

Fig.16.

Fig.18.

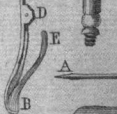

Fig.20.

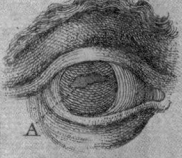

Fig.21.

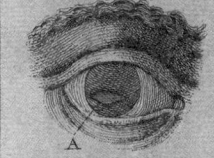

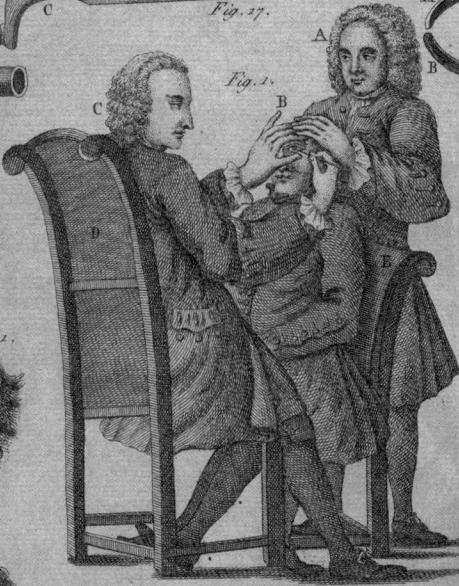

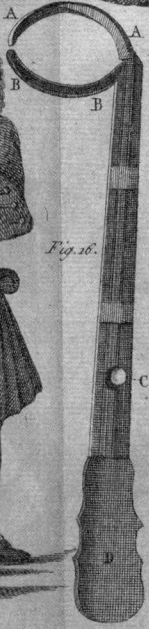

Fig.17.

Fig.19.

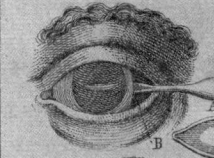

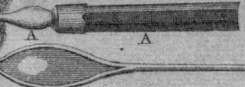

Fig.9.

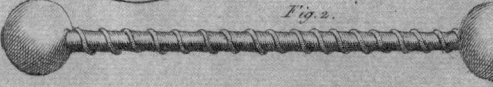

Fig.2.

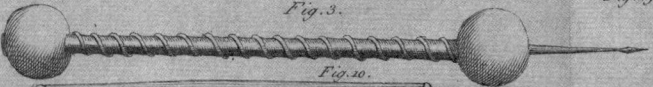

Fig.3.

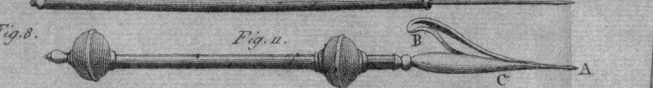

Fig.10.

Fig.11.

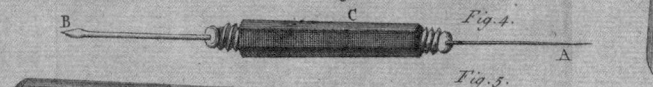

Fig.7.

Fig.8.

Fig.4.

Fig.5.

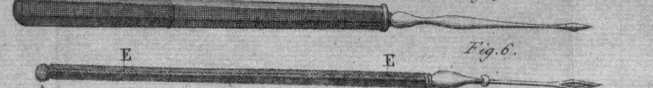

Fig.6.

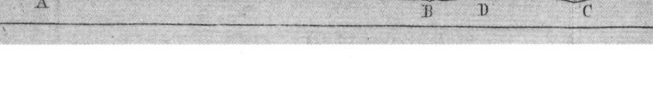

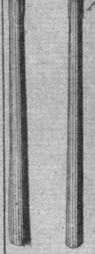

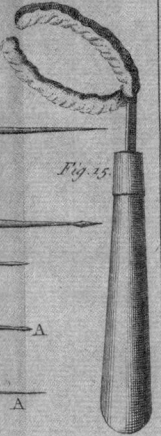

Fig.15.

understood, is among its greatest accomplishments. It was also a goal of 'quack' eyecare, as in 1701 a 'Dr Clark' offered coaching for cataracts 'after a new method, without pain, inflammation of the Eye, or confinement to the Bed, as is usual in the Operations by others'.[18] Pain was inherently associated with eye surgery, as it was not only a pain experienced through the body but literally seen in the process of surgery itself.

Eye surgery was the last resort. Wandering through the English countryside in 1882, the novelist Thomas Hardy met an old man in Lyme Regis who had undergone a cataract operation. He explained to the ever-curious Hardy, in search of anecdotes for his fiction:

> It was like a red-hot needle in yer eye whilst he was doing it. But he wasn't long about it. Oh no. If he haff been long I couldn't ha' beared it. He wasn't a minute more than three-quarters of an hour on the outside. When he had done one eye, 'a said 'Now my man, you must make shift with that one and be thankful you bain't left wi' narn.' So he didn't do the other. And I'm glad 'a didn't. I've saved half-crowns and half-crowns out of a number in only wanting one glass to my spectacles. T'other eye would never hae paid the expenses of keeping en going.[19]

Pain and cost: one function was to be ameliorated in the moment; the other remains a problem of the social inequalities of healthcare today, even it seems, in the British NHS. But, he implies, both are worth the price, to have vision restored. Hardy has notions of pain that 'are attributed to no malign agent, and that hold no hope of prevention or remediation'. They, and that is certainly true in the moment above, 'ask us to experience ourselves less as potentially responsible observers of pain than as fellow sufferers'.[20] No objectivity, only a pessimistic empathy, for that which cannot be changed or altered. For the moment . . .

A surgeon and his assistant holding down a patient while performing cataract surgery, with the surrounding instruments, from Robert James, *A Medicinal Dictionary, Including Physic, Surgery, Anatomy, Chymistry, and Botany, in All Their Branches Relative to Medicine*, vol. III (1745), the most extensive medical dictionary of the eighteenth century, with contributions by James's friend, Samuel Johnson. The surgical tools numbered 19–21 are taken from William Cheselden's *Anatomy of the Human Body* (1713).

The search for means to ameliorate pain *caused* by the physician had been an unattainable goal from the ancient Greeks onwards. By the beginning of the age of chemistry, bench science developed one of the first general anaesthetics.[21] The chemist Joseph Priestley, who first described oxygen and its functions, described nitrous oxide in 1772. And a very young Humphry Davy observed in 1795: 'as nitrous oxide in its extensive operation appears capable of destroying physical pain, it may probably be used with advantage during surgical operations in which no great effusion of blood takes place.'[22] Anaesthesia became slowly accepted and central to the practice of surgery after the demonstration of nitrous oxide as an anaesthetic by the dentist Horace Wells (apprenticed in Boston, MA, 1834–6) in 1844, and then of ether, by yet another dentist, William Thomas Green Morton (Baltimore College of Dental Surgery, 1842), in 1846.

Given the state of dentistry in the age of scientific medicine, 'in the first half of [the twentieth] century, nearly all dentists were regarded as quacks by the medical fraternity.' But it was claimed that 'they were empirics [physicians who rely on observation and experimentation], but not charlatans. There were quacks as there always are in any vocation. But, relatively, there was not nearly so much quackery as exists to-day' in 1900.[23] This is, of course, during a time that Henry James once called the 'undentisted ages'.[24] It is of little surprise that dentists were seen as 'philosophers of decay', 'who gaze into their patients' mouths as raptly as any soothsayer into a crystal ball.'[25] Magic everywhere, pace Max Weber. Indeed, dentistry, seen as quackery before the age of scientific medicine, perhaps because of its marginality, was able to innovate forms of pain mitigation. As late as 1914, Professor Guido Fischer (*Zahnarztliche Prüfung*, University of Berlin, 1900; Dr phil., University of Leipzig, 1904), director of the Royal Dental Institute in Marburg, observed that: 'A certain class of practitioners are in the habit of guaranteeing their patients absolute painlessness, and exploit this fraudulent promise in their advertisements; but such quackery cannot be condemned sharply enough as being unprofessional and unscientific.'[26] And that is dentistry already deep in the age of anaesthesia.

Yet it was the acceptance of such amelioration by the medical establishment that was necessary for anaesthesia to become an acceptable intervention.[27] Chloroform quickly followed when employed by the surgeon Sir James Young Simpson (MD, Royal College of Surgeons,

Edinburgh, 1832) in 1847, following its development by the medical student Robert Mortimer Glover (University of Edinburgh and studies in Geneva, licensed in 1837) in 1840. There was a lot of 'shouting in the marketplace' and thus Wells, Morton and Simpson were given the priority of discovery of anaesthesia even though all the substances employed were well known beforehand.[28] And many others also claimed their priority. But general anaesthesia was a form of death in life; what was also needed was a local anaesthesia that meant that the greater risk of dying under general anaesthesia could be avoided.

In 1884, two years after Hardy's conversation, a young neurologist decided, having been separated from his fiancée for a little bit more than a year, to make a quick trip to visit her, travelling from Vienna to Hamburg, 'hastily [winding] up my investigation of cocaine and . . . [contenting] myself in my book on the subject with prophesying that further uses for it would soon be found'.[29] In doing so he misses the chance to become the 'father' of local anaesthetic for eye surgery. He had staked his claim by authoring a series of well-published papers which he shared with a colleague, who then first used local anaesthetic for eye surgery while he was off on holiday. Or so at least the tale goes.

Had Hardy's informant only been in Vienna when the young Karl Koller (MD, University of Vienna, 1882), having undertaken a series of experiments with cocaine as a local anaesthetic, had a short account of his experiment presented by a colleague in a meeting of German ophthalmologists in Heidelberg, on 15 September 1884. Koller was the product of the scientifically reformed Viennese medical school and clinic; his vacationing friend and colleague was Sigmund Freud. Like Freud, Koller was Jewish and found his academic career so hampered by antisemitism that he soon thereafter, in 1888, emigrated to New York City. But in Vienna Koller was an assistant physician in the ophthalmological division of the university's hospital, which was chaired by the prominent ophthalmologist Carl Ferdinand Ritter von Arlt (MD, German University of Prague, 1839). Arlt bemoaned the absence of local anaesthesia every time he operated, as such surgery was difficult because of the involuntary reflex motions of the eye, which responded to the slightest stimuli. Ether as a general anaesthesia was available in 1846 and was adapted as a local anaesthetic by eye surgeons. And it was still being sprayed into the eyes of Arlt's patients in what was called 'Richardson's ether spray', with limited and very short-term effect. General anaesthesia (ether and then chloroform) was impractical for operations on the eye; Arlt remarked to Koller on the 'unsuitability of general narcotics, even the great danger of their application in eye operations'.[30] Patients died. The first surgeon to employ chloroform, James Young Simpson, having introduced it as an anaesthetic on 4 November 1847, learned quickly of its fatal potential. Two months after first using it, one of his patients, Hannah Greener, a fifteen-year-old, died suddenly under chloroform anaesthesia.[31] Local anaesthetic was much preferable given this risk. New interventions do have magic properties, especially when they arrive with the imprimatur of modern science.

Koller had already 'tried chloral, bromide and morphine and other substances, but without success and gave up these experiments for the time being'.[32] Freud had been exploring the neurological and anaesthetic function of a relatively new drug, cocaine, an alkaloid derivative, which had first been purified in 1855 from the coca leaf. In 1863 the Corsican chemist Angelo Mariani had infused coca leaves in wine, and 'Mariani elixirs' became a staple of the quack medicine market; indeed, coca became linked to healing, with 'Coca-Cola' joining the market in 1886, to treat, it was said, the morphine addiction of its creator, the Atlanta pharmacist John Stith Pemberton. That cocaine numbed was well known, its localized properties had been widely discussed from its purification, but 'up to now cocaine . . . [had] not found any medical use. But on account of its powerfully stimulating effects on the psyche, respiration and the heart and also on account of its anaesthetizing effect upon the mucous membrane, it might deserve experimental trials in quite a number of diseases', as a well-thumbed medical textbook in Koller's library stated.[33]

Koller relates the 'ah-ha' moment when 'another colleague of mine, Dr Engel, partook of some [cocaine] with me from the point of his pen-knife and remarked, "How that numbs the tongue." I said, "Yes, that has been noticed by everyone that has eaten it." And in the moment it flashed upon me that I was carrying in my pocket the local anesthetic for which I had searched some years earlier'.[34] He applied it to the eye of a guinea pig. One of his colleagues continued the tale:

> it was necessary to go one step further and to repeat the experiment upon a human being. We trickled the solution under the upraised lids of each other's eyes. Then we put a mirror before us, took a pin in hand, and tried to touch the cornea

with its head. Almost simultaneously we could joyously assure ourselves, 'I can't feel a thing.' We could make a dent in the cornea without the slightest awareness of the touch, let alone any unpleasant sensation or reaction. With that the discovery of local anesthesia was completed.[35]

Koller then had a colleague read a short paper on the effect of cocaine at the ophthalmological conference in Heidelberg, as he didn't have the money to travel there, and then with much more detail about the function of cocaine as an anaesthetic for eye surgery in a paper on 17 October 1884, at the meeting of the Royal Medical Association in Vienna, where he acknowledged Freud's work.

Word quickly spread across the globe and Koller's innovation was immediately incorporated into the best practices for ophthalmological surgery. The prominent Parisian medical journal *Le Progrès médical* on 29 November 1884 reported:

All medical journals resound at the moment with news of this triumph of healing. It is scarcely two months since Dr Koller of Vienna published for the first time the happy attribute [of cocaine] as a local anesthetic for the eye – and already publications on the subject are so numerous and the results so uniform that there exists a whole bibliography ... As always in such cases one has already taken as reality that which for so long had been only a hope, and one has the thought that cocaine is to be the means of banishing chloroform for operations on the eye.[36]

Local rather than general anaesthetic for surgery of the eyes is now much more possible and safer. It is no longer a choice between vision and agony. Pain had been vanquished and eye surgery no longer feared. And Koller became famous, precisely because new innovations in medicine were front-page news across the Global North. The news was 'shouted in the marketplace'. Others followed suit: novocaine, synthesized by Alfred Einhorn (Dr. phil., Chemistry, University of Tübingen, 1878), a professor of chemistry at the University in Munich, initially as a local dental anaesthetic, quickly sought to replace Koller's tincture of cocaine. While cocaine is rarely used today as an anaesthetic, both because of its addictive potential and because it degrades the cornea, it had a long and useful life; today lidocaine is the local anaesthetic of choice.

Koller was a celebrity. The notion that being a physician-scientist was also a means of social mobility had become engrained by the age of scientific medicine. The rise of science in the nineteenth century paralleled the rise of the educated bourgeoisie. And this was often translated, centrally in the German-speaking world, into the image of the nouveau riche, those who were now able to have the accoutrements of middle-class society but did not quite have the manners for it. The Jews of Vienna and Berlin became the exemplars of this striving for status and wealth, always undeserved and always suspiciously acquired.[37] In the Austrian Leopold von Sacher-Masoch's short story entitled 'Zwei Ärzte' (Two Physicians, 1892) the reader observes the confrontation between the 'scientifically trained' Jewish physician and his miracle-working 'shtetl' counterpart.[38] Only science can win, and magic must bow gracefully to its pre-eminence with all of the disenchantment that Max Weber predicted. Sacher-Masoch's tale of science and the Jews reflects the siren song of the Haskalah, the Jewish Enlightenment, which perhaps even more than the general Enlightenment saw science as the path of escape from the darkness of the ghetto into the bright light of modern culture. It was a modern culture defined very much by the Enlightenment mathematician and philosopher Jean de Rond D'Alembert's assessment of science and technology as the tools for the improvement of the common man. But science, especially applied science such as medicine, implied the ability to enter the mainstream of the so-called 'free' professions, such as medicine. It implied a type of social mobility increasingly available to Jewish men over the course of the nineteenth century. But even with this social mobility, Jewish doctors, even converts to various strands of Christianity, remained labelled as Jews because they came to be understood as part of the immutable or at least identifiable racial category of the Jews.

Koller's experience in antisemitic Vienna accounts for why he, at the height of his fame, moves to New York. In January 1885, Koller's colleague Fritz Zinner, a surgeon in Theodor Billroth's clinic, called him 'a Jewish swine' in public at the hospital where they both worked and Koller struck him across the face. Even though Jews were understood in Vienna at the time as not 'having honour' and could not therefore actually fight a duel, the two men fought with heavy sabres. Koller's opponent received two deep gashes. Having won what was de facto not only an illegal but from the standpoint of the antisemites a morally impudent duel, Koller was blackballed. Seeing no future studying in Vienna, he emigrated to the Netherlands following a meeting with the German American ophthalmologist Hermann Knapp (MD, University of Giessen, 1854) in Strasbourg, as Knapp recorded: 'I saw young Dr Koller, he intends to become an oculist, but is not yet educated in this specialty. He will probably go to [Hermann] Snellen in Utrecht, for being a Jew, as he told me, he had very little chance in Vienna . . . [I made a toast] on the rising generation of oculists, in particular Dr Koller who had made us the greatest gift we had received for many years.' Snellen (MD, University of Utrecht, 1858) had introduced the Snellen eye chart in 1862 (yes, that eye chart which we see every time our vision is tested) and was world-famous.[39] Koller was not the only one to meet with Knapp on his various journeys to Europe. In 1886, Sigmund Freud wrote to his fiancée Martha Bernays from Paris that he was approached by someone who

> said: 'I heard you speaking German. I'd like to introduce myself' . . . 'I am a German, but I emigrated to America long ago.' At last I gave him my card, but it happened to be one without an address. He glanced at it and said: 'Could you be Dr F. from Vienna? I've known your name for a long time, from your publications, especially the one on cocaine.' I was a little surprised and inquired after his name, which turned out to be [Hermann] Knapp. Now, Knapp is the foremost ophthalmologist in New York, who has also written a lot about cocaine and to whom I once wrote a letter in Koller's name.[40]

Indeed Freud returned to Vienna and created 'psychoanalysis' but Koller relocated from the Netherlands to New York after he received his training, and one assumes that Freud's letter to Knapp had to do with supporting his qualifications for a job in the New World. Eventually Koller became chief of the ophthalmology department at Mount Sinai Hospital, a Jewish hospital in New York City, not, we can note, at the College of Physicians and Surgeons at Columbia University where the non-Jewish Knapp had been professor of ophthalmology from 1888 until 1902.[41] And this in the age before Flexner, where European credentials truly mattered, (almost) trumping antisemitism. Who is here the quack; who is the doc?

Sigmund Freud married his fiancée Martha Bernays, became world-famous and remained, of course, in Vienna, until he was driven out by the Nazis after Austria was 'merged' into the Third Reich in 1938. His academic path was somewhat smoother than Koller's but still was impeded by his Jewish identity. He eventually was awarded the title of Associate Professor in 1902, unpaid but required to lecture annually, and the title of Full Professor in 1920, each time after long delays. Freud called himself a 'godless Jew' and spoke with his usual well-honed irony at times about 'our race'. And yet, despite his sharp critique of religion, he joined the Jewish men's club B'nai B'rith and wrote in his autobiography of 1925: 'My parents were Jews, and I have remained a Jew.'[42] But, following the success of Koller and cocaine, Freud shifted the focus from ameliorating surgical pain to the treatment of psychic pain. Both of these, as it turns out, are factors in modern medicine.

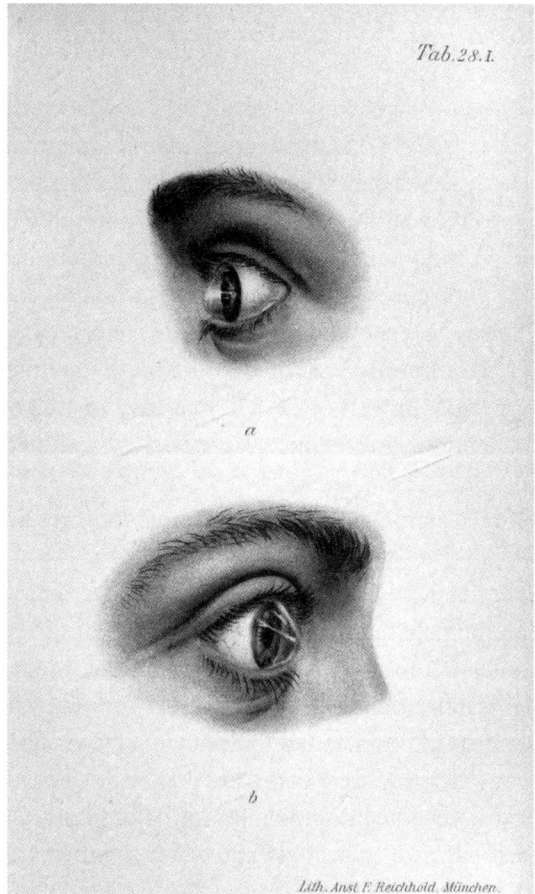

An illustration of keratoconus from Otto Haab, *Atlas of the External Diseases of the Eye*, 2nd edn (1903).

Corneas

Ophthalmology became a medical specialty by the early nineteenth century, centring on the somatic diseases of the eye, of vision, but in trying to limit itself in its therapeutic goals, it reflected the complexity of the worlds in which the newly minted ophthalmologists functioned. Our case study here is keratoconus, a disease once listed as a 'rare' or orphan disease, but today it impacts about 1.4 per cent of twenty-year-olds in the developed world and approximately 7 per cent in developing countries. It is understood as one of the major under-treated diseases of the eye.[43] It can, in its worst cases, eventually lead to blindness.

Keratoconus was and is characterized by progressive thinning and changes in the shape of the cornea, the thin, dome-shaped, clear outer layer of the eye. As the cornea thins a cone-shaped bulge can develop near or below the centre of the cornea. The result is distorted vision, sensitivity to light, and potentially increasing difficulties with seeing, even with glasses. Blurred vision, halos around light sources (as in cataracts), diminished visual acuity, difficulty in seeing things far away (short-sightedness/near-sightedness or myopia), multiple images and other forms of distortion all inhibit individuals from functioning in a world that demands more and more reliance on 'normal' eyesight. It seems, like the ubiquitous nineteenth-century diagnosis of 'dementia praecox', the madness of youth, which eventually evolves into our modern concept of schizophrenia, to be a disease that primarily manifests itself with teenagers and young adults but can appear at any stage of life, though generally, the older the onset, the less rapid the changes. What interests us here is how the disease is imagined and described, what its aetiologies are thought to be, and how treatment becomes a means of observing shifts in standards of care. And in the end, who decides in such cases on the boundary between good medicine and quackery?

Keratoconus was first described by our John Taylor, self-designated 'Chevalier' and doctor of ophthalmology *avant la lettre*. Yet the ophthalmologist George Coat (MB, University of Glasgow in 1897; MD, 1901) after whom Coat's Disease of the retina is named, still dismisses him to his scientific colleagues in 1915, as 'an unparalleled liar, preeminent among charlatans in the arts of advertisement; . . . In professional matters his knowledge was good; he was a shrewd observer and not without original ideas; but his actual practice was deeply tainted with the dishonest arts of the quack.'[44] Taylor described keratoconus in two works published in 1766; he called it 'ochlodes', Greek for turbulent or unruly. Taylor was very specific when he described his classifications of pathologies of the cornea:

> In the second class of diseases of the cornea, the first disease in this class is when all the cornea preserves its transparency and elevates itself in a form of a cone, the point of this is obtuse (blunted) and the base occupies the entire circumference of the cornea. There is another kind of disease, where the cornea is not only high, retaining its transparency, the same as in the previous one, and similarly of a conical shape, but the point is so acute and so heightened, that one at any time fears its breaking.[45]

In an earlier work, written in a crabbed mixture of academic Latin and oddly inflected German, he described 'ochlodes' as 'a change in the form of the cornea by which it takes the form of a cone, whose apex is blunt, but whose base is equal to the diameter of the cornea, which preserves transparency'.[46] Taylor's description simply notes that these are pathological changes in the cornea of interest to the physician, without positing any remedy or cause. He only distinguishes keratoconus from other pathologies of the cornea that impact vision.

While Taylor was the first to propose a clinical categorization of keratoconus, there was already a case description by the London oculist Benedict Duddell (who had had an apprenticeship some 19 kilometres [12 mi.] from Paris in 1718). Duddell found himself in 1736 in London's St Martins Lane, where 'by chance I met at the said Place, and was desired by his Master to inspect his Eyes, which I accordingly did. His patient was 'a Boy of 14 Years of Age . . . 'whose Cornea's is very prominent, like obtused cones, which were sufficiently conspicuous. The Globes were trembling or quivering, which is called Hippos, and the Ruby Pupils were the most Curious of any.' And then he quotes from a contemporary that 'a great many white Rabbitts have their Choroides almost of the same colour of other animals Retina; they cannot well suffer a great light. There is a whole People in [the fabled land of] Darien, who have their Eyes of the same Formation, having white Hair and Eye-lashes.' And he continues that 'this Lad's are also of the same

Colour.' The boy 'could see very well in the Day-time, especially to his Focus, which was about 5 inches to his right Eye: the Focus of his left Eye is something longer than that of the Right, and makes it necessary to hold objects more obliquely towards that Temple.... Certainly his sight is as good as that of many Myopes is in the Day.' Duddell's description seems to be keratoconus. The patient described seemed to have been an albino with nystagmus (random eye movement) and yet with relatively good vision.[47]

Unlike Taylor, Duddell *does* explain the aetiology of the boy's pathologies: 'the cause of this Boys Eyes being so, was that his Mother when with Child of him saw two Cats fighting. She was surprised to see a redness in their Eyes like Flames vibrating, occasion'd by the rarefaction of the Humours over-agitated; which made such a lively Impression upon the Infant, as to turn his Eyes red in her Womb; and perhaps rolling their Eyes in the Battel might cause the Hipposses.'[48] Now, we have been speaking, as my late friend Roy Porter notes, about the complexity of distinguishing between quackery and medical practice in the world of John Taylor.[49] What one can also add into this mix is that for Duddell the cause of the boy's pathology, as with other cases of visual pathologies or blindness, is the result of the mother's *seeing* the world in a frightening or dangerous manner while pregnant. That Duddell's young man is an albino places this discussion into another realm – that of the anxieties about difference and the demand for explanations, all of which also haunted William Cheselden's medical science.[50] Seeing as well as vision demanded the oculists' attention. Taylor's mock-Linnaean description of what comes to be called keratoconus is radical, as it reflected what was believed to be the model of objectivity developed by the taxonomist Carolus Linnaeus at the time. Linnaeus' model rested on the scientists' belief that they were able to sort all species and genera by their appearance, either on the surface, or based on their dissection. They held that what they were doing was 'true to nature', not understanding that their models created or at least shaped the nature they described.[51] Excluded then was how the patient imagined the world they saw and perhaps even its cause. Seeing was truly believing, for patient and for oculist, even though the latter struggled with the work of reducing the complexity of variability to the simplicity of rigid description.

These gaps come to be filled in the age of scientific medicine, for good or for ill. By 1828, the pathology had been named 'keratoconus'

– Greek *keras*, or horn, and *konos*, cone, for the conical-shaped cornea – by the ophthalmologist and surgeon Friedrich August von Ammon (MD, University of Göttingen, 1821) in a paper presenting a case of three sisters seemingly born with the disease. He begins, in good scientific terminological detail following Linnaeus, by listing the names for the 'conical expansion of the cornea': 'staphyloma pellucidum, Hyperceratosis, Ceratoconus, cornea conica'.[52] He too shrugs his shoulders when confronted with the aetiology of the pathology, observing that it 'would be possible to discover the true cause of this phenomenon only when a physician would have the luck to examine a Staphyloma pellucidum on a cadaver'.[53] The living patient narrating what she sees will not reveal the aetiology to the anatomist, whose scientific gaze is knowledgeable and thus objective. By 1828 von Ammon was the director of the Surgical-Medical Academy in Dresden and in 1830 founded the journal bearing the new scientific designation for his specialty, the *Zeitschrift für die Ophthalmologie*. So, the name of both the disease and the specialty were altered, an attempt to rescue both from the world of the quack, of the oculist, like John Taylor, and move them into the new world of scientific medicine in which he found himself a major player. He sealed this with the publication of one of the first systematic handbooks of ophthalmology in German, published between 1838 and 1847. Note that this is not 'merely' a clinical handbook of the illnesses and pathologies of the eyes; it is accompanied, as was the want in nineteenth-century medicine, by an 'atlas', a volume of plates reflecting the objective scientific reality as defined by the new specialist, to train other new specialists in this art of seeing the eye seeing.

As the oculists gave way to ophthalmologists during the opening decades of the nineteenth century more and more cases are entered into the literature, first under the name of 'staphyloma pellucidum conicum', and then as 'keratoconus'. Empirical experiments mapped the pathological cornea, as when the Scottish ophthalmologist James Wardrop (MD, St Andrews University, 1834, after training as a surgeon in Edinburgh in 1800 and studies in Vienna and Paris) asked his neighbour in Edinburgh Sir David Brewster (MA, Theology, University of Edinburgh, 1800; LLD [Doctor of Laws]), Marischal College, Aberdeen, 1807), the Scottish physicist, to examine one of his cases of keratoconus:

When you [Wardrop] first mentioned to me the case of Miss —, I was much surprised at the number of images which she observed round luminous objects. As this multiplication of images could arise only from some irregularity in the cornea, or crystalline lens, which gave their surface the form of a polyhedron, it was completely inexplicable from the shape of the cornea itself, which [has] a regular surface, resembling very much that of a hyperboloid . . . As the disease was evidently seated in the cornea, which projected to an unnatural distance, it did not seem probable that there was any defect in the structure of the crystalline lens. I was therefore led to believe, that the broken and indistinct images which appeared to encircle luminous objects, arose from some eminences in the cornea, which could not be detected by a lateral view of the eye, but which might be rendered visible by the changes which they induced upon the image of a luminous object that was made to traverse the surface of the cornea.

I therefore held a candle at the distance of fifteen inches from the cornea, and keeping my eye in the direction of the reflected rays, I observed the variations in the size and form of the image of the candle. The reflected image regularly decreased when it passed over the most convex parts of the cornea; but when it came to the part nearest the nose, it alternately expanded and contracted, and suffered such derangements, as to indicate the presence of a number of spherical eminences and depressions which sufficiently accounted for the broken and multiplied images of luminous objects.[54]

Brewster had earlier suggested such an experiment to distinguish whether the error of refraction lay in faults in the cornea or the crystalline lens: 'by examining the image of a taper reflected from the outer surface of the cornea, he [the observer] will readily discover whether its form is spherical or cylindrical. If it is spherical, there can be little doubt that the crystalline is in fault and it will remain to be determined whether the differences of refraction in different planes arise from the lens having one or both of its surfaces cylindrical, or what is more probable, from a want of symmetry in the variation of its density, – an effect which is very common at that period of life when the eye begins to feel the approach of age.'[55] After examining Wardrop's patient he becomes fascinated by this phenomenon and seeks out 'a great variety of cases of conical cornea'.[56] He was the first modern scientist to employ such a method in the clinical setting.

Yet the science is even older, as in 1619 the Jesuit astronomer Christoph Schiener, who had co-discovered sunspots, had already become obsessed by the mechanisms of seeing. Schiener then measured the radius of the cornea, comparing the reflections produced by different glass spheres of a known diameter with the reflections produced by the anterior surface of the cornea. With the subject seated opposite a window, the image of the crossbars could be observed in the cornea. Then different marbles could be held near the cornea, and a comparison made of the size of 'reflex', until the sizes of marble and cornea coincided. By a process of elimination, the radius of the cornea could be ascertained.[57] Yet his work had no impact on the 'oculists' of his day. Too much science; not enough medicine.

Brewster's insight is a brilliant example of the melding of bench science and scientific medicine in a world in which both are evolving. Yet each sees the case from their own scientific point of view, and as we shall see, physics tops medicine, as physics already had a claim of being the new science on the block. Brewster, an ordained Presbyterian minister, was one of the most celebrated physicists of his day. Beginning in 1799, as an independent researcher, he undertook a range of experimental work in physical optics, mostly concerned with the study of the polarization of light, resulting in the discovery of Brewster's angle, at which angle light is perfectly transmitted through a transparent, insulating surface, without reflection. When unpolarized light is transmitted at this angle, the light that is reflected from the surface is therefore perfectly polarized. He studied the double refraction of crystals under compression and discovered photoelasticity, thereby creating the field of optical mineralogy. He later became principal of the University of Edinburgh and one of the first serious, scientific opponents of Charles Darwin. Faith and science were seen as being in opposition by him, not because of Darwin's data, which he accepted, but because of Darwin's explanation for evolutionary change, functioning without a prime mover. That Brewster, a pillar of the 'auld Kirk', has no problem with the physics of biblical narrative conflicting with his own research illustrates more than anything how belief functions in disciplinary development in the age of science. That the physicians believe the physicists is a prime example of what Marjorie Garber labelled decades ago as 'discipline envy', thinking that a field perceived as far from one's own is better able to handle questions than the one in which you were trained. As she notes: 'the prestige and power of individual disciplines vary over time. New disciplines develop; others fade away. Envy, or desire, or emulation, the fantasy of becoming that more complete other thing, is what repeats.'[58] And that is what we see with these two disciplines, physics growing out of philosophy and scientific medicine distancing itself from the clinic.

Physics in the Clinic

The introduction of the science of the time in the development of ophthalmology is complicated and often hesitant. In his 1844 essay on keratoconus the Irish physician James Pickford (MD, Trinity College, Dublin, 1841) condemns experiments trying to replicate similar symptoms as those found during the chronic Indian famines in 'emaciated infants . . . with the cornea of both eyes . . . [becoming] thin and prominent', through experiments on dogs. He rejects these as 'revolting

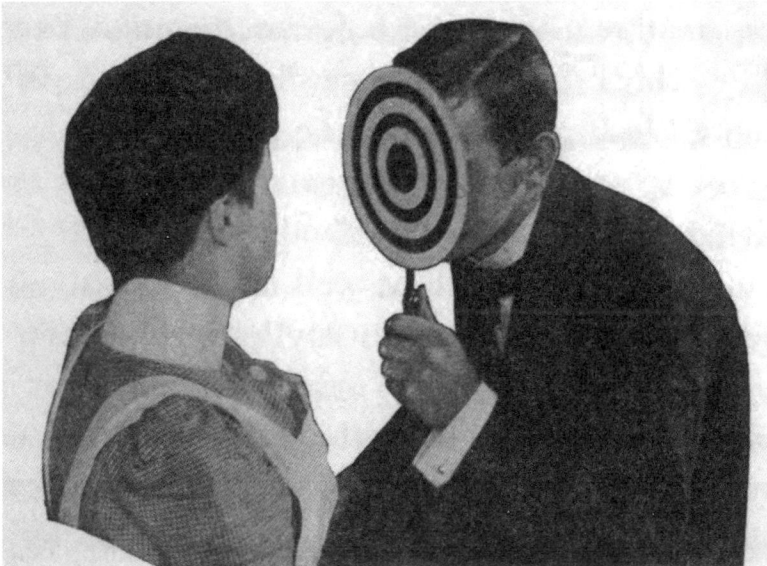

Plácido's disc, a device used to qualitatively examine corneal irregularities and astigmatism, illustration from Simon Snell, *A Practical Guide to the Examination of the Eye* (1898). There is a small convex lens on the back side to enable close examination without needing to accommodate the distortion of the concentric rings projected on to the cornea.

immolations of brute creation at the shrine of science and philosophy, as a disgrace to humanity and the nineteenth century.'[59] Such experiments with dogs to create lesions of the cornea may well be traced to 1712 with the work of the French oculist François Pourfour du Petit (MD, University of Montpellier, 1690), who cut the nerves to the eye in dogs and reduced the blood flow.[60] The Enlightenment fascination with replicating in laboratory animals symptoms found in humans both resulted from and enabled the charting of the sympathetic nervous system. It did little to promote the aetiology and therapy of corneal diseases, as dogs could not say what they saw.

However, Brewster's innovation quickly becomes a new technology, analogous to the stethoscope. Henry Goode (MB, Cambridge University, 1846), in 1847, described the first modern device which used the reflection of a square object from the cornea as seen from the side of the eye. 'In order to ascertain if it were possible to detect any error of curvature on the surface of the cornea, I observed the appearance of the reflection of a small luminous square held a few inches from the eye; but in the central part of this structure the reflected image was perfectly square, while the distortions produced at the circumference were equally produced in the sound eye; and there was no reason to conclude that the defect of vision arises from any defect in the cornea.'[61] In 1867 the ophthalmologist Antonio Plácido da Costa (MD, University of Porto [Portugal], 1879; Professor at School of Medicine and Surgery, Porto) turned what had been bench-science anatomy into a diagnostic device: his keratoscope, using a circular target of alternating concentric light and dark rings with a central aperture (called, needless to say, the Plácido disc).[62] This has stood the test of time and current topographers, mappers of the eye, more or less work on the same principle of assessing the reflection of a concentric set of black and white rings from the convex anterior surface of the cornea. In 1874 Ferdinand Cuignet (MD, University of Paris, 1851) coined the term 'keratoscopy' to describe this technique, which now is called 'retinoscopy'. With the introduction of photography this then took on a further technical shift. Allvar Gullstrand (MD, University of Stockholm, 1888; Nobel Prize, Physiology or Medicine, 1911, 'for his work on the dioptrics of the eye'), in 1896, was the first to analyse quantitatively what comes to be called 'photo-keratoscopic' images of the cornea. He was able to provide qualitative information of the anterior corneal surface as the reflected rings may appear non-circular in cases of high astigmatism or other corneal abnormalities such as keratoconus.[63] Physics vanishes into clinical practice.

What we can see in Brewster's examination of Wardrop's patient is the application of his work on experimental optics and refraction to a pathology of vision. He presents us with a hypothesis based on his assumptions of what is causing the imperfections of the patient's sight without questioning the accuracy of her account. He then, employing his knowledge of refraction founded on his work on crystals, creates an experiment, which provides an answer to Wardrop's question about the cause of the patient's dilemma. This in 1808, the age of amateur science becoming scientific disciplines. Wardrop, trained in London, Paris and Vienna as a surgeon and ophthalmologist and in 1808 elected a fellow of the Royal Society of Edinburgh, sees his claims as an answer to the quacks (perhaps such as John Taylor): 'for it is only in proposition as facts are accumulated, and the various morbid appearances investigated, that the phenomena of disease can be understood, the morbid actions explained, the science of medicine freed from erroneous theories and hypotheses, and its practice liberated from the rash and unskilful hand of empiricism.'[64] The new science is objective and can be replicated; it is not merely the accumulation of experience, experience filtered through non-scientific assumptions.

We noted immediately that Wardrop and Brewster limited their examination to the observation of the eye and not the aetiology or treatment of the disorder. This was not much different from the limitations that John Taylor placed on his description. Wardrop mentions various cases in which inflammations of the brain lead to weakness of the eyes and loss of sight and follows this account with an attempt to limit the population he was dealing with as 'he never found it in persons younger than fourteen or sixteen . . . It is a change . . . which sometimes takes place at the age of puberty.'[65]

It takes until about a decade later, in 1817, that there is an account of the therapy for keratoconus by Sir William Adams (qualified as a physician in 1805 at St Thomas's and Guy's hospitals; elected MRCS, 1807), who states that 'having been hitherto considered by authors as incurable', he had developed a procedure by which 'vision, it will be shown, may be restored nearly to perfection.'[66] This was important; as a physician his goal was to ameliorate disability, for 'vision is destroyed in relation to the useful purpose of life, and he [the patient] becomes nearly as dependent as if totally blind.'[67] As he claimed in the case of a clear lens extraction by 'needling operation' in a young woman 'who, during six years, found her sight gradually decreasing, and, at the expiration of that period, had become so blind, from this disease, as to be unable to continue her employment as a servant, and was in consequence obliged to apply for parochial maintenance.'[68] Surgery allows the individual to return to their function in society and relieves the state of their financial support. He concludes that

> in returning to the consideration of the case detailed of the young woman with the conical cornea, it may perhaps be supposed, that by admitting the susceptibility of the retina to have been increased by its being twelve months exercised after the operation, and the adjusting powers of the eye to have been acquired from the same cause, that I abandon my opinion of the morbid degree of separation of the light in its passage through the thickened cornea, together with the natural refraction produced by the crystalline lens being the cause of the confused and imperfect vision previously experienced by the patient; this however is not the case, as the fact of the girl being capable of seeing after the total removal of the lens, which was not in the slightest degree opaque, after having been blind previously, shows clearly that the refractive powers (the conical cornea and crystalline) were too powerful, and that the cure was effected by the removal of one of them.[69]

That the one eye seemed to function better than the other puzzled Adams, but he put it down in part to her naivety. He records that she commented that 'when she underwent the operation upon the second eye, "that her sight continued to get stronger" (an indefinite mode of expression made use of by poor people in their recovery from almost every species of diseased eye).'[70] That the first surgical intervention is a version of the standard treatments for cataracts and is based on the application of contemporary scientific claims about optics should be no surprise.[71] For they used *both* the new science and the classical technology that was at hand. That it also no longer relied on the account of the patient, dismissed as repeating meaningless platitudes, means that we have entered the age of scientific ophthalmology.

Let me stress that Adams's refusal to believe what the patient says comes to be a hallmark of scientific medicine. Medical science observes, whether it is vision or pain, and is therefore deemed neutral and therefore scientific. In this act the patient vanishes and is replaced by the disease. Listening was part of the oculist's art. In his *Briefe Treatises concerning the Preservation of Eie-Sight* (1586), Walter Bayley (MB, New College, Oxford University, 1559; Regius Professor of Medicine, Oxford) recounts a tale not dissimilar to that told by Hardy, except that as a physician he recounts listening:

> In truth, once I met an old man in Shropshire, called M. Hoorde, above the age of 84 yeares, who had at that time perfect sight, and did read small letters very well without spectacles: he told me, that about the age of fory [*sic*] yeare, finding his sight to decay, he did use [flowers of] Eyebright in ale for his drinke, and he did also eate the powder thereof in an egge three dayes in a weeke, being so taught by his father, who by the like order continued his sight in good integrity to a very long age: I have heard the same confirmed by many old men. Rowland Sherlooke an Irish man, Phisition to Queene Marie, did affirme for trueth, that a Bishop in Ireland perceiving his sight to wax dimme, about his age of fifty yeares, by the use of eiebright taken in powder in an egge, did live to the age of 80 yeares, with good integrity of sight.[72]

Listening to patients was equivalent to reading accounts by medical colleagues as oral transmission of knowledge counted as a primary source of clinical knowledge. These are central to Bayley's medicine, along with the classic medical authorities of the day such as Galen and Avicenna. This prophylaxis could 'do no harm', as Bayley saves any suggestions for treatments of pathologies 'to the professors thereof, by whose helpes they may receive remedy of all infirmities and affectes, which shall happen to the eies'. Listening to the patient has all but disappeared by Adams's medicine.

If you read all these early nineteenth-century accounts, with their description of the specific tools developed and the procedures undertaken, the patient, except as a placeholder for the disease, vanishes. Pain is never evoked, except when it does not occur. Von Ammon, after rupturing the membrane and removing, with some difficulty, the lens of one of his keratoconus patients with a 'cataract needle', treats the wounded eye with cold compresses and 'neither pain nor swelling nor redness appeared.'[73] This seems very much in line with the rhetoric of couching for cataracts, as when a British physician, recently returned from the Raj, describes specialty instruments that he brought home with him from India, where 'their operation is tedious, it requires a long time, but it seems not to give any material degree of pain or uneasiness.'[74] 'Pain', if mentioned in the multitudinous case studies of conical cornea, is attributed to the disease, never to the cure: 'he suffered from headache, dizziness, ocular and orbital pain.'[75] Hardy's old man still stands in the shadow of the doctor's unwillingness to acknowledge pain as a primary response to surgery.

Surgical therapy becomes a fallback for the ophthalmologist. Firstly, they prescribed, both Wardrop and Adams note this, spectacles of the type normally employed by individuals who had had cataract removal, but when the effectiveness waned over time surgery came to be employed more and more. Though their contemporaries are often sceptical of both the interventions and the theories behind them.[76] It is only in 1854 that a comprehensive monograph appears on keratoconus, the Liverpool ophthalmologist John Nottingham's *Practical Observations on Conical Cornea*. Here we are well into the age of science. Nottingham was particularly well trained, first at Guy's Hospital in London and then in Paris with the noted surgeon Guillaume Dupuytren, one of the first generation of teachers at the newly established École de médecine. Nottingham became an MRCS in 1832.

What is vital is that Nottingham's study appears when the members of the Royal Society of Physicians are debating the classifications of diseases, the boundaries between them, and as a result what is appropriate care in each category. And ophthalmology remained at the periphery of the scientific nomenclature of the day:

> A good classification ought to be inclusive – that is, it should include all forms of disease. The official classification by no means fulfils this condition. How poor, for example, is the nomenclature of diseases of special organs, as those of the eye . . . But nowhere the official classification does succeed in naming the known conditions of an organ or part, it is rather by the method of simple enumeration than by a rigid adherence to methodical arrangement.[77]

Nottingham's monograph attempted to undertake this and more.

One of the striking features of Nottingham's work is that he surveys the totality of the existing literature, indeed from the eighteenth century through to the medical science of his day and across most of the medical cultures in Europe and North America. His claim is that retrospective analysis is necessary because

> the causes, nature, and treatment of conical cornea have not yet been illustrated by observations sufficiently numerous and varied to enable us to consider that this ocular malady is as well understood as are many other complaints that attack the organ of vision, hence it is obvious, that additions to our store of materials for the study of this affection seem to be more in request than are attempts at anything like systematic treatises on the subject: the morbid anatomy of the disease is the department in which accurate information is most scanty; having, in itself, no tendency to destroy, or to shorten life, opportunities for observing its vestiges, post mortem, have hitherto been exceedingly rare.[78]

But he does contribute one such post-mortem, undertaken by Richard Middlemore (apprenticed, 1820; St Bartholomew's Hospital, 1823; MRCS, 1827), whose unillustrated 1,600-page study on the diseases of the eye was the expansion of his 1831 Jacksonian prize awarded after 1800 by the Royal Society of Surgeons for the best essay on a surgical topic. This remained in print in various improved editions until 1935:

> I have had one opportunity of examining, after death, the state of the cornea, in a person who was affected with Conical Cornea in an extreme degree; and in that instance, its laminæ were less moveable upon each other, its circumference was of a natural and ordinary degree of thickness, but its apex was much thinner than usual, and rendered opaque on its exterior only, for its neural surface, even at the apex, was perfectly transparent; in other respects it did not appear to have undergone any change, unless I mention that alteration in the evenness and equality of its surface discovered by Dr Brewster, but which was not visible to the naked eye.[79]

Here again the invisible science made clear what the visible autopsy could not. Brewster's work is joined now with that of the anatomist, autopsying the dead, as both are necessary for even a basic description of the disease. The problem of linking the science of physics to the science of anatomy was that over time the ophthalmologists trusted the narratives of their patients less and less. Cadavers absolutely cannot tell you what they are seeing, which seems should be the first priority of ophthalmology.

As for therapy, Nottingham is agnostic about virtually all surgical and pharmaceutical interventions available to him. In the decades before his book, they included leeches applied to the lower lid or temple, systemic calomel for fluid absorption, emetics, purgatives or silver or iodine or zinc sulphate ointments. Surgical procedures concentrated on corneal flattening, resection of the cone and optical bypass, through piercing the cornea.[80] Nottingham describes a wide range of these, but he is not convinced:

> medicine, surgery, optics, and mechanics have been taxed for the production of therapeutic agents, capable of lessening or removing the serious defects of vision which this formidable disease of the eye, even in its earlier stages, or minor forms, is capable of producing; in the application of these, success has been various, and disappointment by no means rare; with one practitioner, general treatment has been fortunate; with another, local applications; a third has been gratified by the favourable results of a surgical operation; a fourth, with the improvement of vision effected by some optical or mechanical contrivance; in the hands of some, various combinations of these means have been wisely and usefully adapted, in accordance with the special conditions or particular forms of the malady; while others, having met with cases of unfavourable character, have tried, without any satisfactory results . . .[81]

We stand, he implies, on a bare shore, where all quackery has led to little progress and real science has yet to accomplish much.

Here we need to provide an alternative voice, the voice of the surgeon. Nottingham's contemporary, Sir William Bowman (apprenticed at the Birmingham General Hospital, 1832, to the surgeon Joseph Hodgson, who had founded the first eye clinic there in 1824; MRCS,

1839), also saw himself as one of the first of the scientific explorers of ophthalmological surgery dealing with keratoconus. One of the leading histologists of his age, he also pioneered the use of the microscope in the realm of anatomical research, identifying, at the age of 25, 'Bowman's Capsule' in the nephron in the kidney. His primary training was as a surgeon, but as his biographers noted: 'When patients presented themselves at King's College Hospital, and asked for the "oculist", he declined the appellation, saying he was a surgeon; but, partly owing to his success in the treatment of the affections of the eye, and partly owing to the [staffing] circumstance . . . the tide of ophthalmic practice became too strong to be resisted, and he gave himself up to it.'[82] Not as an oculist, but as an ophthalmologist. And in 1844 he became part of the staff of the Royal Ophthalmic Hospital, London, where he introduced the ophthalmoscope developed in 1851 by the world-renowned physicist, Hermann von Helmholtz (a student of Johannes Müller; see also Chapter One). This innovative technology enabled the new world of ophthalmology to view the fundus, the back of the eye, much like our first sight of the back of the moon, an extraordinary feat. Three years later, in 1854, Helmholtz developed keratometry to measure the corneal radius of curvature based on the light reflected off the surface of the cornea. This led to an avalanche of technical innovation to photograph and measure corneal reflections and then the corneal curvature over the next decades.

Brewster's surgical procedures for keratoconus concentrated on corneal flattening, resection of the cone and optical bypass. In 1859, regarding surgery on the eye for keratoconus, he described his procedure:

> I cannot say that this expectation has been borne out in any marked degree, but nevertheless the vertical slit is much more slightly than the horizontal, and certainly equally good for vision, so that at present I prefer it. The improvement of vision from a first iriddesis downwards has been in almost every case decided, the patients being delighted with the result. In some the second iriddesis upwards has not seemed further to increase the precision of view, in others it has certainly done so, and in the present state of the inquiry I am disposed to continue to practise it in cases of considerable conicity.[83]

As Sir William Adams noted, every patient seems happy with every procedure no matter its rate of success and Bowman reported a complication rate of some 20 per cent. Any discussion of pain, in terms of the actual surgery, is missing from Adams's early papers; indeed, pain existed only to be ameliorated by the surgeon, successful or not. Indeed, Adams's conclusion is that 'no reliable testimony exists as to the success of any measures hitherto adopted for the restoration of the cornea to its natural curvature; though possibly, it would be wrong to say that it is not an object to be aimed at in slight and early stages.'[84] Here we have a good reason for Nottingham's careful evaluation of surgical interventions. The Swiss ophthalmologist Johann Horner (MD, University of Zurich, 1854; studied in Vienna and Berlin), who wrote his dissertation on keratoconus in 1869, advocated chemical cauterization of the cornea to alter its shape, following the German ophthalmologist Albrecht von Graefe (MD, University of Berlin, 1847), who in 1866 proposed radically cauterizing the cone with silver nitrate to produce a flattened scar.[85] In 1872 a Dr Bader described an innovative technique that involved excising an elliptical piece of full-thickness corneal tissue at the apex of the cone.[86] All were reported as 'successful', as with Bowman's cases, but with ever smaller numbers of long-term reduction of symptoms because of infection and inflammation and, without stating it, the painful experience of the procedures. Pain never figures in their accounts of their procedures.

Nottingham is equally sceptical of pharmaceutical interventions, either in the form of poultices on the eye or those taken internally as well as the latest fad of electrotherapy, of which the young Sigmund Freud too quickly becomes disabused.[87] As Nottingham observes: 'Imponderable agents have been tried, especially electro-magnetism. In. collyria [eyewash], acetate and sulphate of zinc, as well as preparations of lead. Infusion of tobacco dropped upon the eye, has been recommended. In unguents, the nitric-oxide of mercury has had a place. In cases where the apex of the cone had become opaque, the employment of the vapour of prussic acid has been followed by the diminution of the opacity.'[88] Such radical and painful interventions are dismissed as often more harmful than not.

What Nottingham advocates are the least intrusive (and painful) treatments, various forms of spectacles, variants on those already employed for post-operative treatment of cataract surgery. Such eyeglasses should alter the conditions under which vision might be exercised, by allowing the light to fall only upon a part of the cornea. To attain this end, a piece of black wood, in form more or less like the one-half of a walnut shell, was taken and perforated, so as leave a circular opening, beyond and around which a small nipple projected on the exterior, thus converting this hole into a very short tube, standing on the outer surface of the shell of wood, the aperture being, not in the centre, but a little to the inner side of this point; these black goggles being held before the eyes, the axes of their tubular apertures were convergent, more or less, as the axes of the eyes are when near objects are contemplated.[89]

If this description of the 'pinhole' effect shouts out that it was also analogous to the construction of telescopes of the day, we should not be surprised. Science, from optics to lens-making to physics, is linked here by the ophthalmologist as scientist, as William Bowman's own work with microscopy illustrated well. And Nottingham notes that less is more: 'It is obvious that, before proceeding to surgical operation, the different forms of optical contrivance should be resorted to, and their various combinations carefully tried when the simpler ones fail to assist vision.'[90] If not 'do no harm', at least 'cause no pain'.

Nottingham is most suspicious, though, of technical innovations in such therapies that are harmless in and of themselves. He decries the work done by his German colleague Moritz Nussbaum (MD, University of Bonn, 1874; Professor of Ophthalmology in Bonn), which Nottingham dismissively labels 'glazing the cornea'. Nussbaum, experimenting on rabbits, had implanted

a sort of glass button . . . with two little off-sets, or folds, to enable it to hold on, and be steady in the cornea; a short transverse incision is made in the cornea, and the glass piece, as it were, buttoned in and that this can be done without any after and long-continued irritation of the eye, the bit of glass remaining fixed and steady, is proved, as Nussbaum says, by his living rabbits but we feel satisfied that, in the human subject, the glazing of the cornea would not be tolerated; so that it need not here be proposed as a remedial agent in cases of conical, or conical and opaque cornea.[91]

Indeed, he mocks Nussbaum's claim that 'Das Ansehen eines also bewaffneten Auges ist kein besonderes hässliches.'[92] An eye so armoured is not ugly. We, of course, see here the precursor, crude and still surgical, of what comes to be a standard treatment for keratoconus in the twentieth century, the contact lens, which becomes practical only with the work of the Swiss physician Adolf Fick (MD, University of Berlin, 1851) and Eugène Kalt, a Paris optician, in 1888. They had developed a blown glass shell over the entire visible eye to reshape the cornea but soon abandoned them because the patient could not tolerate them for long periods of time and each lens had to be hand-crafted at great cost and with great difficulty.

As for the aetiology of keratoconus, Nottingham works through all the suggestions, from prenatal impact to infection to its appearance because of other malformations, such as a 'conical skull'. He is suspicious of all, providing counter examples for the negative of each case. But one aetiology stands out, hysteria. 'Amongst the various constitutional, general, or nervous affections, that have been observed in connection with conical cornea, hysteria is perhaps worthy of more attention than it has hitherto received; increased accumulation of the aqueous humour, or hydrops oculi, with alteration in the form of the cornea, has been observed along with severe cases of hysteria.'[93] Some of the treatments, such as purges, seemed to work on at least a 'patient of twenty-one [who] had suffered from hysteria; the conical cornea affected the left eye only, and was perfectly cured after twelve months' treatment; but after the lapse of thirteen months more, the malady again returned, and the treatment was repeated with equal success.'[94] Here hysteria is seen as a 'nervous disease' of women, but Nottingham sees the interventions employed as somatic treatments. The creation of specific classes of patients, with specific aetiologies, that define the class itself was commonplace. When Sigmund Freud returned from Paris to Vienna in 1886 and lectured on male hysteria, that category was seen as incomprehensible, as hysteria defined the feminine and the feminine was defined by hysteria.

One pitfall of classification that Nottingham self-consciously avoids is that linked to the close relationship in the nineteenth century between the new scientific medicine, colonialism and race. Nottingham's was the world in which all the human sciences from medicine to anthropology to education (indeed, every arena of scientific thought that classified human beings) were informed by racial science.[95] He reports in his introduction that: 'It [keratoconus] has been observed and treated of as occurring in the Mongolian and Caucasian branches of the human race, and in greater proportion in the former, as observations made in China tend to show; in the other varieties of mankind it has yet to be studied; it has been said not to occur in savages, but whether or not it affects them may very well be left for another generation to decide.'[96] But when he turns to the data, he begins by dismissing this as a reflex of race. 'Conical cornea, as occurring in China, has been alluded to as possibly connected with the "pyramidal" or "conical" head of the Chinese people; in connection with which the question might well be asked, – Have the Chinese generally, a conical or pyramidal head, in those parts of the empire where conical cornea has been observed?'[97] His answer is a resounding no. What is the cause of the heightened rate in China? Quacks, of course, as he ascribes keratoconus

> to the injurious effects of an every-day practice of the Chinese barbers, who cleanse or 'wash' the eyes of the people with an ivory or bamboo instrument, shaped like a small scoop, which they pass under the lids and deeply into the canthi; this 'operation' leaves the eye red and irritated, and as if to make the worst of it, the irritation of the eye is but too often attributed to an inadequate cleansing, whence the repetition of the barbarous process, and the additional mischief which follows it.[98]

Indeed, while he never actually employs the word 'quack' in his monograph, the practice of the Chinese eye 'doctors' and their 'operations' are only the extreme end of those medical colleagues of his whose treatments are haphazard and whose science is retrograde. In reporting on all the theories and all the interventions proposed by his medical contemporaries for keratoconus, he is careful to comment on them as within the scope of practice of ophthalmology in his day, but he is also very careful to distinguish between what he understands as adequate scientific argument and what he sees as limited, situational cases.

With Nottingham, keratoconus enters the world of scientific medicine. It is still a world of medicine at risk of doing harm when surgery is performed, a sub-theme of his book. His is a world without anaesthesia that would make those interventions he dismisses as dangerous possible. His is a world in which even the best surgeons are remarkably resistant to the innovations of Lord Lister and antisepsis, even waiting for a patient to become 'purblind' before proceeding with surgery from fear of infection.[99] It is only as the century ends that surgery comes into its own. And it is accompanied by even more complex questions of the aetiology of keratoconus and its therapy.

Down's Corneas

When William Cheselden undertakes in the 1720s his experiment to answer his query of what a previously blind person understands about the colour black when, with his sight restored, he is first able to see a Black person, he concludes that his terror was a physiological response to a fear of darkness made manifest. In the shift from the oculist's examining how we imagine the world when we see it to the ophthalmologists' limiting themselves to the physics of optics, other sciences of the time appear asking whether human difference is also not manifested in the very physiology, and therefore the optics, of the eye. Race science and eventually eugenics come to play a role in the history of keratoconus.

In the *London Hospital Reports* of 1866 John Langdon Down (MRCS and LSA, London Hospital, 1856; MB [London], 1858) published his 'Observations on an Ethnic Classification of Idiots'. It is this essay which makes Down's name part of twentieth-century medical vocabulary, the eponymous 'Down's syndrome'. Down uses 'Mongolism' and 'idiocy' to describe this form of development; in 1965, wishing to distance post-Second World War medical science from a racial label, the World Health Organization adopted the name Down or Down's syndrome. After the genetics of the disorder seemed to have been discovered shortly thereafter, it also came to be known as 'trisomy 21', as it seems to result from an extra copy of chromosome 21. We shall use Down's own classification here and then shift to other terms for cognitive difference as we move into modernity.[100]

Down's argument engages one of the central themes of race science, whether all human beings belong to the same genus or whether they constitute different species, to be ranked on a hierarchy of development. Race was defined almost universally in terms of the visible difference among groups. Beginning with the monogenist Johannes

Blumenbach in the eighteenth century, whose category of 'Mongol' Down adapted, the advocates of the view that all human beings, no matter the skull shape, skin colour, height or posture, belonged to *Homo sapiens sapiens*, stressing similarities rather than differences. What defined the Mongol more than any other visible sign was the epicanthal (monolid) fold of the eyelid and the shape of the Mongol skull, which Nottingham had rejected as a cause of keratoconus based on his own collection of data from informants in Asia.

Down, as a physician, postulated that one could describe pathologies of cognitive development by using racial stereotypes. He writes of Malay, Caucasian, American and Ethiopian 'idiots', but it is Blumenbach's category of the 'Mongolian variety' that became paramount in medical and popular thought. Central to this is skull and eye shape as well as skin colour, forming one of the two poles of race with the 'Caucasian'. The key to Down's views is that he believed that if pathologies could reveal visible racial difference, then such difference was merely a sign of the variability of the species rather than a sign of radical, inherent difference. The Mongolian 'family has numerous representatives, and it is to this division, I wish, in this paper, to call special attention. A very large number of congenital idiots are typical Mongols. So marked is this, that when placed side by side, it is difficult to believe that the specimens compared are not children of the same parents.'[101] In one case: 'the boy's aspect is such that it is difficult to realize that he is the child of Europeans, but so frequently are these characters presented, that there can be no doubt that these ethnic features are the result of degeneration. The Mongolian type of idiocy occurs in more than 10 per cent of the cases which are presented to me. They are always congenital idiots, and never result from accidents after uterine life.'[102] They constitute thus a disease entity that can be seen as such:

> they present such a close resemblance to one another in mental power, that I shall describe an idiot member of this racial division, selected from the large number that have fallen under my observation. The hair is not black, as in the real Mongol, but of a brownish colour, straight and scanty. The face is flat and broad, and destitute of prominence. The checks are roundish, and extended laterally. The eyes are obliquely placed, and the internal canthi more than normally distant from one another.

The palpebral fissure is very narrow. The forehead is wrinkled transversely from the constant assistance which the levatores palpebrarum derive from the occipitofrontalis muscle in the opening of the eyes.[103]

Race is defined by appearance, and appearance determines not only the way the 'race' is *seen* but how the 'race' *sees* the world.

Later, Down provides a differential diagnosis of Mongolism with the other public scourge of the time, congenital syphilis, as 'very few have had syphilitic teeth; but where I did discover them, I always had confirmatory evidence of the syphilitic history of the case, and the condition of the teeth was always associated with the chronic inflammation of the cornea to which Mr Hutchinson has called attention. I have therefore been led to the conclusion that syphilis is not by any means an important factor in the production of congenital mental disease.'[104] The question of the vision of the Mongoloid idiot becomes a point of differentiation between congenital syphilis, with its heavily moral tone of disapprobation, one of the fascinations of the medical and popular world of the nineteenth century, and the idiot. But that does not mean that Down does not stress the symptoms of impaired sight as a means of defining the idiot: 'Lesions of sight are very frequent. Congenital cataract is very commonly associated with congenital feeble-mindedness. Several cases have also come under my notice of blindness as the result of arrested development of the globe. Strabismus is very common, and nystagmus, though less common, is not infrequent. Myopia, but especially hypermetropia, is a frequent accompaniment of congenital mental lesions. Colour-blindness is occasionally met with, but it is difficult to say in how many cases it is from a want of mental power.'[105] That Down ascribed to the eyes a particular importance brings us back to Nottingham's discussion of the putative conical skull and keratoconic eyes of the Chinese.

Down's use of race theory stressed both the universality of the pathology across collectives but also highlighted the role that diseases of sight, indeed non-infectious malformations of the cornea, play in his categorization. But being able to see the patient's physiognomy of disease is a strong argument even into the twentieth century, when the famed Swiss ophthalmologist August Siegrist (MD, University of Bern, 1892), who had early used contact lens for the treatment of keratoconus, in 1912 describes the typical patient with keratoconus as 'nervous, with a feminine build, often pale. With many you find extreme dry skin, little disposition to sweating, and weakness of memory and loss of hair.'[106] He attributes this physiognomy of keratoconus to a thyroid insufficiency, but four years later returns to his own argument to dismiss it as having little diagnostic power, as it is clear that such a profile shifts over time.[107] Seeing difference may not have the power to define difference in such cases.

Aetiology or Therapy?

Today it is claimed that the incidence of keratoconus in patients with Down's syndrome, now labelled 'trisomy 21', ranges from 0.5 per cent to 15 per cent to as high as 71 per cent, yet there are studies that even deny such a linkage.[108] Some of this is certainly due to better screening options and improved technology; some of it certainly to the population examined. The earliest discussion of the linkage comes at the beginning of the twentieth century and asks whether this specific, defined population is unique in its predisposition for keratoconus or whether it presents with the anomalies at simply a greater rate than the general population. In other words, is the higher rate a by-product of the genetic difference of people with Down's syndrome or is it because of the actions of the individuals in the group, activities that could also have some genetic component? Thus, its aetiology could be behavioural, as 'eye-rubbing has been thought to play a role in developing keratoconus, which patients with Down syndrome may be more prone to due to the higher rate of chronic blepharitis.'[109] But is this because 'chronic blepharitis' could also have a genetic cause? How does one isolate a population that may or may not have higher rates? As has been claimed: 'In the vast majority of cases of conical cornea the lesion occurs in apparently healthy persons; disregarding the cases associated with mongolism and vernal conjunctivitis, one may consider the etiologic theories as of two types: The first type endeavored to explain conical cornea as a partial symptom of disturbance of the glands of internal secretion; the second looked to inheritance to furnish the unknown cause of the development.'[110] You make them into a subclass that is different in essence from all others, but then you need to propose an aetiology that seems to work for all: here they are hypothyroidism and/or genetics? Are these associations chromosomal translocation so that the disorder aligns with keratoconus revealing some type of genetic substrata, at least in those cases where some type of familial pattern is discernible?

In the late nineteenth and early twentieth centuries the search for an aetiology of keratoconus, including among those with 'trisomy 21', is as wide-ranging as the evolving, cutting-edge science of the time. In the age of race science, it was not only the question of whether one or the other of Blumenbach's races had a higher incidence of keratoconus but, closely linked, whether the incidents of both 'trisomy 21' and keratoconus were to be found in families. Indeed, as with virtually every pathology at the time (and since), twin studies were undertaken as the ultimate scientific proof of such claims.[111] (By the way, they are not – as our ability to isolate environmental from genetic aetiologies is still quite limited, except in those cases where the patterns are consistent and overt, as with Huntington's disease.) Even the question of race reappears, as there are several recent studies that returned to the debate that Nottingham and then Down triggered about racial difference (now read as genetic cohorts or haplotypes). Does racial predisposition exacerbate or heighten the prospect for keratoconus?

Today, with the return of 'race' under the guise of an oddly ahistorical genetics, we now have studies reported that record a significantly higher incidence and prevalence in Asians compared with whites, suggesting the influence of 'ethnicity' (a poor substitute for 'race') on keratoconus. Whether this is genetic or behavioural or a mix (remember Nottingham) seems to elude the researchers, depending on their model of the 'Asian' and the medical culture in which this term is employed. For 'Asian', as we note, means something very different in British medical culture from what it does in the United States.[112] The new race science, as I have argued for decades, seems still encumbered by the problems of classification, now masked with arguments about genetic differentiation or the employment of terms from the social sciences (such as 'ethnicity' or 'identity'), which are then treated as biological realities. The supposed predisposition to keratoconus, it was proposed, was the result of higher rates of thyroid insufficiency in those with 'trisomy 21'. This assumed that the higher rate of both keratoconus and hypothyroidism was inherent in this population.

'Mongolism' is often, in this age of scientific medicine, discussed with reference to disturbances of the thyroid and the pituitary gland, as it is the age when the implications of thyroid disease are first made evident. By the 1880s the work of Felix Semon (MD, University of Berlin,

1873) and Victor Horelsey (MD, University College London, 1881) and, in the 1920s, the work of David Marine (MD, Johns Hopkins School of Medicine, 1905) had documented the relationship between thyroid deficiency and specific pathologies, such as Grave's disease, defined by the physical appearance of the patient's eyes.[113] Researchers extrapolated this also in the case of 'mongolism', and thus the heightened rate of keratoconus. Indeed, one proved the other. Ferdinand Siegert (MD, University of Strasburg, 1889), professor of paediatrics in Cologne, made an intensive study of the literature of 'mongolism' and keratoconus in 1910 and reported that usually normal findings were found on both macroscopical and microscopical examination. He personally felt that in most cases of 'mongolian idiocy' there is 'at certain times a disturbance of function of the thyroid gland independent of the presence of demonstrable manifestations of hypothyroidism . . . .' Yet 'in the majority of cases in the older literature pathologic changes in the glands were absent; nevertheless, Gordon expressed the belief that at times a functional disturbance of the thyroid is present in mongolism, independent of the presence of demonstrable manifestations of hypothyroidism.'[114] No proof; good enough.

This desire to see aetiology and diagnosis as linked in defining keratoconus both in the general and the limited populations can be seen after Casimir Funk (PhD, Organic Chemistry, University of Bern, 1904) 'discovered' the 'vitamine hypothesis' in 1912. It hit scientific medicine like a bomb, explaining virtually 'everything'. In 1928 the Nobel Prize for Chemistry was awarded to Adolf Windaus 'for his studies on the constitution of the sterols and their connection with vitamins' and the next year the Nobel Prize in Physiology or Medicine for 1929 was awarded to Christiaan Eijkman and Frederick Gowland Hopkins for their contributions to the discovery of vitamins. Everything, in this age of discovery between 1913 and 1945, became the result of a vitamin deficiency; some claims accurate, many more far off the mark.

When vitamin B is shown to be the cure of beri-beri, a vitamin B deficiency, quacks soon invent vitamin 'P' as an aphrodisiac.[115] But this was true of actual vitamins, as they were uncovered as being at the cause of a wide range of pathologies. The word itself 'evoked glamorous reverberations of buoyant health'.[116] This led to major public health interventions in the United States, such as the mandating of the inclusion of folic acid and B_{12} in commercial bread to reduce neural tube defects (such as spina bifida) in infants. And that worked. But ophthalmologists sought the origin or the therapy for keratoconus, too. From vitamin A in 1939 to the employment of oral vitamin B (riboflavin) as a dietary supplement, there was the assumption that vitamin deficiencies were and are closely linked, correctly or incorrectly, to therapies for keratoconus.[117] This is very different from the use of vitamin B (riboflavin) as an energy transfer material (and not a dietary supplement) in contemporary surgical procedures, as we shall discuss at the close of this case study. Likewise, the question of the role that vitamins played in the development and lives of people with Down's syndrome looked at vitamin A absorption levels in the 1950s (and well before) as a symptom of the disorder to ask whether such children have a higher risk of autoimmunity because of lower vitamin D levels.[118] Individuals with Down's syndrome seem to frequently exhibit impaired olfactory function, which may be an early clinical symptom of Alzheimer's disease. Would vitamin D_3 have a prophylactic function in this population?[119] Whether these are chromosomal variations, strongly suggested in the twenty-first century, is still not clear. Or perhaps there is not an anatomical or genetic cause at all. One size fitting all is one of the problems of applying bench science innovations to therapeutic and diagnostic categories.

Keratoconus and Scientific Medicine

Indeed, what is striking in the debates about the aetiology of keratoconus is the number, even in 2022, of unknowns: 'The cause of keratoconus is unknown; however, it is usually linked to genetics, environmental variables such as eye rubbing, atopy, ultraviolet exposure, hormones, the inflammatory response and pregnancy. Aside from these often-reported connections, there is a substantial volume of literature on keratoconus comorbidities such as Ehlers–Danlos disease, Marfan syndrome, mitral valve prolapse, floppy collagen syndrome and Down syndrome.'[120] To this we can add: the use of hard contact lenses, Leber's congenital amaurosis and osteogenesis imperfecta, like Ehlers–Danlos disease, a non-inflammatory connective tissue disorder, vernal keratoconjunctivitis and a slew more.[121] We are tempted here to simply quote the American Secretary of Defense in the 1970s (and later) Donald Rumsfeld that 'reports that say that something hasn't happened are always interesting to me, because as we know, there are known knowns; there are things we know we know. We also know there are known unknowns; that is to say we know there are some things we do not know. But there are also unknown unknowns – the ones we don't know we don't know.'[122] In other words, if we cannot find a cause for keratoconus so that we can intervene in advance and prevent the occurrence, perhaps our focus should be on therapy, and that therapy would not target any specific group defined as different, such as those with 'trisomy 21'. How we link these categories is vital, as many more people in our age of air pollution and poor air quality chronically rub their eyes than just those with Down's syndrome.

So, the shift comes slowly to begin to abandon the search for the aetiology of keratoconus and to focus on symptom interventions to slow or reduce its pathological impact. By the close of the nineteenth century these included prolonged pressure patching with drugs that constrict the pupil as well as glass contact shells to arrest, retard or cure the changes by pressure. Optical treatments included spherocylindrical spectacles, stenopaic slits, blocking lenses, multiple pinholes, hyperbolic lenses and for a brief period the use of the 'hydrodiascope'. This was introduced in 1896 by Theodor Lohnstein (PhD, Physics, University of Berlin, 1891; MD, University of Berlin 1895), a physician in Berlin who suffered from bilateral keratoconus, as a potentially superior alternative to contact lenses available at the time as an effective means of optical correction. His surgery had failed; he had had galvanocautery (electrical excision) on his keratoconic left eye in November 1895 and other instruments seemed ineffectual.[123] So, he developed a new form of spectacles. His 'hydrodiascope' resembles a swimming goggle for a single eye. It was filled with liquid and fitted with a plano-convex lens with its plane surface nearer the eye.[124] It worked, even if you looked weird wearing it, even in the age of the monocle, but was out of fashion as soon as contact lenses became easily available and relatively inexpensive in the early twentieth century. An earlier version had been suggested by the prominent laryngologist Johann Nepomuk Czermak (MD, University of Würzburg, 1850), who had developed a water-filled goggle strapped to the front of the eye to correct keratoconus, a device that he called the orthoscope, but which had never been used in therapy. Spectacles at least do no harm.

The shift from a specific for keratoconus to a general acceptance of contact lenses by the public was shouted in the marketplace by physicians as a non-invasive, new technology. In 1915 the optical company Zeiss produced the first trial set of contact lenses especially for keratoconus. By 1920 they had begun to produce a four-lens pre-formed fitting set primarily for keratoconus. It was introduced and developed by Wolfgang Stock (MD, University of Tübingen, 1899; Professor of Ophthalmology, University of Jena), who was a sufferer of the condition. Two years later Zeiss were granted a U.S. and German patent for plastic (Cellon or celluloid) contact lenses.[125] But as late as 1930 a letter to the editor in a California newspaper queried 'whether there is an eye glass which is worn in direct contact with the eyeball?' The editor answers that 'there is such a lens, but it is worn only to relieve a condition known as keratoconus, as conical deformity of the cornea. It is worn with extreme difficulty and is not practical for correction of ordinary errors of refraction.'[126] Technology in the service of the twentieth-century ophthalmologist but creating 'discomfort' and tolerated only because of its therapeutic effect in very limited cases. By 1939 a physician can counter that 'invisible spectacles are practical and efficient and recommended by competent oculists . . . They were introduced for a condition known as keratoconus, a thinning of the membrane of the eyeball which causes the cornea to protrude at the center . . . But about three years ago Carl Zeiss, the great optical instrument maker in Jena, was able to grind these lenses so that they can be accurately and properly fitted to any ocular defect.'[127] No longer painful, they were able to be worn after a period of acclimation, without discomfort. And no longer to be used specifically for the treatment of keratoconus. Today, specialized (gas-permeable) contact lens, for one or both eyes, is the therapy of first choice. They are effective with early onset keratoconus. Yet we slowly see the paradigm shifting (and so it should be, for changing technology expedites this by changing risk/benefit and the outdated 'let's watch the patient get worse before we actually treat them') and move toward surgical procedures, which we shall discuss below, before they can no longer wear their contact lenses. As they seem ever less effective as the disease progresses, for with younger patients they may well also exacerbate the progress of the illness, leading to the need for surgical intervention.[128]

Lohnstein's role as a patient persuaded him that surgical intervention in the age before local anaesthetic was less than ideal. But electrotherapy, now using electricity to cauterize the eye, rather than as a form of direct treatment, became a surrogate. At the time there were three commonly used procedures: thermal cauterization with perforation of the cornea, without perforation and a non-contact application of heat to the eye. All modified corneal shape, using electrotherapy since it was the most modern form of surgical intervention. Each had immense drawbacks, leading 'to devastating complications (for example, a case reported by Mr Killick, whose patient developed phtisis bulbi [end-stage eye disease leading to blindness] after a total of six procedures).' A 23-year-old medical student from Moscow requested a surgical intervention from his mentor, Sergei Semjonovic Golovine (MD, University of Moscow, 1895), chair of the Department of Ophthalmology at the New Russian University of Odessa, because of rapidly progressing bilateral keratoconus. Golovine performed cauterization of the corneal apex three times. 'Stubborn complications have existed,' he reported.[129] Scarring the cornea following surgery to flatten the apex of the cone without entering the anterior chamber could also be accomplished with silver nitrate applied to the cut surface to promote the flattening of the corneal cone by the contraction of the resulting scar. But the randomness of the resulting scar meant that the surgeon could not deliver reasonable visual results. We need to imagine both the surgery and the application of the acid as from the standpoint of a patient. And these, of course, are the published accounts of the relatively successful interventions! All are abandoned because of 'poor predictability'.[130] (Though they get revived again with better technology and pain management in the 1970s, without better outcomes.)

Alternative therapies and such invasive attempts to restructure the cornea more and more give way to surgery after Carl Koller and the introduction of local anaesthetics. Prior to 1904, operative treatment for keratoconus principally comprised cauterization by electricity or heat to flatten the corneal apex, as in the case of Dr Lohnstein, both painful and often ineffectual. Keratotomy, a surgical intervention cutting into the cornea to alter its shape, in this case for correcting astigmatism, was made by the Norwegian Hjalmar Schiotz (MD, University of Kristiania, 1877) in 1885 and other surgical innovations for keratoconus followed, yet all had meagre outcomes because of infection and inflammation.[131] It became rare enough that the provincial American press could announce such procedures in 1902 as: 'Mrs Edmund Tardy . . . was operated upon by Dr Pond Thursday morning for keratoconus. The operation was very successful and Mrs Tardy is doing well. Keratoconus is a very common trouble but seldom recognized, usually being taken for near-sight.'[132]

But shortly after Koller's intervention, surgery of all types became more and more plausible. Penetrating keratoplasty, full-thickness corneal transplant, is one of the first of the post-Koller procedures, developed by Eduard Zirm (MD, University of Vienna, 1891) in his landmark 1905 surgery.[133] Zirm's patient suffered catastrophic burns to both eyes through the lime used to clean chicken coops. The procedure was in the end effective only in one eye due to the problems with antisepsis and inflammation – a problem that continues today even with routine modern sterile technique and eye banking, for rejection down the road leads to a poor prognosis of microsurgical transplants. Zirm's model had been, of course, the first successful modern transplant, a thyroid allograft performed by Theodore Kocher (MD, University of Bern, 1865) in Switzerland in 1883. By 1936 Ramón Castroviejo (MD, University of Madrid, 1927) successfully corrected keratoconus in a very advanced patient with a corneal transplant.[134] Given the dangers associated with the procedure, he saw this as a last resort. Castroviejo presented his results at a major scientific meeting and was greeted with scepticism by his peers. The next year he presented the same thing but with a twist. At his own expense, he rented slit lamps, hired a bus and transported his patients to the meeting room. Seeing was believing. In the following decade he repeated the procedure with over two hundred patients and claimed a success rate of 80 per cent. But such procedures remained dangerous and costly.

Transplantation ruled but the older methods only slowly passed out of use. Thus in 1914 there was a meeting of the ophthalmology section of the Royal Society of Medicine. The presenter was Charles Wray (studied at London Hospital, MRCS, 1881), who as of 1887 oversaw the newly opened Ophthalmological Department at Croydon General Hospital and became the same year a fellow of the Royal College of Surgeons. He documents a number of cases of superficial cauterization early in the earliest stages of keratoconus, for to 'wait until thinning is as dangerous as the initial softening is unsound practice and needs justification in view of the efficiency and safety of operative treatment by means of the cautery in the early stages.' Wray was to change the refractive focusing properties of the peripheral cornea with cautery. What he undertakes is 'a rather deliberate burn 2½ mm. long ... made at right angles to the correcting cylinder so as to involve about 1½ mm. of the cone.'[135] Directing 'heat' using electro-cauterization at specific locations of the cornea led to contraction of the tough sheets of collagen in the cornea, producing a change of its shape. This treatment was used to treat keratoconus; while some improvement was achieved, low predictability and significant regression after that initial improvement was also the case. The case material that Wray presented documented few positive changes, but, as he is convinced of the relation between keratoconus and hypothyroidism, which is associated in two of his five cases, admonishes his listener thus: 'special vigilance is called for in young subjects when the eye affection is associated with hypothyroidism.'[136] This is an unexceptional paper in its time, defending older interventions for the reshaping of the cornea in an age where more and more radical surgical interventions, post-Zirm, are being introduced.

What is of interest is the discussion that followed Charles Wray's presentation of his cases at the Royal Society of Medicine. In the chair at the meeting is Sir George Anderson Critchett (MD, Middlesex Hospital, 1872; Ophthalmologist Royal to both Edward VII and George V). In 1912, when a new section for ophthalmology was started in the Royal Society of Medicine, he was its first president. He had qualified in 1872, quickly becoming one of the leaders of this evolving field. In 1881 he was selected ophthalmic surgeon to St Mary's Hospital, and it was his work there that finally established his reputation and incidentally built up one of the most extensive eye clinics at any of the general hospitals in London. But his world is quickly fading. He opens the discussion about Wray's presentation with the following observation:

> the subject of this communication [Wray's paper] was always an interesting one to him [Anderson Critchett] personally, but he could not avoid taking a prejudiced view, because a parent always liked his own child best. He invited views on the operation (kindred to his own) which had been brought forward to-night, or on his own. Though it was now twenty years since he introduced his operation, he still continued to practise it at intervals when these rare cases came into his care, and, what was even more gratifying, he was frequently receiving letters from confreres, foreign as well as those practising in the United Kingdom, saying they continued to do the target operation with considerable success and with great confidence.[137]

And yet the question remained, how could such minor interventions provide long-term relief? How could such insignificant cautery strengthen the cornea? One explanation is not only of the time, but very much in line with the anxiety about harmful interventions that could (and did) over the long-term damage vision:

> his experience was that if a very superficial scar were produced, so that little more than the corneal epithelium were burned, it practically vanished. Members must have seen instances of these burns when it was the fashion for ladies to wear fringes. He had had five or six in which ladies had been curling their fringes, and there remained one hair, and, in turning the handle of the cautery to break off that single hair, the cautery accidentally touched the cornea. In one case to which he was called there was a dense white streak, and he gave a cautious prognosis, but in forty-eight hours it had cleared up. He had not seen any such burns which led to any serious consequences.[138]

We can think of Nottingham's assumptions about hysteria and keratoconus, but even more the notion that such interventions 'do no harm'. His analogy is striking because it speaks of how minimal interventions were being defended in the new age of ocular surgery. As early as 1844, well before Thomas Inman, who was said to have coined the phrase, evoked the spectre of 'doing no harm', the Parisian oculist Charles Deval (MD, University of Paris, 1834), trained in Vienna in the newest surgical techniques, warned that 'we must above all conform to the adage "*primum non nocere*" [do no harm], which, as Boyer says, is the first precept of our art, [as] we would never advise the operation to a person with a unilateral cataract.'[139] *Don't risk surgery if the patient has one good eye!* Deval's admonition echoed that of Alexis Boyer (trained in Paris as a surgeon with Antoine Louis and P. J. Desault), Napoleon's household surgeon, in his two-volume *Traité des maladies chirurgicales et des opérations qui leur conviennent* (1814–26), where he urged patience in couching for cataracts at too early a date: 'By operating [at this stage] one would act against the first precept of the art: *primum non nocere*.'[140] In the debate about the risk of harm to the patient's sight eventually Wray responded that 'His cases spoke for themselves.'[141] But of course what they undertook as treatment was of a world prior to Koller, indeed, prior to Zirm's innovations, a decade after they had been widely accepted.

Yet from 1906 on to the end of the twentieth century, lamellar keratoplasty, where diseased corneal tissue is removed and replaced by a layer of corneal tissue from a donor, and for a brief period epi-keratoplasty, where a lens made of human corneal tissue is sutured onto the anterior surface of the cornea to change its anterior curvature and refractive properties, were employed, but penetrating (perforating) keratoplasty, itself a variant of transplants, dominated the field. At the beginning of the twenty-first century there was a resurgence of more and more extensive forms of transplants, the emergence of intracorneal rings, small plastic rings that are inserted into the cornea to flatten the conical shape of the cornea caused by keratoconus, and, of course, the application of lasers (specifically, holmium and other heat-inducing lasers), no longer electro-cauterization, to treat kerato-plasty.[142] Technology changes; procedures adapt; more and more focus is on therapy, less and less on questions of aetiology and/or classifications. Here John Langdon Down's general objective seems to have been accomplished: treat all people who have keratoconus for their difficulties with their vision; stop classifying them as inherently different, and thus as a special class predisposed to this problem.

The Twenty-First Century

At the very beginning of the twenty-first century, we find ourselves at the ophthalmological clinic at the Carl Gustav Carus Technical University in Dresden, whose new chair was Annelies Frühauf (MD, University of Leipzig, 1960). She had assumed the leadership of the clinic when her predecessor, Theo Seiler, had taken the chair in ophthalmology at the University of Zurich. She found several major research projects under way at what was one of the oldest (and yet also most recent) academic programmes in ophthalmology. Having its roots in late medieval practice, it was reconstituted at the beginning of the age of scientific medicine. The Dresden programme had a long and rather distinguished path, or at least was the home of some of the best-known 'oculists' at one of the richest courts in Europe, that of the electors and kings of Saxony. The court in Dresden funded individuals such as the sixteenth-century Georg Bartisch (apprenticed at the age of thirteen to a barber-surgeon), who became the royal oculist and the author of the first German-language handbook of ophthalmology, the *Ophthalmodouleia, der Augendienst* (1583). This was also the first Renaissance account of the state of eye surgery. By the nineteenth century the city hospital's eye clinic under the leadership of Friedrich August von Ammon, who has already appeared in our tale, saw Dresden as one of the centres of treatment and research in the field. In 1828 the Technical University was founded in Dresden and von Ammon came to direct the Surgical-Medical Academy in 1828. By 1837 he was the royal physician to Friedrich August II.

This pre-eminence in the field continued through imperial Germany into the Weimar period. With the establishment of the German Democratic Republic, the models for medicine, research and treatment shifted more and more to those practised in the Soviet Union. The clinic expanded, took in ever more patients, but faded from the attention of those engaged in the most important innovations in the field – a fact in general reflecting medicine in the GDR, except for the great public hospital and research centre of the Charité in (East) Berlin. After 1990 and German (re-)unification, depending on your politics on the day, the universities in what was the GDR were suddenly stripped of their leadership: they were too politically compromised, they were political hacks, their science and their methodologies were corrupted by the ideological compromises of Soviet science and, pragmatically, a lot of marginally employed West German (BRD) academics needed jobs as there had been a massive overproduction of physicians with their habilitation compared to the number of jobs available.

By 1993 Theo Seiler, who had held the position of *Oberarzt* (senior physician) at the ophthalmological clinic (Charlottenburg) at the Free University of Berlin, in what had been West Berlin, was appointed to the chair at Dresden. Theo Seiler had rather unusual credentials as he had received his MD (in Ophthalmology) as well as his PhD (in Physics). Beginning as a physicist, with a dissertation on 'Modulated Dynamic Nuclear Polarization of the Nuclei of Smaller Gyromagnetic Ratios' in 1975, he then commenced his medical studies, which he concluded in 1981. He completed his habilitation in 1984 with a dissertation on 'Linearity of Tonometry', the study of how intraocular pressure was measured, a field in flux because of new and rapid changes in the available technologies. He quickly moved up the ranks in West Berlin until, in 1993, he moved to Dresden, replacing the East German-trained Ernst Marré. What Seiler brought with him was an interest in the intersection between technology, bench science and clinical practice, a sort of combination of Nottingham and Brewster.

This, in the jargon of contemporary medicine, is now labelled 'translational medicine', from the bench to the clinic. But here it is not *the* science shaping clinical practice: rather specific clinical problems were referred, not to bench researchers working on basic scientific problems, but to other clinicians, whose interest was focused on resolving specific clinical difficulties in the laboratory. Not basic science but applied clinical practice. Seiler modernized the surgical reach of the clinic, introducing refractive laser surgery (LASIK, PRK) among other innovations. (Ironically, at the same time, iatrogenic cases of keratoconus were reported in patients precisely having these interventions.) His research palette reached from biomechanics to one of the most important innovations in the treatment of keratoconus since Zirm and corneal transplants a century prior, the use of riboflavin (B_2) together with ultraviolet light exposure to stop the development of the symptoms.

Now the science here was new and the technological innovations important, but they brought together knowledge that was already available. Johann Ritter (studied medicine at the University of Jena, 1796) had identified ultraviolet light in 1801, following William Herschel's discovery of infrared the year before. Suddenly there was the possibility of emanations beyond visible light. By the twentieth century UV light had been explored as a potential antisepsis, when its anti-bacterial quality was discovered. When 'seasonal affective disorders' were first described UV light seemed a mild antidepressant. UV (in all three spectra: A, B and C) began to take a more important role in potentiating other biochemical interventions. As we discussed, the twentieth century was already the age of vitamins. One of the earliest discovered was B_2 (riboflavin), discovered in 1922 by Richard Kuhn (PhD, Chemistry, University of Munich, 1922; Nobel Prize in Chemistry, 1938, for 'his work on carotenoids and vitamins') in Germany and Theodor Wagner-Jauregg (PhD, Chemistry, University of Munich, 1926), the son of the Nobelist Julius Wagner-Jauregg, in Austria. Although, in 1879, an English chemist, Alexander Wynter Blyth, had already isolated a water-soluble material with yellow-green fluorescence from cow-milk whey, the vitamin present in it was isolated in 1933 by Kuhn and Paul György (MD, University of Budapest, 1915) in Germany. Though not linked to any of the more evident vitamin deficiency diseases, it was soon discovered that it plays a central role in the metabolism of other vitamins, such as niacin and B_6.

Linking the two was one of the undertakings by Theo Seiler in Dresden (and a team from 'Vide Infra', created by the ophthalmological entrepreneur, Michael Mrochen (PhD, Dr rer. medic. [Doctor of Medical Science, a research degree], University of Dresden, 1999). Beginning with animal experimentation in 1995, Seiler's laboratory realized that there was a significant increase in corneal biomechanical stiffness found after collagen cross-linking by combined riboflavin and ultraviolet-A treatment. One did not need to use extra-ocular devices, such as a contact lens, or indeed surgical scarring of various forms, to increase the rigidity of the bands of collagen in the cornea. The procedure seemed to increase corneal tensile strength and resistance to collagen corneal fibres for enzymatic degradation over time. Now, this was the application of a discovery in polymer chemistry using 'photopolymerization' that showed increased inflexibility. This was first applied to the treatment of the eye in creating injectable lens replacements.[143] What Seiler's laboratory, spurred on by Mrochen, realized was that this could be applied directly to the collagen in the cornea itself. When riboflavin is administered together with ultraviolet-A, it serves as a photosensitizer. The ultraviolet-A-excited molecules of riboflavin produced by this interaction convert oxygen to reactive oxygen species as well as resulting in a cross-linking effect causing mechanical stiffening of the cornea. Most of this 'cross-linking' occurred within the collagen molecules themselves and the corneal matrix.

The Dresden group then undertook a study on human subjects with keratoconus. The procedure was quickly labelled CXL (Corneal Collagen Cross-Linking). By 2003, treating 23 eyes with advanced to severe damage, the progression of the disease was uniformly halted in all patients.[144] A subsequent study from Dresden in 2008 increased the number of eyes to well over two hundred, and it was found that not only was the progression of the disease halted but there was some measurable improvement in visual acuity. The progress of the disease was halted, vision improved somewhat, and the potential risk of major surgery, such as transplants, seemed to have been reduced. Suddenly larger and larger studies were undertaken across the globe, all with the same results.[145] This was even true of patients with Down's syndrome, where if keratoconus was detected early and CXL treatment performed it appeared that the progress could be halted. When such patients reached advanced stages of the disease in the past they needed corneal transplantation, as did others with the same impairment. For complex reasons, some social, some medical, the long postoperative follow-up was particularly complicated in Down's syndrome patients.[146]

Sounds perfect but, and there is always a 'but', since there was never any consistent definition of what 'progress' of the disease meant over time in keratoconus, the fact that CXL slowed the progress of the disease seemed a claim too far. Also, it seemed that the earlier the disease was identified the more successful the procedure became. The technical equipment to identify the disease (autorefractometry, auto-keratometry, as well as corneal topography and tomography) was new and expensive and not generally available, even though it was a major improvement to earlier forms of corneal imaging (think MRI rather than X-ray). And (and there is always an 'and') there seemed to be serious side-effects of the process, such as stromal haze (increased opacity), higher complication rates in older patients and our old bugbear, infection.

Why infection? Because CXL, approved in its roughly twenty-year-old original form by the FDA in 2016 as a treatment for progressive keratoconus, remained a surgical procedure. It was deemed necessary surgically to remove the corneal epithelium that covers the front of the cornea as it acts as a barrier to protect the cornea, resisting the free flow of fluids from tears, and prevents bacteria from entering the epithelium and corneal stroma. If it would not permit bacteria from entering, it was reasoned, it might inhibit the entry of riboflavin. The researchers tried it and tried it without removing the epithelium, but they could not get adequate riboflavin into the corneal stroma where it was needed. It turned out that three reagents – riboflavin, O_2 and ultraviolet-A – must be in the right place at the right time in the right concentrations for penetration. And anyway the epithelium regenerates quickly, usually within seven to ten days post-surgery. The longer it takes, the greater risk for negative outcome ensues. The procedure, reminiscent of the older scarring techniques, often used a motorized scrub brush. Always with the appropriate local or topical anaesthetic, of course. The protocol followed the traditional one for cataract surgery: one eye, complete rehabilitation, and then, after documenting the healing in the first eye, usually about three months later, the second eye. This quickly becomes the treatment of choice, even though, and here we listen to the echoes throughout our case, of the risk of post-operative pain and infection, with some risk of damage to the cornea.[147] Again, the trade-off seems clear: short-term pain and risk of infection against the progression of a debilitating illness. And in 2011 a study showed that this procedure seemed to be less effective when the protective epithelium was left intact in a control group.[148] 'Epi-off' becomes the standard of care.

This is a breakthrough in the treatment of keratoconus. The century-long debate about reshaping the cornea by surgical or various non-surgical means, from scarring to wearing specialized contact lenses to function; the eventual need to undertake transplantation when the disease progressed to a point where the patient was unable to function – all are replaced by a relatively simple procedure whose bio-molecular explanation was relatively clear. All was good. But ophthalmologists were concerned about the simple inherent risks and challenges of 'epi-off' while acknowledging its basic success. It was also relatively expensive, because of the pricing of riboflavin and the UV device necessary (from Avedro, the privately held pharmaceutical and medical device company), and it was an office-based procedure, which limited its availability outside of tertiary care or specialty clinics' facilities. And, at least in the United States, the moment you recognize 'risk', even as we discussed in our opening chapter, you are setting yourself up, if not for potential litigation, then for a heightened expense in malpractice insurance. All were deemed appropriate, if this procedure could not be improved, as this was now the 'standard of care'.[149]

Roy Rubinfeld was the first ophthalmologic surgeon to perform the 'epi-off' CXL procedure in the Washington, DC, area in 2009 under IRB ethics board approvals. He, like his colleagues globally, had to deal with the pain and challenges of the treatment (including the need for opioids, which would quickly become a social problem nationally) while recognizing the real benefits to his patients. Rubinfeld had first been a scientist trained in microbiology and immunology on an NIH (National Institute of Health) fellowship before his medical training at SUNY Downstate Medical Center in 1982. He then trained in ophthalmology at Georgetown University Hospital (Washington, DC), where he eventually served as chief resident, then came a fellowship subspecialty in cornea at the Wills Eye Hospital in Philadelphia. In private practice he formed a keratoconus research study group, initially with a range of both researchers in private practice, as well as at academic institutions from Miami to Chicago and Cambridge, Massachusetts. This research group was designated as CXLUSA, eventually growing to include 36 research investigators. By 2012, he and his team had developed an effective, non-invasive CXL ('epi-on') without corneal scraping, for those with early-onset keratoconus. What made this possible was an improvement to the combination of drugs applied to the eye. They increased the riboflavin concentration, adjusted the tonicity and pH and added sodium iodide 0.015 per cent to the riboflavin 0.5 per cent.[150] This, combined with novel disposable sponge delivery devices, further potentiated the vitamin, allowing it to better penetrate the intact epithelium. He also headed the design of novel UV delivery devices that used less UV light but achieved better results, as they could treat both eyes at the same time.

His group began to publish their findings, and Rubinfeld went on the hustings advocating for this variation of the 'standard of care'.[151] This was registered at the United States patent office in 2013, followed up by an expanded version the following year. He stressed that, while the original epi-off 'Dresden Protocol' was a huge leap forward, the existing protocol had real-world medical and social consequences simply because of its surgical component. Certainly, the risk of infection remained a central problem but the possibility of 'haze' was a factor in all corneal surgery. Equally important was that there was also a social dimension because of the multi-week period necessary to undertake surgery in both eyes, as we noted: one eye and then, weeks later, the second eye. This meant, and here the American context is vital, a loss of income, and, he noted, many patients, quite happy with the procedure, felt that they could not invest both the time and the cost for the second eye. Shades of Thomas Hardy's friend! But also 'epi-on' meant that this procedure could be undertaken conveniently worldwide.

We used to speak of 'Third World' medicine in the 1980s, assuming that we, in the Global North, were the definition of 'First World' medicine. The truth was and is that there are areas of the United States and the United Kingdom with much less access even to basic care than in developing nations. That the maternity morbidity and mortality rate in some of the American states is higher than in areas of sub-Saharan Africa may be an index of this. Rubinfeld's innovation treated both eyes simultaneously and there was only a one-to-two-day rehabilitation period. And, yes, the pain (usually designated as 'discomfort') following the epi-off was present in the healing process for epi-on but was minimal and brief. Think opioids for a week versus one dose of Tylenol. The results seemed to be equivalent.[152] Yet the secondary impact on the patient seemed not to be included in the calculus of success or equivalence.[153] Pain, as we have noted repeatedly, should always be a factor and while it is clear that local anaesthesia ameliorates pain during the procedure, the removal of the epithelium causes protracted pain. And protracted pain means a longer period of recuperation, during which only very limited activity is possible. Here speaking with the patients would play a major role in the comparative evaluation of the procedures.

If epi-off is the standard of care, it is even FDA-approved, and it is 'real' medicine based on 'real' science, why change it? More than that, the research took place in a real laboratory in a real university by celebrated, widely honoured researchers with a worldwide reputation. In 2018 Seiler finally responded to one of the papers documenting the effectiveness of epi-on. Rubinfeld's team had published their first detailed account of a two-year clinical trial conducted in Atlanta, Georgia, of this unique version of epi-on, on 308 patients (512 eyes) with keratoconus (and others with similar pathologies of the cornea following LASIK surgery). The patients were followed up regularly until two years post-surgery. They also tracked paediatric patients, whose disease traditionally has been shown to progress more readily, and found that even in these patients the progress of the disease ceased and vision actually improved. They concluded that 'Epithelium-on CXL using this new protocol halted the progression of keratoconus and ectasia after LASIK. It was safer and provided more rapid visual recovery than CXL with epithelial removal, allowing routine bilateral, simultaneous treatment.' And that 'the increased safety, enhanced patient convenience, rapid return of visual acuity, lack of complications, and possibility of retreatment, if necessary, make this technique preferable to epi-off CXL for the treatment of ectatic [diffuse] corneal disease.'[154] Here the research group placed their work as being a substantial improvement, but not a rejection of, the Dresden findings. They were 'standing on the shoulders of giants'. This is the historical cliché so elegantly documented in 1963 by the medical sociologist Robert K. Merton as reaching back into the shades of written records.[155] But Merton cleverly subtitled his very funny book 'A Shandean Postscript', and in an odd way that is what occurred now.

Theo Seiler, by 2018 the recipient of dozens of major awards from ophthalmological and scientific societies across the world, sitting at one of the premier universities by everyone's rankings, responded to

Rubinfeld's paper (as I shall refer to it here) in a letter to the editor. He began with the rather startling claim that, unlike the group's earlier studies, with this one, 'despite clear editorial guidance from this journal and international standards bodies, the trial was never registered with a clinical trials database.'[156] And it did not have 'an epi-off control arm', as other epi-on studies did. This is bad medical science because it is 'bad' science.

The trajectory of medical research over the past decades (and the introduction of massive, public databases of research-in-progress) meant that public knowledge of experiments in human medicine has radically shifted. Until the late twentieth century, the way you found out whether an experiment was even undertaken (unless you were on the Institutional Review Board, mandated by the FDA, that approved using human subjects at your university or clinic) was to read the results of the (always successful) experiment years later in your disciplinary journals. There was no central listing of what experiments at any given time were being undertaken, so failed experiments were rarely (and that is kind) reported. The situation was little different elsewhere in the Global North.

What the researchers relied on was on the one hand 'control groups', which often in medicine meant approximating but never duplicating *all* the genetic and experiential variabilities of subjects in any given study, and on the other 'replicability': other researchers basically redoing the experiment and seeing whether the findings would come out the same. That always sounded like 'science', but unlike physics or chemistry, when you are dealing with human subjects you can never know every single difference between each subject. So, one tack has been to suggest (and in some cases to mandate) making the basic data of the experiment available to other researchers, so that one did not need to run the entire experiment again but simply see if the same conclusions would be found. If not, one always had the ability to simply run the entire experiment again. Seiler concludes his letter as follows: 'Per the basic tenets of the scientific method, if others were allowed to replicate their work (perhaps under a nondisclosure agreement to protect commercial sensitivities) to validate their claims, this would help alleviate many of our concerns. Unfortunately, every request to date (by us and others) has been refused. Ultimately, we believe that the claims made by Stulting et al. cannot be substantiated by this study because of serious flaws in the methodology.'[157] We do not want to duplicate your experiment in our labs, but we want to have access to your data to rerun it, the riboflavin, the delivery sponges as well as the patented uv devices to see whether we get the same outcomes.

Having access to raw data too has been a new claim of evidence-based medicine since it is substantially easier to access computer-generated materials. Give us your statistics and we will see if we get the same results. But rerunning the data is not merely a mechanical undertaking. Again, the old truism 'Gi-Go', 'garbage in, garbage out', applies. Each rerunning of the data based on specific statistical models can indeed give you radically different outcomes. But it is part of what the pioneer X-ray crystallographer and sociologist of science J. D. Bernal claimed in 1939 as an intrinsic feature of scientific medicine: 'the growth of modern science coincided with a definite rejection of the ideal of secrecy.'[158] Unless, of course, it is your proprietary secret.

But Seiler also claimed that the basic structure of the design was flawed: 'It is standard clinical practice to perform cxl on adults with keratoconus only when progression occurs. Instead of using Scheimpflug images [achieved by producing multiple cross-sectional scans of the cornea to provide detailed three-dimensional images] to determine progression, the current study relied on medical records and a highly unusual definition of progression.'[159] He also claimed that what looked like a robust study, based on the numbers of patients (and eyes), turned out to be skimpy: 'Five hundred ninety-two eyes started the study. However, the rates of loss to follow-up and dropout were enormous, on the level of 39 per cent to 41 per cent year on year. Although this is a more robust dataset, only 19.4 per cent of the patients were enrolled.'[160] On top of this the rhetoric of these claims was hyperbolic: 'Observations such as "no eyes progressed" (clearly, they did), "no vision-threatening events were observed" (1 case of hydrops that required keratoplasty), and "the new technique avoided the potential complications of epithelial removal for cxl" (30 eyes had epithelial defects) are, we believe, inconsistent with the data the authors present.'[161] But this then begs the question: other than showing what 'bad' science the study shows, what could be achieved by rerunning the data set?

Following *the* science becomes complicated when you do not know at what point 'change' becomes 'progress'. The historical metric of progression of keratoconus is called 'Kmax', the single steepest point on the cornea, that is, the more exaggerated the distortion of cornea, the worse the disease. Repeatedly in peer-reviewed publications the percentage of eyes that 'progressed' used Kmax as the base line without defining progression at all. Rubinfeld turned to Roxanne Littner, an epidemiologist who had worked at the American Health Foundation and then a multinational oil company looking for disease clusters near refineries. Littner analysed some of Rubinfeld's data and concluded that vision and Kmax were in no way correlated. This begged the question of why it had been used. The answer was evident: because it could be documented through technology and its impact reduced to a statically defined scale, irrespective of the patients' accounts of their inability to see. By changing the metric to gauge vision, that is, function, before and after intervention in order to assess the results of treatment of a disease that caused vision loss was deemed 'radical'. Thus, the claim that 'no eyes progressed' rested on change in corneal shape as the measure of progress rather than the patient's statement of their improved vision.

Rubinfeld publishes a rejoinder to Seiler in the same issue.[162] No, he writes, our study was registered with 'clinicaltrials.gov' and the approval of two ethics boards, giving the registration number: data point one. Two, none of the 'epi-off' studies to date have an epi-off control arm. Your data is wrong, and yet you created the field. Three, because our procedure is (virtually) risk-free, we 'believe that an effective epi-on procedure without these risks can be appropriately offered to young patients at the time of diagnosis and to older patients with at least a subjective history of progression, as we did in our study'.[163]

Subjective accounts, as we have found over and over again in this world of evolving evidence-based medicine, have been discounted because they can never be scientific even though they recount the experiences of patients' decline in visual acuity. (Recently the FDA encouraged 'PRO', patient-reported outcomes, and these questionnaires have been validated.) Here we are back to Cheselden and Adams and their accounts of their patients. And this in a world of twenty-first-century medicine that has claimed more and more to include the patient's perspective (pun intended). Rubinfeld's rejoinder continued as follows, stating that no, we have not breached scientific protocols since 'our inclusion criteria are not "highly unusual"', as they are 'virtually identical to those used in the U.S. Food and Drug Administration clinical trials of epi-off CXL'.[164] Rubinfeld further states that even Seiler admits that 'our new procedure even with these false assumptions . . .

consider our results to be similar to every other published epi-off trial to date. With "similar" results, epi-on CXL with our protocol provides significantly less risk and significantly faster visual recovery than epi-off CXL, making it a more desirable technique.'[165]

But remember this is a Shandean postscript to the claim that the researchers stand on the shoulders of giants: 'We respect past contributions from Dr Seiler and others. We hope that one day Dr Seiler and others will accept the possibility that epi-on CXL using our protocol might improve the original Dresden protocol by producing results that are at least as good but without the risks associated with epi-off CXL.'[166] In 2022 Rubinfeld's group, after years of looking for funding to undertake the sort of wide-scale final study demanded by the FDA (and implicitly Seiler), received 'a $32 million Series A funding round led by AXA IM Alts through its Global Health Private Equity strategy plus a syndicate of individual investors, including leading cornea specialists. The new investments will support the advancement of CXL Ophthalmics' (CXLO) transformative cross-linking system, EpiSmart®, through Phase 3 trials on the way to a New Drug Application with FDA.'[167] What will come of this lies in the future, but it is a case of trying to change the boundaries for medicine even ever so slightly, which is also part of this narrative. And the process itself is of interest.

Now, priorities matter in science and in medicine. But today it is the follow-up that leaves the greatest impression. Few of us received the Sabin live-virus polio vaccine when it was first on the market, as the inactive vaccine developed by Jonas Salk (MD, New York University, 1939) quickly eclipsed the priority of Albert Sabin (MD, New York University, 1931) and his earlier vaccine. (One can note here that both were Jewish, and that New York University was one of the few medical schools on the East Coast that did not have a quota for Jewish students.) Sabin found it difficult to get funding (just like Rubinfeld) for a mass trial, so undertook it in the USSR. When he showed its successes in 1960, the vaccine was approved in the United States. Status matters. And while work in the USSR seemed adequate in the Cold War, it nevertheless had a bit of a stigma to it. Salk's innovation was vital to the mass production of the vaccine. But Salk could not patent his invention for the same reason he never received the coveted Nobel Prize for Medicine, because his lawyers at the National Foundation for Infantile Paralysis held that it was not 'novel' enough for a patent. In a 1955 interview with Jonas Salk, Edward Murrow asked him who owned the patent for the vaccine and Salk replied: 'Well, the people, I would say. There is no patent. Could you patent the sun?' A side note: at one point Salk suspected that Parke, Davis & Co., the pharmaceutical company that was to manufacture his vaccine, was sabotaging his proposals for creating an inactive vaccine, as he believed that they wanted to use ultraviolet radiation, on which they held the patent. They weren't and they didn't.[168]

In the end Salk's name is remembered (and honoured), even though his intervention was not 'novel', it was impactful. And out of it arose the Salk Institute for Biological Studies, where he spent the rest of his life.[169] We need to remember that historically 'the medical profession . . . has usually frowned upon patents taken out by medical men . . . The regular profession has . . . maintained this stand against private monopolies ever since the advent of patent law in the seventeenth century.'[170] After the Second World War such a socialization of medical practice was rejected in the very same circles where the socialization of scientific knowledge went unchallenged.

But we noted, also in the first chapter, that growing apace with the rise of scientific medicine in the nineteenth century was the world of the pharmaceutical industry, a global, economic power in the twenty-first century equivalent to coal and steel at the close of the nineteenth century. So, one sub-theme of this account of where we are in the treatment of keratoconus today is that the inventors of these innovations have, in good American tradition, trademarked the epi-on formula as 'RiboStat' and its developers created a for-profit entity, CXL Ophthalmics LLC, in which R. Doyle Stulting and William B. Trattler, two of the collaborators, and Rubinfeld had a financial interest. Their economic as well as scientific interest lies in innovation. We need also to note that Theo Seiler is a scientific consultant to Avedro, Inc., and Schwind eye-tech-solutions GmbH & Co. KG, and that, regarding the following colleagues and co-authors of the reply discussed above, Paolo Vinciguerra is a consultant to Oculus Surgical, Inc., Nidek, Inc. and Schwind eye-tech-solutions GmbH & Co. KG and Farhad Hafezi is chief scientific officer and shareholder of EMAGine AG. How do we know this? Because all reputable scientific publications require that the authors 'disclose' their financial interest in the research they are presenting. A practice unknown in the rise of scientific medicine, where such interrelationships between capital and science were commonplace, but still a bit embarrassing. Usually, the capital came from the state, but the expanding world of pharmaceuticals certainly also played a major role. But this seemed to put the scientist-physician beyond the pale of 'pure' science or the 'healing arts'.

Big business plays a role too in debates about 'standing on the shoulders of giants'. We often hear today that after Frederick Banting (MB, University of Toronto, 1916; Nobel Prize, Physiology or Medicine, 1923, for the 'discovery of insulin') discovered insulin in 1923, he refused to put his name on the patent. He felt it was unethical for a doctor to profit from a discovery that would save lives. Banting's co-inventors, James Collip and Charles Best, sold the insulin patent to the University of Toronto for a mere $1. Today the high cost of insulin is one of the most debated problems in the United States. Prices have become literally unaffordable for many individuals who rely on their daily doses (or, indeed, multiple daily doses). Modern insulin is a far cry from the pharmaceutical developed in Toronto, but it has a huge global market that differentiates between countries that control its price and those that do not. Not surprisingly, those that do not have had a radical spike in costs over those that do control pricing. If 'epi-on' means that this procedure will become the standard of care and that it could then be safely undertaken worldwide, what will this mean for the marketplace? Should we assume that ophthalmology should be any different? Perhaps Roy Porter really was right: 'Historians want doctors to fit tidily into today's categories. Was a particular practitioner skilful, or a bungling quack? A pillar of the faculty or a coxcomb adventurer? A philanthropist or an opportunist?'[171] In the end these are distinctions without a difference as they meld and merge throughout the history of medicine.

4

Backs

I N THE SPRING OF 2009, the National Institute for Health and
Clinical (now Care) Excellence (NICE), the British equivalent to
the USA's Food and Drug Administration (FDA), approved alternative treatments for relieving the symptoms of low back pain to be
used in the British National Health Service. This followed the recommendations for these interventions a few years before, in July 2001,
by the British Medical Association (BMA), the official organization of
allopathic medicine in the UK. (We can note that officially the BMA is
'the trade union and professional body for doctors and medical students in the UK'.) They 'concluded that acupuncture should be made
more widely available to British people through the NHS and that general practitioners should receive training in it'. The association based
its conclusion on three things: evidence showing that 'acupuncture is
more effective than control interventions for back pain, nausea and
vomiting, migraine and dental pain'; the fact that 47 per cent of general
practitioners have arranged for their patients to receive acupuncture;
and the wish of 46 per cent of those professionals to receive training
in acupuncture to treat their patients. Vivienne Nathanson (MD,
University of London, 1978), head of health policy at the BMA, said:
'We need to see more high-quality research into the effectiveness of
acupuncture. Greater use of acupuncture would save the NHS millions
of pounds each year.'[1] NICE's subsequent job was to evaluate efficacy
against cost, and they felt that up to nine sessions with an osteopath,
chiropractor or physiotherapist who was trained in manipulation, or
an acupuncturist, was effective in pain management. Professor Steve
Field (MD, University of Dundee, 2001), the chairman of the Royal

College of General Practitioners, said: 'It's good that GPs are finally being given what appears to be authoritative and well-researched guidance. I have found osteopathy and chiropracty helpful with some patients, and become more convinced about acupuncture, having previously been sceptical.'[2] Field's scepticism seemed a small caveat.

The British Medical Association had controversially approved acupuncture's use for pain reduction, among other symptoms and addictions, in 2000.[3] But the response of their membership was quick and negative, at least from more traditional quarters, as a letter to the BMJ stated quite clearly in November 2001.

> The BMA report on acupuncture is regrettable. It suggests, among other things, that acupuncture is effective for back pain, dental pain, and migraine. Three recent systematic reviews show the importance of basing judgments on high quality information. For back pain, four randomised and blind studies showed no benefit; five open studies showed benefit. The BMA's conclusion that acupuncture was effective in back pain was based on all nine studies . . . Doctors should beware. There is no useful evidence showing that acupuncture helps; there is evidence that it harms. Perhaps the important point is that we should not deceive ourselves, or people who trust our recommendations. There is no gold standard evidence that acupuncture improves pain or anything else. The BMA report is quite simply wrong.[4]

Note that both the pro- and contra- views relied on claims of 'evidence', but evidence understood in the tradition of what was called 'evidence-based medicine': randomized trials, comparative evaluations, and so on. Thus Sir William Asscher (MD, University of London, 1954), then the chair of the BMA's Board of Science and Education, one of the authors of the BMA's positive report, noted that: 'The BMA calls for substantial research funding, the production of guidelines, and a formal appraisal of acupuncture.'[5] In the same issue, Mike Cummings (MB ChB, University of Leeds, 1978), the director of education of the British Medical Acupuncture Society, agreed but proposed a caveat: 'There is a dearth of randomised control trials with positive results, but this may be due more to methodological difficulties than a lack of efficacy. The positive results in lower quality trials may not be attributable solely to bias. The pain community would be done a disservice if acupuncture techniques were not tested in both a logical and methodologically sound manner.'[6] Evidence is at the core of determining not merely efficacy but the scientific claims of acupuncture.

Now, given that there were more than 5,500 acupuncturists in the United Kingdom at the time, of which 3,500 were licensed health professionals, and that, according to William Asscher, 'acupuncture is the complementary therapy most used by general practitioners, with most patients being referred for pain relief and musculoskeletal disorders. Acupuncture is now reported to be used routinely ahead of physiotherapy and drug delivery systems in 86 per cent of chronic pain services,' it only made sense to test this out in practice under the umbrella of the NHS. By the beginning of the new millennium the initial medical assumption was to at least attempt to provide a medically defined therapy desired by a range of potential patients and supported by an existing network of providers that could eventually fulfil the need for scientific evidence to show why it was efficacious.

British politics had made complementary and alternative medicine (CAM) (that is, non-allopathic medicine) a cause since the beginning of the millennium.[7] Indeed, the House of Lords had in 2000 published a complete vindication of CAM, arguing that acupuncture presented 'a credible evidence base'. Although the acupuncturists' claims are 'based on theories about their modes of action that are not congruent with current scientific knowledge. That is not to say that new scientific knowledge may not emerge in the future. Nevertheless, as a Select Committee on Science and Technology we must make it clear from the outset that while we accept that some CAM therapies, notably osteopathy, chiropractic and herbal medicine, have established efficacy in the treatment of a limited range of ailments, we remain sceptical about the modes of action of most of the others.' Not their efficacy, but their 'modes of action'. And therefore they 'recommend that CAM should attempt to build up an evidence base with the same rigour as is required of conventional medicine, using both randomised controlled trials (RCTs) and other research designs'. Quackery is not here a risk in and of itself in the application of CAM but rather the possibility that 'patients could miss out on conventional medical diagnosis and treatment because they choose only to consult a CAM practitioner. We recommend that all NHS provision of CAM should continue to be through GP referral.'[8] This model had been developed to deal with psychoanalysts, specifically lay analysts, who could treat only in consultation with licensed medical practitioners. Trust but verify was the motto. The key was, however, the mode of evidence that was produced to show the efficacy of CAM, especially Steve Field's bugbear, acupuncture.

As it turned out, there seemed to be a lot of evidence for CAM therapies already present. Beginning in the 1980s the establishment of professional organizations and professional journals began to mimic the various organs and associations of allopathic medicine. Here we need to remember the views of Robert G. A. Dolby, who was interested in how what he labelled 'deviant science' establishes itself as 'a deviant form of medicine [that] must compete with orthodox medicine, which claims to be science based'. Such 'deviant systems of belief, which compete with orthodoxies appealing to the authority of science, thrive best if they also claim to have their own scientific basis.' And how this can be accomplished by creating a 'belief system . . . directly modelled on orthodox science or scientific medicine, [with] institutions . . . which offer quasi-educational facilities for training and research'.[9] Dolby is not speaking of the truth-values of heterodoxy, but rather how it needs to refashion itself in the world of scientific medicine.

The British Medical Acupuncture Society was founded in 1980 by medical practitioners interested in employing acupuncture within their practices. The gold standard was to develop randomized, double-blind trials in concert with other forms of treatment for pain such as nerve blocks and opiates; the use of various means of scanning the activity of the brain, such as fMRIs; and the use of sham or 'placebo' treatments: shallow needle insertions as opposed to 'varum' (real) acupuncture therapies. One can note here that technology also plays a real role in the assumptions of the efficacy of a treatment. Sham insertions are simply of greater assumed efficacy than sham pills, as 'placebo needles can exhibit therapeutic effects relative to placebo pills [as they employ] enhanced touch sensations, direct stimulation of the somatosensory system and activation of multiple brain systems.'[10] In other words, needles, a more complex technological delivery system, employ their own physiology as well as meaning attached to them.

In most of the studies of the time, as we noted above, there were either equal or relatively weak responses to acupuncture as pain relief. But researchers also found that those patients who were actively seeking such pain relief showed higher rates of response than those who had simply been assigned to the study. Indeed, it was also clear that the 'social nature of patients', their 'experiences of treatment, and [their position] . . . as embedded in both their own personal social networks and also those relationships involved in treatment (e.g., with practitioners)' contributed to the efficacy of the procedures. And whether positive outcomes could be different 'according to whether that treatment is received in usual care or in a research setting'.[11] But in general psychosocial factors were not taken into consideration. Overall, the model used for proof was to be identical to that in allopathic medicine and the notion that an intervention had radically different responses based on the desire of the patient seemed to weaken the case for its claims. Indeed, even pain researchers at the time who did not advocate the use of acupuncture, and whose approach was limited to prescribing opioids, did 'not have an explanation for, so far, the reason its effects last so long in some patients'.[12] What was the reason it seemed to work and why was it present?

Traditional Chinese Medicine and Scientific Evidence

To understand the claims of acupuncture within CAM as well as modern allopathic medicine, we need to examine the question of evidence and the creation of what is now labelled 'Western-style acupuncture'. While medical or 'trigger point' acupuncture is the form usually practised within the NHS, it is clearly an adaptation of what is labelled 'traditional Chinese acupuncture'. The latter claims to be 'holistic' and applies its principles to the entire body and all pathological conditions; the former is usually employed for pain relief, primarily for musculoskeletal pain.[13] Now, such a distinction seems to reinforce our understanding, in our age of 'evidence-based medicine', of the chasm between traditional or folkloric systems of medicine and allopathic therapies. Alternative medicine may well have by chance stumbled onto some valid modalities of treatment, which bench science could then verify and turn into recognized therapies. For we can only imagine well-managed, well-monitored and scientifically validated therapies as coming out of the laboratory (which they did) and therefore not to be found randomly in 'nature'.[14] This replicated itself over and over in the age of scientific medicine, from antibiotics to anti-inflammatories. Luck versus science.

In evaluating the efficacy of some CAM therapies in the United States in 2009 the key was

> the quality of the evidence cited in the evidence-based CAM curricula of the fifteen organizations that received National Institutes of Health National Center for Complementary and Alternative Medicine (NCCAM) grants. We do not consider the large, complex issues concerning the role of CAM in health care. Evidence-based medicine (EBM) requires a critical analysis of the quality of research, use of an up-to-date database and continuing revision of evaluations as new data become available. It also requires the integration of the best research evidence with clinical expertise and each patient's unique values and circumstances.[15]

In other words, science, not luck. But that is, in the case of acupuncture, a difference without a distinction.

To understand this, we need to return to the immediate post-Second World War era and the rise of the People's Republic of China as a global medical soft power. One of the striking moves on the part of Mao Zedong was quickly to recognize that both internally and externally the role of public health and medical therapy would strengthen the new revolutionary state's claims for improving the daily life of the Chinese population, ravaged by decades of war and civic conflict. But he also understood that, given the realities of Chinese economics and politics, healthcare could also fashion a space for the PRC's claims to provide a model for healthcare on the global stage. Most of the internal histories of acupuncture published by its advocates (certainly for those in the Global North) see it as an indigenous, anti-modern Chinese traditional system with its roots in the distant past: 'from a few hundred years leading up to the Common Era. Sharpened stones and bones that date from about 6000 BCE have been interpreted as instruments for acupuncture treatment . . . The first document that unequivocally described an organized system of diagnosis and treatment which is recognized as acupuncture is *The Yellow Emperor's Classic of Internal Medicine*, dating from about 100 BCE.'[16] The reality, however, lay with the new revolutionary state that sought to place indigenous traditions on a par with allopathic ones, and created, more or less out of whole cloth, what came to be labelled 'Traditional Chinese Medicine' (TCM).[17]

That there were multiple, conflicting, often secret systems of health interventions in East Asia over millennia is without a doubt accurate, but that there was a systematic medical practice with its roots in a specific moment is a creation of twentieth-century global politics, one that Mao's China took advantage of in the 1950s.

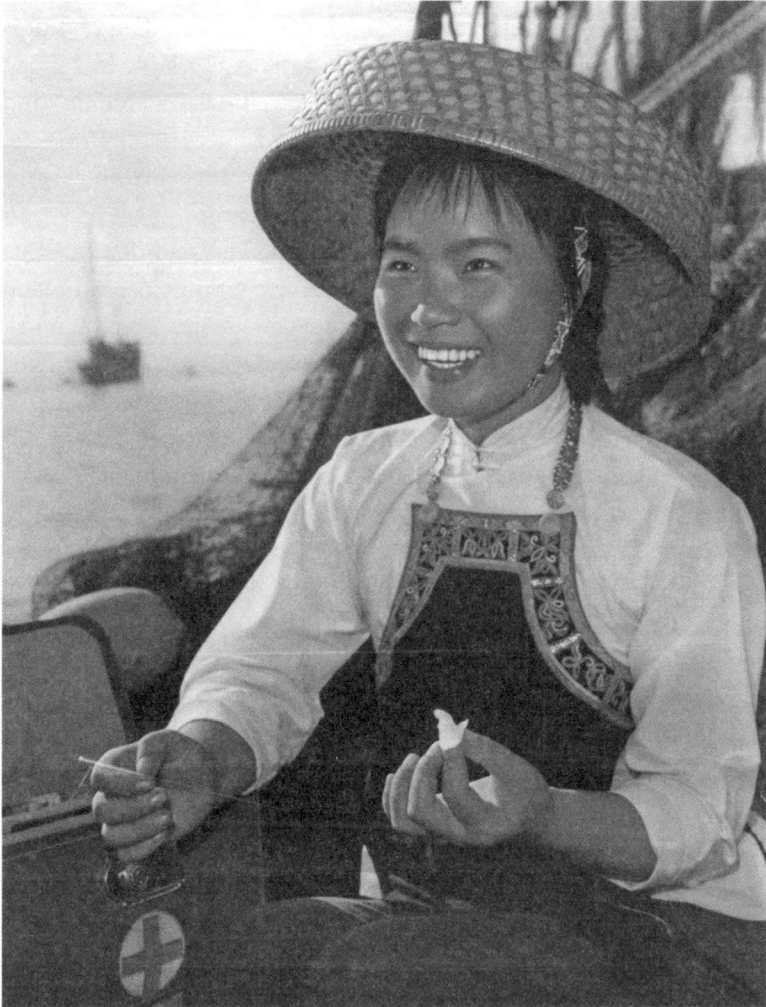

China during the Cultural Revolution, 1975, lithograph after Peng Yuzhang. A young woman doctor in a fishing village is preparing acupuncture needles by taking cotton from a first aid box to clean them. This is a typical fishing village on the South China Sea, and the woman doctor is one of the 'farmer doctors,' so-called barefoot doctors (*chi jiao yi sheng*) in the 1970s. These doctors were also local fishing or farming people and sometimes also members of 'educated youth' (*zhi shi qing nian*) from urban areas. Their motto was 'use a silver needle to cure hundreds of illnesses; use a red heart to warm thousands of families'.

In 1958, Mao issued his dictums that 'Chinese medicine and phar-macology are a great treasure-house' and to 'weed through the old to bring forth the new', that would shape the development of TCM (*zhongyi*) as a unified, specific medical system.[18] *Zhongyi* translates simply as 'Chinese medicine'. The addition of 'Traditional' and capital-ization of the phrase in English is meant to indicate that, as opposed to 'traditional medicine', TCM was a new, more simplified and uni-fied system. In 1959, during the Great Leap Forward, Mao had urged that 'Doctors of Western medicine study Chinese medicine', and having observed that acupuncture could be effective in stopping pain, Western-trained doctors asked, 'can it also produce anaesthesia for operations?'[19] The answer, of course, was yes.

What was vital was that it be understood as *scientific*. At least as scientific as the Soviet medicine of its day, with its deep roots in nineteenth-century German bench science and medical therapy, much of which had been corrupted by Stalin for ideological reasons, as in the Lysenko affair, or was radically out of date by the 1950s.[20] As one of the Chinese reformers of the day stated, Soviet science provided 'a new sci-entific medicine to judge the scientific level of Chinese medicine, and see which parts of it were insufficient'. It would give the new Chinese medicine 'a new medical scientific theory, a scientific basis, so that after they [the doctors] have learnt it, they can [use it] to explain the origin of disease, pathology and make a reasonably accurate scientific diagnosis and [use this] to analyse and determine treatments'.[21] Relying heavily on Ivan Pavlov's proto-behaviourist theory of the higher function of nerves, they specifically reinterpreted the 'new acupuncture' as a means of treat-ing the nervous system, which the Soviet behaviourists saw as central to all manifestations of illness within the body and thus all theories of therapeutics and methods of prophylaxis. It created a parallel system to allopathic medicine, synthesizing the claims of evidence-based medi-cine into therapeutics adapted from older systems of treatment. It was an invented tradition, in the sense of Eric Hobsbawm, created in the present while simultaneously creating its own past.

But the present was dominated by allopathic medicine and a scien-tific ethos very different from the medical traditions amalgamated by Mao. The 'standardization of TCM' consisted of institutionalizing edu-cation and practice in TCM colleges and of writing TCM textbooks from 1956 to 1964. The first set of eighteen textbooks was completed by 1962. The model was allopathic medicine with a Soviet flavour; its focus was on the nervous system rather than on Qi, the circulating life force that underpinned most earlier forms of East Asian medical praxis. And one of the prime therapies to illustrate this was the 'new' acupuncture. It set itself against the 'acupuncture currently being practised in the countryside', which 'does not stress cleanliness and sterilization . . . they do not understand physiology and anatomy, some of them are not even sure how to find acupuncture points.'[22] The local practices needed to be systematized and regularized, mirroring allopathic medicine in the age of scientific medicine.

There are a few key moments in the global reception of the new unified TCM through the reformed therapy of acupuncture. In 1971 James 'Scotty' Reston of the *New York Times*, at the same time as Henry Kissinger was secretly preparing Richard Nixon's 1972 trip to China that captured the world's attention, experienced TCM at first hand when he had an emergency appendectomy at the Anti-Imperialist Hospital in Beijing on 17 July 1971. Although the doctors successfully removed his appendix under local anaesthesia (he received conventional anaesthetics, xylocaine and benzocaine), he experienced lingering pain in his stomach. Dr Li Chang Yuan, the hospital's acupuncturist, alleviated his discomfort by inserting three needles below his right elbow and kneecaps 'that sent ripples of pain racing through my limbs and, at least, had the effect of diverting my attention from the distress in my stomach'. But the claims were much broader than that: 'Judging from the cables reaching me here, recent reports and claims of remarkable cures of blindness, paralysis and mental disorders by acupuncture have apparently led to considerable speculation in America about great new medical breakthroughs in the field of traditional Chinese needle and herbal medicine. I do not know whether this speculation is justified and am not qualified to judge,' Reston wrote to his American readers.[23] But the prime example, with press photographs in the various illustrated magazines and even some footage on the weekly news, was the use of acupuncture for pain relief.[24]

This became a standard stop for the physicians visiting Mao's China after Nixon's visit. In 1972 ten members of the National Medical Association travelled to China as guests of the government for a ten-day tour of major medical facilities. One member, Emerson Walden, Sr (MD, Howard University, 1953), a surgeon from Baltimore and then president of the NMA, observed the 'use of acupuncture for anesthesia . . . on the afternoon of October 18, 1972, I was taken to the Chou Yang

Hospital in Peking. There I learned that three patients were scheduled for surgery under acupuncture anesthesia.' He then describes the course of the surgery:

> The patients had been exposed to acupuncture to acquaint them with the procedure and to determine effective sites of insertion. They were also told what feelings to expect during the procedure . . . a 34-year-old male had a bleeding duodenal ulcer and had been admitted 30 days previously . . . The male was photographed on the operating table. All were photographed while receiving acupuncture anesthesia induction, during and after surgery. All patients were aware during surgery, were free of pain and talked freely with us through interpreters. Technique was superb. During the question and answer period, we learned that more than 2,000 cases have been done under acupuncture anesthesia at the Chou Yang facility since 1965.[25]

Walden's central interest was reimplantation surgery, a field that the Chinese had developed during the early 1960s with a successful hand reimplantation in Shanghai. He reports that none of these procedures that he observed were done under acupuncture anaesthesia.

The group's trip was highly structured, as were all such visits, to highlight the 'reorientation of the entire medical profession toward the recognition that its controlling and perennial duty was service to the people'. The result was that 'the NMA delegation returned to the United States greatly inspired by what it had witnessed of the colossal achievements of the People's Republic of China in a scant 23 years under their political system and with a deep sense of challenge to produce under our system matching accomplishment in the parallel areas of medical education, training and recruitment of workers in all the health related areas, community medicine, family planning and the provision of adequate health for all the American people.'[26] One can only assume that the elite African American physicians in the age of the struggle for civil rights had to claim global interest ('all the American people'), even though the need clearly was simultaneously local to the African American community.

With all this interest in the 1970s in medical innovations in the PRC, we need to stress here that the use of acupuncture as anaesthesia was part of the modernization of indigenous medical practices now reinvented in Mao's China as TCM. In the late nineteenth century Chinese medicine had been, in the eyes of the Global North, a sign of barbarism. The editors of the *Boston Medical and Surgical Journal* in 1841 wrote that 'The Chinese are more ignorant of medicine and surgery than of most other things which confer direct physical benefit on the race,' and that 'knavery and quackery of the most ingenious and yet of the most absurd character' were rampant among China's physicians.[27] Yet there is always the counter-image that is present in the Global North, the idea that 'exotic' cultures are 'closer to nature' as they are far from the technological burden of scientific medicine. By the post-Second World War period what in the nineteenth century seemed 'primitive' to physicians and missionaries in the age of 'heroic medicine' came to be seen as a more benign alternative to the regimentation and technological distance imputed to allopathic medicine.

This new perception dominated the awareness of acupuncture in the Global North during the 1970s. Reston had observed acupuncture anaesthesia during open-heart surgery, images of which circulated throughout the American media.[28] Only decades later, in 2006, was it claimed that acupuncture anaesthetic, observed by visitors from beyond the PRC, was supplemented, as, in one case, 'the patient had been given a combination of 3 very powerful sedatives (midazolam, droperidol, fentanyl) and large volumes of local anesthetic injected into the chest. The acupuncture needles were purely cosmetic.'[29] But this was the speculation already when E. Grey Dimond (MD, Indiana University School of Medicine, 1944), founder of the University of Kansas-Kansas City School of Medicine, who brought the first physicians from the PRC to the United States in 1972, asked for the first time about 'acupuncture anesthesia': 'I carefully inquired whether this means a hollow needle with procaine and it does not. My instincts tell me that they were actually needling a nerve itself and that the shock of the needle in the nerve area simply sends signals back to the spinal cord and shuts that nerve down so to speak.'[30] Simple quackery? But he also admitted that 'placing a sharp needle in the skin for a few minutes could well be impressive psychosomatic therapy. The fact that acupuncture treatment programs often go on for two weeks or a month and often for such obscure problems as backache, rheumatism, and tired liver makes one highly suspicious that time plus the doctor's attention have a great deal to do with most results.'[31] Or not?

Acupuncture in the Global North

Acupuncture, we can add, already had a complex history in the Global North, quite invisible to commentators in the 1970s. As a system of therapy, it had been introduced by fleet surgeons Willem Ten Rhijne and Englebert Kaempfer with the Dutch East India Company in the late seventeenth century, who learned about acupuncture while stationed at the company's trading post in Japan. Knowledge of the practice spread through the aegis of the Dutch East India Company's wide-ranging network of colonial stations in Japan and Indonesia. Early practitioners included Erasmus Darwin, who treated intense cramps in the calf muscle as analogous to

> the colic of Japan . . . and that that disease was said to be cured by acupuncture, or the prick of a needle; I directed some very thin steel needles to be made about three inches long, and of such a temper, that they would bend double rather than break; and wrapped wax thread over about half an inch of the blunt end for a handle. One of these needles, when the pain occurred, was pushed about an inch into the painful part, and the pain instantly ceased; but I was not certain, whether the fear of the patient, or the stimulus of the puncture, occasioned the cessation of pain; and as the paroxysm had continued some weeks, and was then declining, the experiment was not tried again.[32]

Darwin imagined that the pinpricks (perhaps) allowed air to escape and thus relieved pain. By the late Enlightenment there was a consensus that it worked more or less like homeopathy – that is, 'like cured like'. It was seen as a form of counter-irritant.

When early nineteenth-century physicians such as Louis Victor Joseph Berlioz (MD, University of Paris, 1802) in Paris and Bordeaux turned to it as a general therapy for a range of disorders, he had quite another explanation: acupuncture worked 'by dissipating the symptoms [of illness], [which] demonstrates that disorder of the nervous system only had given rise to them'.[33] Indeed, he opined that: 'it is never more successful than in cases where it produces little or no pain.' To the contrary, Berlioz believed that acupuncture's effects were not achieved by reducing inflammation, but that it 'acts by stimulating the nerves, or

Acupuncture needles,
plate from James Morss
Churchill, *A Treatise on
Acupuncturation* (1821).

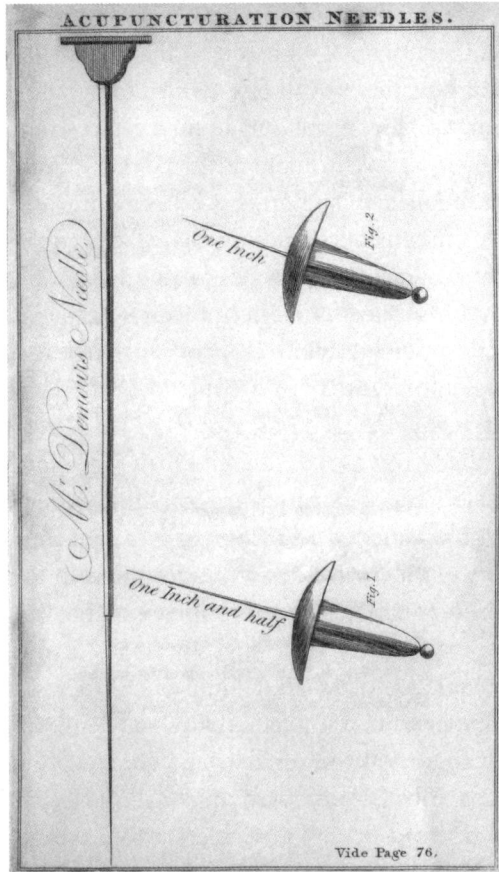

ACUPUNCTURATION NEEDLES.

Mr Demours Needle

One Inch

Fig. 2

One Inch and half

Fig. 1

Vide Page 76.

by restoring to them [that] of which they [were] deprived through the effects of pain'.[34] After his initial success he quickly turned to treating whooping cough, back pain, headaches, muscle pain and paralysis.

In London Berlioz was read and his approach implemented by James Morss Churchill, who claimed to be a member of the Royal College of Surgeons as well as 'consulting surgeon-accoucheur to the Westminster Lying-in Institution'.[35] He treated patients with acupuncture and in 1821 published the first book-length English-language work with the method. Churchill, however, was more limited in his use of acupuncture and restricted his treatment to 'local diseases of the muscular and fibrous structures of the body', such as rheumatism, muscle strains and pain in the back, neck and shoulders.[36] As a therapy for lower back pain he set the standard in British medicine and grounded it, to no surprise, in the scientific claims of the time, as he 'would not admit the fables which are promulgated by these people, as evidence of its efficacy, had not this efficacy been witnessed by European spectators on its native soil, and at length experienced in our own hemisphere; and even, latterly, in our own country.[37] By 1828 'acupuncture [was] now employed, not only in the Eastern Hemisphere, in France and in America, but throughout the British dominions, and in our London hospitals, under the auspices of men, who stand deservedly high in the ranks of literature and science.[38] No quacks here. The perfect summary of colonial attitudes to all innovations found beyond the world circumscribed by Western medicine.

Importing medical techniques in the eighteenth century from the colonies was not unique. Major innovations in the use of facial flaps for reconstructive surgery were imported into Britain from India.[39] But in the Global North they had to be sanctioned by the established medical profession. If not, they became quackery. At the same moment, in the very early nineteenth century, a home-grown form of using needles to pierce the skin to alleviate a wide range of diseases had developed in the United States, where Churchill's work was well received among physicians. It was quickly subsumed into other forms of quackery, unlike in Europe. The *Atlantic Magazine* published an anonymous satirical article in defence of 'quacks' in 1824. The author listed 'amulets and abracadabras, cobwebs and camphor bags, robs [*sic*] and rusty nails, skullcap, cubebs and sarsaparilla, tar water, tractors and acupuncturation' among the contributions quack doctors had made to the practice of medicine.[40] Two years later, the editors of the *Ohio Medical Repository* wrote: 'At present, it is the fashion among the knowing ones of this metropolis to rank acupuncture and moxibustion with metallic tractation and animal magnetism.'[41] But why did people flock to it? George Bacon Wood (MD, University of Pennsylvania, 1818), a professor of medicine at the University of Pennsylvania and onetime president of the AMA (and a close friend of Franklin Bache, who conducted the first clinical trial of acupuncture on American soil), answered in his 1856 textbook on therapeutics and materia medica. Wood equated the effects produced by acupuncture needles with 'painless dentistry'. He wrote that in most instances, acupuncture 'acts through the mind, as the cold steel of the dentist will cure the toothache before the tooth has been pulled, or as the metallic tractors.'[42] In other words, acupuncture did not work by producing any verifiable physical effects, but only created an impression on a patient's mind that caused the pain to go away. Mere quackery.

Franklin Bache, whose MD from the University of Pennsylvania in 1814 was under the prominent American physician Benjamin Rush, translated one of the first studies of acupuncture by J. M. Morand, employing Berlioz's ideas, from the French in 1825.[43] He then undertook a series of treatments, most of them (according to him) successful, using acupuncture on inmates at the Walnut Street State Prison in Philadelphia, treating more than twenty prisoners between 14 June and 2 December 1825. He focused on four specific conditions (neuralgia, chronic pains, muscular rheumatism and ophthalmia), supplementing acupuncture with procedures such as cupping and blistering as needed. Bache, for example, treated all the prisoners in his trial in the same manner: in patients with back pain, he inserted needles into the back; in patients with shoulder pain, he inserted needles into the shoulder, and so on. It still functioned as a type of localized counter-irritant. Bache published the results in 1826, making him the first American physician to conduct clinical trials of the procedure.[44] The paper was recognized but the practice remained unusual within allopathic medical circles as well as traditional dentistry.

It is with the American physician-novelist and essayist Oliver Wendell Holmes, Sr (MD, Harvard, 1836), the father of the jurist, that acupuncture becomes part of a discourse of healing in the public sphere. Holmes's status in the Americanization of scientific medicine was beyond question, as he was one of the first to advocate for antisepsis, echoing Lord Lister's views.[45] But he was also a popular and widely read author. Holmes's bestselling *The Poet at the Breakfast Table* (1885) reflects on the need for the physician simply to act: 'When a person is sick, there is always something to be done for him, and done at once. If it is only to open or shut a window.'[46] The promise of the new scientific medicine is bogus for 'the men that have science only, begin too far back, and, before they get as far as the case in hand, the patient has very likely gone to visit his deceased relatives.'[47] It is 'science out of place'. Yet Holmes was one of the physicians who had been trained in Paris in the new clinical approach and then introduced the new technology of the stethoscope into American medicine. He evokes quite an alternative practice:

By far the larger part of the facts of structure and function you find in the books of anatomy and physiology have no immediate application to the daily duties of the practitioner. You must learn systematically, for all that; it is the easiest way and the only way that takes hold of the memory, except mere empirical repetition, like that of the handicraftsman. Did you ever see one of those Japanese figures with the points for acupuncture marked upon it? You see they have a way of pushing long, slender needles into you for the cure of rheumatism and other complaints, and it seems there is a choice of spots for the operation, though it is very strange how little mischief it does in a good many places one would think unsafe to meddle with. So they had a doll made, and marked the spots where they had put in needles without doing any harm. They must have had accidents from sticking the needles into the wrong places now and then, but I suppose they didn't say a great deal about those. After a time, say a few centuries of experience, they had their doll all spotted over with safe places for sticking in the needles. That is their way of registering practical knowledge.[48]

Not exotic but rather scientific: a mapping of the body not unlike that of the anatomists and physiologists. Not quackery at all; just an alternative way of understanding the body beginning with clinical experience, not science.

Holmes understood Rudolf Virchow's revolutionary claims that medicine, of all sorts and locations, was political in its essence. In 1861 Holmes observed:

The truth is, that medicine, professedly founded on observation, is as sensitive to outside influence, political, religious, philosophical, imaginative, as is the barometer to the changes of atmospheric density. Theoretically it ought to go on its own straightforward inductive path, without regard to changes of government or to fluctuations of public opinion. But look a moment while I clash a few facts together, and see if some sparks do not reveal by their light a closer relation between the Medical Sciences and the conditions of Society and the general thought of the time, than would at first be suspected.[49]

But that notion, that social forces, for good or for ill, shaped medical understanding, did not marginalize acupuncture as therapy in the age of scientific medicine.

With the rise of scientific medicine at the end of the century one would imagine acupuncture being sent into the outermost bounds of medical quackery. Yet exactly the opposite takes place. No less a figure than Sir William Osler, whose presence has and will continue to serve as a litmus test for scientific medicine in the first generation in the United States and the United Kingdom, advocated for the practice. In his definitive *The Principles and Practice of Medicine*, the bestselling medical textbook of its time, Osler made several references to the efficacy of acupuncture. For acute cases of lumbago, he wrote that acupuncture is 'the most effective treatment' for pain relief. He recommended inserting needles into the lumbar muscles and leaving them in place for five to ten minutes. 'In many instances the relief is immediate.' For patients with sciatica, Osler stated that acupuncture 'may also be tried', with the needles 'thrust deeply into the most painful spot for a distance of about two inches' and left in the body for fifteen to twenty minutes.[50] As Osler's textbook remained in print until 1947, it exposed hundreds of thousands of American physicians to the idea of using acupuncture for conditions such as low back pain and sciatica well into the mid-twentieth century. Osler's echo was heard when American physicians, quite shocked by his prescience, referred to Osler's entries on acupuncture in *The Principles and Practice of Medicine* when James Reston's story appeared in the *New York Times* in 1971.[51]

Osler reads acupuncture as a therapy within modern, allopathic medicine, not as an indigenous Asian approach to healing. In 1889 he had condemned the non-scientific training of physicians in the 'Wild West' of American medicine as 'the unrestricted manufacture – note the term – of doctors, quite regardless of the qualifications usually thought necessary in civilized communities – of physicians who may never have been inside a hospital ward, and who had, after graduation, to learn medicine somewhat in the fashion of the Chinese doctors who recognized the course of the arteries of the body, by noting just where the blood spurted when the acupuncture needle was inserted'.[52] This set the pattern for allopathic medicine through the post-Second World War era. Allopathic medicine under the influence of Osler still used acupuncture into the 1970s as part of scientific medicine. When acupuncture was the therapy discussed, the concern was raised that chiropractors might adopt it, risking 'acupuncture's possible misuse . . . by quacks'.[53] Another author points approvingly to law cases which restrain the practice of acupuncture by lay acupuncturists while

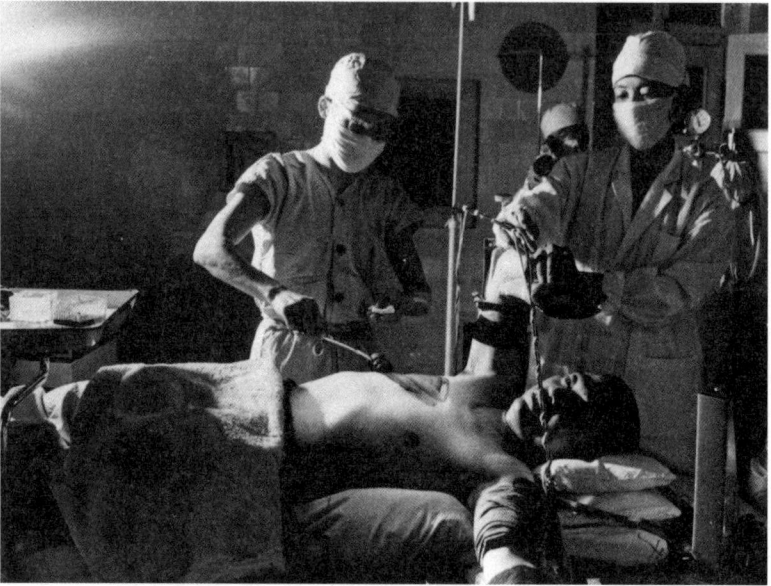

A patient being prepared for surgery under acupuncture anaesthesia, 1979,
World Health Organization photograph by D. Henrioud.

permitting licensed physicians to perform the treatment.[54] So the path
of its reception in the Anglophone medical world was already paved
by the professional interest in it as a form of treatment.

Visitors from abroad who observed the use of acupuncture as
anaesthesia had also been prepared by a wide range of media accounts
in the Global North of the new, radical medical interventions in the
PRC. The New York physician and president of the American Public
Health Association Victor Sidel (MD, Harvard Medical School, 1957)
and his medical sociologist spouse Ruth (PhD, Sociology, Union
Graduate School, 1978) promoted the innovations that they found
in Maoist China.[55] He was in one of the earliest groups of prominent physicians to visit China in September 1971, which included Paul
Dudley White, E. Grey Dimond and Samuel Rosen. As their visit came
a mere two months after Reston's appendectomy, it meant that the two
events would be linked in popular memory. Media coverage of their
visit focused especially on their observations about the use of acupuncture, which 'Scotty' Reston had made famous. It was acupuncture
– especially acupuncture anaesthesia – that captivated the public. Was
acupuncture truly a medical marvel that could circumvent many of the
problems of conventional anaesthesia? Did the procedure carry any
risks or side-effects? How did it actually work? The answer was that

acupuncture was ancient (read: not modern) and potentially could provide fixes for the problems of life in a modern society. This assumption
glossed over nearly two decades' worth of research and experimentation by Chinese scientists and physicians as well as the established
research agenda in the Global North in this practice. Acupuncture,
American observers found, was worthy of (further) investigation but
should be approached cautiously, using methods accepted by the scientific community.[56] A new health miracle seemed to be on the verge
of being introduced (again) into the Global North from the medical
fringe, needing to be sanctioned by the medical establishment.

From 1971 to the WHO's Alma Ata Conference on Primary Health
Care in September 1978, the global enthusiasm for the 'Chinese
Approach to Health' increased exponentially over time. This had come
about somewhat more slowly in the PRC the decade before. By the 1960s,
the new collective communes began to offer training courses at less
busy seasons to villagers on how to treat minor illnesses, elementary
acupuncture and some basic knowledge of common diseases and their
prevention. This quickly became the core of the other selling point for
Mao: cheap, effective, local healthcare, the barefoot doctors and their
acupuncture therapy. But, as the historian of modern China Zhou Xun
notes, 'the propaganda image of Barefoot Doctors delivering health care
with a "Bunch of Herbs and One Acupuncture Needle" that adorned
village health centres, further hindered individual barefoot doctors'
competence to deliver care that addressed villagers' actual health
needs.'[57] She also noted that some of these lay healers were with their
patients much longer than allopathic healers and 'were also empathetic
and always willing to spend time with . . . patients and listen to their
troubles'.[58] In 1967, for example, a medical delegation from Tanzania
visiting China was said to be 'impressed by the stage of development
of health services, which have been revolutionized and transformed
by the new China'.[59] The PRC leadership quickly capitalized on this,
viewing health cooperation with these developing countries as 'inexpensive but profitable' undertakings that could help its effort to promote
a new international order – a 'people's revolutionary movement in
Asia, Africa and Latin America' against 'colonialism, imperialism and
hegemonism'.[60] Beginning with sending medical teams to 'aid' newly
independent Algeria in 1963, the PRC continuously dispatched medical
teams to more than 22 countries in Africa in the next decades. Different
provinces in China were twinned with African nations. For instance,

teams of doctors of both allopathic medicine and the newly created
TCM from Shandong went to Tanzania.[61] Acupuncture imported from
the PRC as part of the newly created 'Traditional Chinese Medicine'
became widely popular. In September 2017 the Ministry of Health in
Mozambique announced plans to introduce acupuncture into main
provincial hospitals in parts of the country.[62]

The central focus was on the exotic and autarkic nature of TCM,
when in fact it was not only shaped in all its form by the model of
bench science and its approach to medical therapy but laid claim to
the same level of scientific evidence. Using a Pavlovian model of excitation, inhibition and equilibrium of cortical nervous processes in the
nervous system, the mechanistic nature of acupuncture in this model
had clear neural pathways and direct, observable results. Anatomically
it was clearly not based on named or known nerves or neural pathways, although similar pathophysiological explanations were (and
are) posited.

It was not so much an alteration of the pathways of Qi but the neural
pathophysiology of Soviet behaviourism that had merged Pavlov with
Marx. Prior to the break between Mao and Stalin's heirs, as of the 1950s
the 'Soviet Academy of Sciences deified Pavlov, elevating his "teaching"
above criticism, committing all Soviet neurophysiologists and psychologists to the task of "elaborating the Pavlovian heritage".'[63] Chinese
acupuncturists, too. So, the science of acupuncture was already well
committed to nineteenth-century models of laboratory science and
their claim of what acceptable evidence could be. And this had been
true already in scientific medicine from Osler on. Simultaneously,
acupuncture was also seen as an antidote to scientific medicine; the
'ancient' status of these preparations rendered them closer to 'nature'.
TCM, moreover, offered a system of medicine that seemed analogous
to scientific medicine: methods proven through millennia of use that
had been validated by science.[64] You couldn't lose. This underpinned
the claims that led to the NHS recognition of the practice:

> Debates over the legitimation of acupuncture also have led to
> interesting re-classifications, as in the UK, where mechanistic
> biomedical models and statistical evidence have made possible
> the recognition of acupuncture as a 'professionally organ-
> ised alternative therapy', for which there is scientific evidence
> of its efficacy, in contrast to TCM, for which no convincing

evidence of efficacy was reported as in the House of Lords Select Committee on Science and Technology Report of 2000. The science invoked by the UK legislative bodies is a globalised form of the biosciences, while practitioners, anthropologists and historians emphasise Chinese–scientific continuities, as acupuncture and moxibustion (*zhenjiu*) were historically considered a sub-category of Chinese medicine.[65]

But if the core of the argument is that the 'new' acupuncture was now science, and a science well grounded in the model of evidence for allopathic practice in the age of evidence-based medicine, there were certainly many who not only objected to these claims of evidence (as we have seen in the responses to the BMA approval of acupuncture), but dismissed it as quackery.

David Colquhoun, a pharmacologist at University College London, and his co-author, the neurologist Steven Novella (MD, Georgetown University, 1991) of the Yale School of Medicine, labelled acupuncture and its training in the UK as training 'in subjects that aren't true, and that's largely restricted to various forms of quackery'.[66] Colquhoun and Novella denounced acupuncture as merely 'a theatrical placebo'. There is no scientific evidence, in their terms, of the efficacy of the procedure. As there is

> no point in discussing surrogate outcomes, such as functional magnetic resonance imaging studies or endorphin release studies, until such time as it has been shown that patients get a useful degree of relief. It is now clear that they do not. We also see little point in invoking individual studies. Inconsistency is a prominent characteristic of acupuncture research: the heterogeneity of results poses a problem for meta-analysis. Consequently, it is very easy to pick trials that show any outcome whatsoever. Therefore, we shall consider only meta-analyses.

And these turn out to disprove the very claims underlying the procedures.

This view looks like the science of the 'new' acupuncture. But they also dismiss the underlying claims attributed to the autarkic practice of acupuncture as 'somehow more holistic, or more patient-centered, than medicine . . . All good doctors are empathetic and patient-centered. The idea that empathy is restricted to those who practice unscientific medicine seems both condescending to doctors, and it verges on an admission that empathy is all that alternative treatments have to offer.' Their conclusion is clear from the title of their essay, that it is a 'theatrical placebo': 'The outcome of this research, we propose, is that the benefits of acupuncture are likely nonexistent, or at best are too small and too transient to be of any clinical significance. It seems that acupuncture is little or no more than a theatrical placebo.'[67] Acupuncture studies had, in spite of such criticism, tended to follow along two general models that reflected biomedical concepts in the Global North. One was the neurogenic interpretation, in which acupuncture was thought to work through an electrical action via the nervous system, or perhaps acted on the endocrine system and affected hormone levels. The other was the psychogenic interpretation, in which it acted as a form of hypnosis or otherwise invoked some kind of placebo effect. Either way, its truth was to be found in scientific models from the Global North, not traditional Asian models of treatment. And even the placebo effect seemed, as we have seen, to run against some practitioners' sense of what was 'real' scientific medicine.[68] But expectations matter; expectations shape how therapy is received and equally importantly how it is offered. Is 'empathy' hard baked into modern clinical medicine?

The Face of Acupuncture

Early in the post-Second World War fascination with acupuncture at least one physician attributed the efficacy of acupuncture anaesthesia in China to a combination of hypnosis and 'Chinese stoicism', asserting that American patients could not (or would not) bear the pain of an operation with only acupuncture to dull that pain. Racial difference becomes a central means of explaining the efficacy of acupuncture if it is not merely quackery and sleight-of-hand.

> Most of them believe that Chinese stoicism plus hypnosis are what makes acupuncture anesthesia seem to work. One writer told of his experience some years ago with a patient afflicted with a painful axillary abscess. The patient, a young psychologist, was told that a general anesthetic was indicated

for the necessary surgery. 'I won't need that', he replied. 'I'll use self hypnosis.' When preparations for the operation were completed, the patient asked for a brief delay. For a few minutes, he seemed lost in deep thought. Finally, he said softly, 'I'm ready.' During incision and drainage of the abscess, the patient's face remained immobile, eyes closed, his body perfectly still. Dressings applied, the surgeon said, 'That's all.' The patient opened his eyes, smiled, and thanked the physician . . . Although skepticism is a valuable trait in scientists and although no one has a sound explanation for the mechanism of acupuncture anesthesia, there have been enough anecdotal reports from reliable observers to justify research.[69]

This is merely a continuation of the stereotype of the inscrutable visage and therefore soul of the 'Oriental'. Such a view has a long history.

Before the American Civil War, the writer (and translator of Goethe's *Faust*) Bayard Taylor observed that the 'Orientals' had 'dull faces, without expression', filling him 'with an unconquerable aversion'.[70] They are inscrutable; as Senator John F. Miller's speech introducing the bill that would become the Chinese Exclusion Act (1882) states: 'It may seem strange that the apparently insignificant, dwarfed, leathery little man of the Orient should, in the peaceful contest for survival, drive the Anglo-Saxon from the field', but 'the American people are far more impressible than the stoical Chinese.'[71] What is at the core is

the challenge posed by the Chinese 'face'. By 'face', I refer to the Chinese concept that brings together individual composure and social relations, an alternative taxonomy of affective expression that troubles the colonial ruse of universal true feeling. The slippage between the Chinese face as concept and embodiment [evokes] the optical logics of American race science that was obsessed with faces, heads, and skulls and its confluence with sentimentalism as an ideology that lingers in white Anglo-American philosophical, scientific, and cultural considerations of feelings. Chinese faces and Oriental inscrutability . . . are intertwined in the genealogy of American-Chinese encounters.[72]

Pain and the inability or undesirability of showing pain is central to this image of the Chinese face.[73] But are these habits of culture, which could be learned by anyone, or is it a racial quality of the Chinese?

When Peter Parker (MD, Medical Institution of Yale College, 1834), in 1836, the first American medical missionary to arrive in China, began his treatments, they were part of the 'heroic age of medicine', especially surgical interventions, which were dangerous and painful: no antisepsis and certainly no modern anaesthesia. From then until he resigned from the 'Ophthalmic Infirmary' in Canton, he and his colleagues treated some 50,000 patients for a wide range of injuries and disease, from cataracts, which is why the hospital was so named, a procedure unknown beforehand in China, to tumours and leprosy. The English name of the hospital reflected the upcoming field of ophthalmology; its Chinese name was quite different, it was 'Pu Ai Yi Yuan', or the 'Hospital of Universal Love', which reflected Parker's sense of the missionary work his hospital was doing for its Chinese patients and Anglophone funders. The English name gestured as well to Christ's miracle of making the blind see and, as a missionary, Parker's role in making the 'heathen' Chinese into Protestants. His argument, when soliciting funds to create the hospital, was that the infirmities and the pain of the Chinese are no different than they would be if found in England. China's 'fevers are as burning – insanity as raving – leprosy as polluting – blindness as great – its cancer and stone as painful, and gout as excruciating', Parker told the readers of his fundraising letter,

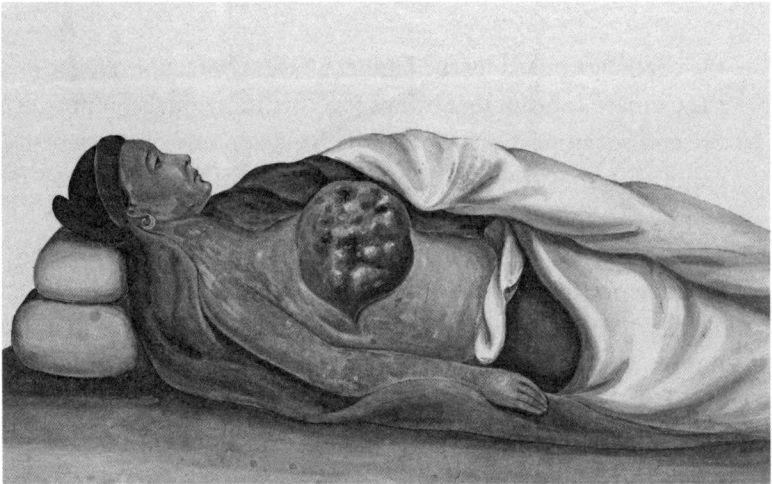

A 'stoic' patient with a breast tumour, c. 1837, gouache after Lam Qua.

'as they would be, if only the Mersey or the British Channel separated them from the skill and charity that could relieve them'.[74] This is a vital claim for the humanity of the Chinese, for the American S. Weir Mitchell, certainly one of the most visible physician-authors of the nineteenth century, had bemoaned that 'in our process of being civilized, we have won, I suspect, intensified capacity to suffer. The savage does not feel pain as we do'.[75]

Of course, we have seen this argument before concerning African Americans. Are the Chinese 'savages' or are they merely human beings with the same need for the amelioration of pain? Parker's notes on the patients' responses to surgery, prior to the introduction of anaesthesia, bear some attention: 'Woo She (case no. 4016), for the removal of a cancerous breast: "Her fortitude exceeded all that I have yet witnessed. She scarcely uttered a groan during the extirpation, and before she was removed from the table, clasped her hands and, with an unaffected smile, cordially thanked the gentlemen who assisted on the occasion."'[76] Is this 'Chinese stoicism' as observed in the reading of the efficacy of acupuncture as an anaesthetic or is it the social relationship between the colonizer and their patients, with the former in a position of power over the latter, analogous to that of the royal court or any other authority?[77] We note that Parker's mention of the man who says that 'It hurts, doctor' reflects a rupture between our expectations of how a patient should respond and 'the insouciant coolness of its "coolly" delivered form. The phrase calls attention to itself as a representation of pain that does not call formal attention to itself as a representation of pain'.[78]

Peter Parker undertook interventions over the next decades that were for the most part more extensive than the superficial removal of growths on the body that he began in the 1830s, well documented by the series of paintings of his patients by the Cantonese portraitist Lam Qua (Guan Qiaochang).[79] They, as Eric Hayot commented, 'present a Chinese relation to pain defined by the representation of a startling and quasi-heroic stoicism. And like the paintings, they generate that stoicism by presenting a startling disjunction between tumour and person, representation and likeness. The patients' "natural" voices, like the expressionless faces of the portraits, communicate again and again the act of non-translation (the non-act of translation?) whereby the objective evidence of pain does not appear in the subjective response to it'.[80] Pain is literally in the eye of the beholder.

We have a good account of this in a review of the Lam Qua paintings when they were shown in Boston in 1845, the reviewer no less than Oliver Wendell Holmes, Sr:

> These monstrous growths are very serious things to our fellow-creatures of the Celestial empire. But they are so out of all reasonable proportions, and sprout up in such strange shapes and places – and China is so far off, and a China man is so much an abstraction to our minds – and the almond-shaped eyes, the pigtail, the brown-sherry complexion and the Oriental environments of the sufferers, so blind us to the naked fact of the existence of an unsightly or devouring malady, that we cannot help looking at them with a little twitching about the levator anguli oris [the facial muscle which allows us to smile], which if not inhuman is at least highly unbecoming.[81]

How alien is the Chinese patient as seen in the paintings by Lam Qua? Frozen in space and time, no hint of discomfort while presenting with the most extraordinary tumours, they are distanced and exotic, so very different from Holmes's patients that all he can do is smile. His dead colleagues whom he mourns 'start from their slumbers no more at the cry of pain; they sally forth no more into the storms, they ride no longer over the lonely roads that knew them so well'. This is the ideal, the country doctor, and his 'good patient is one' who, 'having found a good physician, sticks to him till he dies'.[82] So very unlike Peter Parker's stoic patients.

But we have a remarkable way of testing this hypothesis, as Parker is the one who introduced ether into China after 1845. Parker notes that he had obtained 'a good supply of sulphuric Ether, with a letter from the latter gentleman' (Dr Charles T. Jackson, MD, Harvard Medical School, 1829, who had claimed to have discovered the aesthetic properties of ether) explaining particularly his mode of procedure, which he tested on a farmer: 'In forty-three seconds, the muscles of his arm suddenly relaxed and he ceased simultaneously to inhale the ether, and in a state of insensibility he was laid back upon the table his head still being elevated . . . [he] had no recollection of the incisions during the operation.'[83] He wrote further about his initial patient: 'The patient declared that though he knew the operation was being performed, he was scarcely sensible to the presence of the knife or needle. The same afternoon the tumor was extirpated, which weighed about a pound, he walked about the room, and as if nothing had happened. He slept quietly the following night.'[84] Medical practice in China had disavowed any opening of the body for religious reasons (and perhaps because of a perceived heightened danger). But there was always a contrast between missionary and indigenous medicine, upheld by both sides. And straddling them, the line between real medicine and the quack, is suspicion.

By the age of scientific medicine, prior to the First World War, the notion of 'Chinese pain' toleration became a question of class. The British missionary-physicians William Hamilton Jefferys, based in Shanghai, and James L. Maxwell, in Tainan, a small city on Taiwan, begin their account of contemporary medicine in China by disabusing readers of the 'very general impression among foreigners that the pain sense of the Asiatic, particularly the Mongolian races, is not nearly so highly developed as in other races of men. The statement is made that this is so, not only by laymen, but widely by physicians.'[85] And:

> Surgeons will, if they differentiate in the matter, observe that the Chinese, with the exception of practically all but the coolie class, suffer mentally and physically, are as restless and impatient, as fussy and exacting as the average white patient, and the Chinese patient of the upper classes will compare favorably in difficulty of control with the pampered neurotic and passé fad-indulged food hypochondriac of Boston. It is the coolie classes that give the opposite impression, and with them it is not a question of suffering less pain, but of bearing it better. They are inured to lives of want, hard conditions, struggle, and cheerful submissions. They expect to suffer and expect little relief and care.[86]

Now, the argument is not that 'they are just like the rest of us', but that the extremes reflect the extremes in American culture; not the most wealthy and self-indulgent, but 'the coolie's mechanical indifference to pain' is a quality of the lived experience on the margin of society. And they comment that this may be shifting as 'the nineteenth-century term coolie has been retired by more politic regimes of racial governance.'[87]

The doctor's obliviousness to pain unseen or unheard remains: 'We read once of a certain clinic in China, which had better remain nameless, where the surgeon opened so many abscesses, even amputated fingers, without using any anæsthetic, "because the patients seemed to suffer so little pain." Our private opinion is that the imagination and mental acumen of the said surgeon would have fitted him for transmigration into the future habitation of a pincushion."[88] That stoicism, that oft-misused term, becomes a reading in the Global North for obliviousness of the structure of the world that the Western physicians and their patients inhabited.

During the Cold War, the idea of 'Oriental inscrutability' was easily adapted to the political rhetoric of the time, where 'suspicion' was the hallmark of that to be feared when in 1971 acupuncture came into Western focus.[89] Thus 'if suspicion contoured the cold war paradigm of evidence, then the inscrutable Oriental offers a unique opportunity to explore how racial perception informed the parameters of credible intelligence and the benchmarks for reliable friends.'[90] Or, indeed, our conflicted readings of acupuncture. For suspicion and trust is also the line between quack and doc. While acupuncture had its advocates, especially among those who wished to alleviate the suspicions of the Cold War, others flatly refused to consider acupuncture as something other than communist indoctrination. 'I am appalled by the fact that physicians . . . would go to Red China and come back sounding like converts to Mao Tse Tung's teachings,' wrote one doctor to the AMA's Bureau of Investigation. 'Certainly if acupuncture is a reality then who are we to say that chiropractic and naturopathic teachings are not correct.'[91] Quacks all.

Placebos

But what nonsense, we all *know* that acupuncture is merely a placebo! And therefore, pure quackery! This is the most damning claim that the opponents of acupuncture believed that they could make.[92] If acupuncture is 'merely' the placebo effect writ large, then no empirical evidence had any value, as 'it was all in their minds.'[93] Very early on in the debates about the efficacy of acupuncture, the charge was lodged that acupuncture is quackery because it is *merely* the placebo effect. And the placebo effect was an artefact of the bad old days before 'real' (scientific, bench-science-based) medicine proved that it was quackery. Indeed, it seemed, even in Greco-Roman medicine, to have its roots in the most 'primitive', and therefore least scientific, medical traditions.[94]

While European medicine became more 'scientific' and secular from the mid-seventeenth century onwards, residues of Christian/magical medicine remained outside of (and sometimes within) elite practices well into the nineteenth century. Following Max Weber, magic, and the fear of deception attendant on it, coloured medical responses to placebos.[95]

In that awful age of 'therapeutic nihilism' before we had *real* medicine based on *real* science, placebos were a consistent form of bad practice on the part of healers and the gullibility of the patients, is the claim in our age of scientific medicine. No quacks here anymore; no more marks. As the Pulitzer Prize-winning physician-author Siddhartha Mukherjee (MD, Harvard School of Medicine, 2000), contributor to the *New Yorker*, faculty member at Columbia University School of Medicine, widely cited popular historian of medicine, stated quite boldly in the printed version of his TED talk on modern medicine:

> We tend to forget that much of 'modern medicine' is, in fact, surprisingly modern: before the 1930s, you would be hard-pressed to identify a single medical intervention that had any more than a negligible impact on the course of any illness (surgery, in contrast, could have a transformative effect; think of an appendectomy for appendicitis, or an amputation for gangrene). Nearly every medical intervention could be categorized as one of three P's – placebo, palliation and plumbing. Placebos were, of course, the most common of drugs – 'medicines' that caused their effects by virtue of psychological or psychosomatic reactions in patients (elixirs for weakness and aging, or tonics for depression). Palliative drugs, in contrast, were often genuinely effective; they included morphine, opium, alcohol and various tinctures, poultices and balms used to ameliorate symptoms such as itching and pain. The final category – I've loosely labelled it 'plumbing' – included laxatives, purgatives, emetics, and enemas used to purge the stomach and intestines of their contents to relieve constipation and, occasionally, to disgorge poisons. These worked, although they were of limited use in most medical cases. (In an epic perversion, the tool and the therapy were often inverted. Purging was a common medical intervention in the nineteenth century not because it was particularly effective, but because it

was one of the few things that doctors could actually achieve through medicines; if you had a hammer, as the saying goes, then everything looks like a nail.)[96]

No wonder scientific medicine today is dismissive of anything that smacks of a 'placebo' (meaning 'I please'), a term from exactly this age of the three Ps, of heroic medicine, in the late eighteenth century to describe 'commonplace', potentially inert substances given to placate the patient, so one theory went, while the healing power of nature was allowed to take its course.[97]

Remembering how William Blackstone noted that one could sue if one was called a quack, in 1789 the British politician Warren Hastings, who de facto governed India and was impeached for his actions, was labelled by 'his contemporaries . . . flatterer, liar, sycophant, placebo, snake in the grass'.[98] 'Placebo' here is the equivalent to 'quack'. That this term of opprobrium had its origin in the public sphere of Hastings's day was clear. But medicine in the Enlightenment took on a slightly more benign cast. George Motherby's *A New Medical Dictionary* of 1785, from the age of Hastings, simply defined the term for the very first time in a medical context as 'a common-place method or medicine calculated to amuse for a time, rather than for any purpose'.[99] Another medical dictionary of the day defined placebo thus: '*Placebo* . . . an epithet given to any medicine adapted more to please than benefit the patient'.[100] It was, by the age of Sir Walter Scott, seen as so: 'nothing serious intended – a mere *placebo* – just a divertisement to cheer the spirits, and assist the effect of the waters'.[101] The first mention of 'placebo' in *The Lancet* is in 1825 in regard to the use of 'the compound decoction of the sarsaparilla. Some think it a placebo; others have a very high opinion of its efficacy' regarding the treatment of 'irritable ulcer' of the skin.[102] And even the Americans at the time of the American Civil War knew that 'to secure the moral effect of a remedy given specially for the disease, the patients were placed on the use of a placebo, which consisted, in nearly all of the cases, of the tincture of quassia, very largely diluted. This was given regularly and became well known in my wards as the placeboic remedy for rheumatism'.[103] Such placebos may well have fooled a patient in the age of 'therapeutic nihilism', but by the 1930s medicine knew better, and it knew that such interventions lay in the past and with more 'primitive' peoples.

Doctors' goals in that distant past and among the 'primitives' sought 'by words of cheer and comfort . . . to please the patient . . . [The doctor's] medicines were merely symbols to reinforce this purpose.' The placebo is an answer 'to gratify the patient's desire for active intervention, but which is understood by the doctor to be inert and useless. For example, a bogus puncture.' But the internist W. R. Houston, addressing the American College of Physicians in St Louis in 1937, argues there is 'a second sort of placebo, which seems to be no less a placebo, in the employment of which the patient's attitude is the same, but where the doctor's attitude differs in that though the procedure is valueless, the doctor esteems it to be valuable. For example, an ovarian tablet.' In other words, resting on the ignorance of the physician, but not quite quackery. And this, seen from the 1930s, hypes the kind of intervention

which the doctor fancies to be an effective medicament but which later investigation proves to have been all along inert, . . . [and] is the banner under which a large part of the history of medicine may be enrolled. The herbs of the Indians, the pharmacopeias of the Orient, a large part of the contents of our older books on medicine are made up of these placebos in which doctors erroneously had faith. Their usefulness was in direct proportion to the faith that the doctor had and the faith that he was able to inspire in his patients.

Most lethal is a third type of placebo, which, 'while it is believed in by the doctor, is no longer harmless but harmful, sometimes very dangerous. It would seem peculiarly contradictory to speak of the painful and dangerous placebo, yet men are so constituted that they feel the need in dire extremity of resorting to dread measures. Nervous patients, in particular, feel that a certain standing and sanction is bestowed on their maladies.'[104] Mental remedies for mental illnesses?

By the 1930s, in the age of Flexner, medicine knew better than the 'Indians' and the 'Orientals', knew much better than the physician before the age of scientific medicine. And yet the tradition that placebos pleased the patient, made them happy, rather than curing them, that it was a form of quackery, persisted well into our own era. 'The emergence in the late eighteenth century and, especially, in the nineteenth century of the phenomenon of pathological pleasure that resembled non-pathological pleasure threatened to overturn – in the form of a consolation withheld – centuries or millennia-old assumptions about the recognizability of degrees of health through pleasure.[105] Placebos seemed to make this danger concrete.

Oliver Wendell Holmes, Sr, denounced homeopathy, which appeared to him the most evident form of quackery, in several essays running from 1842 to the 1860s.[106] But Holmes also recognized, in a talk of 1860 given as an address to the Massachusetts Medical Society at their annual meeting on 30 May 1860, that the practice of all medicine is largely faddish; this idea elicited outcry in the medical community, which he takes as proof that it had touched a 'weak spot in a profession'.[107] As for the therapist, Holmes was convinced that after a time those advocating such interventions would be forced by the pressure of the professional world to rejoin allopathic practice, for good or for ill, for 'the ultra Homeopathist will either recant and try to rejoin the medical profession; or he will embrace some newer and if possible equally extravagant doctrine; or he will stick to his colors and go down with his sinking doctrine'.[108] But was it professional to use such interventions in the age of scientific medicine?

Holmes wanted to discount the new objective role of the medical scientist as the distant observer par excellence in the light of the ever-greater role that technology played in diagnosis and therapy thereafter. Yet as Stanley Joel Reiser in his groundbreaking *Medicine and the Reign of Technology* noted about the introduction of non-invasive technology into medicine, patients associated such medical tools with the unfortunate results attributed to the surgeon in the age of heroic medicine: pain and infection.[109] Physicians shied away from such technology for they feared it would lower their social standing compared to that of their surgical colleagues. Only as the techniques became more and more common and the ability to differentiate the subtle changes within the body increased, did such technology come both to be accepted and to be expected. And when it did its impact was explosive, as Reiser notes: 'the effects of the stethoscope on physicians were analogous to the effects of printing on Western culture. Print and the reproducible book had created a new private world for man . . . Similarly, auscultation helped to create the objective physician, who could move away from involvement with the patient's experiences and sensations, to a more detached relation, less with the patient but more with the sounds from within the body . . . sounds that he believed to be objective, bias-free representations of the disease process.'[110] Technology – isolated from pain and infection – literally created distance, and distance reinforced notions of objectivity.

In an early lecture, 'Position and Prospects of the Medical Student' (1844), Oliver Wendell Holmes, Sr, had written that 'A just classification, like the lens in an optical instrument, converges and brings into a clear image the scattered and refracted rays of individual observation.'[111] But he also cautions, 'beware how you commit yourself in a too confident prognosis! . . . Remember that the errors of stethoscopists spring much oftener from the faults of their brains than of their ears.'[112] The trouble, he suggests, is the move from 'observation' to 'inference'. A prognosis, then, is at best an observationally based narrative, and at worst a total fiction. His contemporary, the British neurologist Sir John Russell Reynolds (MD, University College London, 1852), concurred about the pitfalls of modern, scientific technology placed in the wrong hands (and brains): 'I have known distinguished surgeons go down into the country to say whether or not a patient with rheumatic fever had endo- or pericarditis, when neither of them would know which end of the stethoscope to use.'[113] Technology, it is argued, is never a substitute for 'hands-on' clinical experience.

Superstitions abound in medicine, and doctors and patients alike are too likely to have faith in the curative power of pills – Holmes speaks about what would be called the placebo effect, in which people's beliefs about whether a cure will work decide whether it will work. In a lecture to Harvard graduates in 1858, he advocated in some circumstances to 'medicate' the truth 'with the deadly poison of honest fraud'.[114] The oxymoron of 'honest fraud' highlights the conundrums facing allopathy's attempts to distance itself from the quackery of homeopathy, a quackery which rests on the general assumption of a placebo defrauding patients and removing them from the care of allopathic physicians who could at least apply their sense of the scientific to each case. By 1890, in *The Lancet*, Frederick Simms (MB, King's College, London, 1866, MRCP) picked up the discussion raised earlier by Oliver Wendell Holmes, Sr, on homeopathy and quackery, using placebos as his example. Homeopaths, according to Simms, are 'honest, though irregular, professional men'.[115] Alternative therapies understood now as placebos, if practised by licensed and regulated physicians, seem to be tolerated. Perhaps in the case of homeopathy because it does no direct harm, though as other critics at the time noted, it discouraged patients from seeking other therapies. And because we as physicians understand that some of our therapies are indeed placebos.

We can see here that the notion of 'quackery' has been employed by those holding a dominant position (in any realm of medical science or its political overseers) as a rhetorical weapon against those who threaten their dominance. Because the empirical foundation of that dominance is, at best, always shaky and as science inherently desires to be a corrective process, even the corrections are always at risk of revision. This shakiness is more common than many acknowledge – even in handsomely rewarded and culturally venerated 'established' fields or specialties, where in a denotative (rather than connotative) sense, everyone is a quack. But it's the 'quacks' with the most power who wield that power to label their opponents/competitors 'quacks'. What was it Sigmund Freud said at the end of his 1927 work *Future of an Illusion*: 'No, our science is no illusion. But an illusion it would be to suppose that what science cannot give us we can get elsewhere.'[116] While, of course, understanding psychoanalysis as a science.

At the same moment, Alexander Wilder (MD, Homeopathic Medical College of New York, 1867), writing in one of the anti-science periodicals of the day and taking exactly the opposite stance to Holmes on the issue of homeopathy, argued that every such claim is

> hated on sight and denounced; then it is endured from familiarity, afterward pitied, and sympathized with, and finally embraced and accepted. Many are the remedies and methods which were scouted and denounced, and the advocates fined and imprisoned; after which some member of the dominant party perceiving merit in the innovation, and perhaps some hope of profit and reputation, ventured to 'introduce' it to the 'regular' profession. It then became 'scientific', which, in conventional usage, means orthodox. The real introducer, however, is all the time ignored or belied, and generally denounced by the slang-term of medical men, 'quack', – a term that only a time-server, without the instincts of a gentleman, ever employs.[117]

Wilder notes that one cannot condemn these new interventions that rely on human psychology, for 'some procedures of physicians, like administering bread pills, are analogous tricks.'[118] Placebos all.

The opponents of a radical scientific medicine that excluded the psyche, or the soul, had a broad and attentive public audience by the 1920s. Erwin Liek, the surgeon, homeopath and popular writer about such topics in Weimar Germany, bemoaned the objective role that had frozen the 'natural' relations between physician and patient and had to 'be such that the physician has always and under all circumstances the feeling that he stands above the patient, that he occupies a position of authority and that he confers benefits upon him'. What enabled all medicine, including placebos, to work was the impact of the physician's charisma and personality. Most disease was cured through the influence physicians had on the patients' souls rather than on their bodies. Liek stressed that he was all in favour of true science, but due to the rise of a scientific establishment and the infatuation of modern medicine with technology, he argued, many medics had lost or never acquired the ability to use the magic which characterized the true physician. He preferred to use the German word *Zauber* – magic – over the technical term 'Suggestion'. In contrast, he argued, heterodox healers or 'quacks' cured disease exactly because they believed in their own magic abilities.[119]

What is interesting – at least to me – is the 'confidence game' that not only quacks but (in the case of modern medicine) mainstream physicians play in seeking to win their patients' trust in all therapies, not just acupuncture. Every healing encounter involves, if not a shared understanding, then certainly a trusting relationship between, at a minimum, two people: a suffering soul and an authority laying claim to the expertise believed necessary to quiet that suffering. Whether that expertise is deserved or rooted in some underlying empirical foundation matters little so long as trust exists between the one who is suffering (or those involved in his or her care, such as family) and the one who promises relief. All therapies reflect the belief of the patient in the status of the physicians, as 'whatever happens when a patient gets better after ingesting a sugar pill also happens to some degree whenever the patient receives a pharmacologically potent treatment within a supportive healing relationship; that at least some of the symptom relief that follows administration of the active treatment arises from emotional and symbolic factors. That is, the placebo effect pervades much of medical practice even when no placebo has been used.'[120] It helps, of course, if a positive outcome results from the interaction. But a positive outcome is rarely, if ever, required to maintain that trust. As poet Emily Dickinson quite correctly claimed in the age of modern science, the age of Oliver Wendell Holmes, Sr, faith surpasses science 99 out of 100 times, but in the end trust *the* science:

> Faith is fine invention
> When gentlemen can see
> But microscopes are prudent
> In an emergency.[121]

Homeopathy remains the test case for alternative medicine throughout the nineteenth century and the changing status of such medical practices. Beginning as a non-invasive alternative to heroic medicine, which was characterized by bleeding the patient, it came in the Third Reich to be transformed, as we discussed in our opening chapter, into a segment of the 'New German Therapeutics' as the Nazi state's answer to allopathic medicine. By the 1960s it came to be part of the anti-allopathic counterculture. Chiropractic and osteopathy, which arose in the 1880s, were often paired with homeopathy in the world of scientific medicine. Yet their trajectories reflect how the boundary of quackery shifts and shifts again as allopathic medicine becomes defined and then redefined during the nineteenth and twentieth centuries.[122]

Chiropractic remains self-consciously a form of alternative medical therapy, while, as we noted, osteopathy blended its training function into those demanded by the Flexner Report. 'Traditional Chinese Medicine' too is based on the model of allopathic medicine and becomes first a part of the counterculture in the Global North and then integrated into allopathic medicine by the end of the twentieth century, following the lead of osteopathy. Homeopathy remains consistently beyond the pale of allopathic medicine, to be found by the twenty-first century not in medical clinics but in health food stores.

As acupuncture was being touted as a cure-all in the 1970s, suddenly psychiatrists and psychoanalysts began to wonder whether the impact was not physiological but psychological, whether placebos, 'faith', were 'real' medicine after all. As one paper of the day claimed that the success of acupuncture is a 'placebo effect' owing to 'the power of suggestion' for 'it is "well known that some patients are readily suggestible" and will respond to almost any remedy, including acupuncture'.[123] Granted that acupuncture may one day be proven to have a specific value that is scientifically explainable; as a New York acupuncturist admits, 'a psychological factor is indeed involved in any medical treatment.'[124] He argues that, in this age of antibiotics and the beginning of psychotropic pharmaceuticals, 'Those who make the greatest use of placebo suggestions often deny their existence. The apparent resistance to understanding the nature of the placebo response is understandable. Physicians certainly would rather not understand a phenomenon that showed that many of their treatments were effective not because of their knowledge, skill or ability, but because of a universal power of suggestion.'[125]

But 'faith' and 'science' seem actually to be linked in the case of acupuncture, linked if only by the claims of TCM to the status of modern medicine. In the 1970s the sense was that one could not withhold experimental treatment such as acupuncture if there was a chance it could be effective. Indeed, the moral claims against such double-blind studies remain always close to the surface. When an intervention is seen to have markedly positive outcomes, such studies are often dissolved, and all the participants given the 'real' intervention rather than the inert alternative. What if the placebo is the real thing? Indeed, the demand that acupuncture fulfil the criteria for 'real' bench science leads the authors of studies which seem, using a double-blind test, to verify that acupuncture is effective to claim that 'in view of the many unsubstantiated claims made about acupuncture, it is essential that it be investigated by objective factors. Contrary to other reports, our results suggest that acupuncture may be more than a placebo phenomenon.'[126] But this is in the light of the necessary assumption that a placebo is not real medicine but rather a sort of parlour trick, a trick that seemed at the moment not to be proven using the claims of evidence-based medicine.

Yet acupuncture takes on the mantle of scientific psychology explaining placebos, as in one particular randomized controlled trial, based on a series of experiments with fibromyalgia patients, which claimed that a placebo functioning as an analgesia was the result of prior experience of pain relief, and that a social interaction with a trustworthy clinician may have added to its efficacy.[127] In addition, this study examined the relationship between placebo analgesia and the time (months, years) a person had been exposed to chronic disease, by assessing placebo responses in a pharmacological trial in patients with fibromyalgia. The earlier the intervention, the more effective the placebo effect, as in chronic diseases such as fibromyalgia expectations of relief diminish over time. And this impacted on the efficacy of drug therapy for pain relief in chronic sufferers of fibromyalgia. The irony was that when all the participants in a clinical trial with a control group that knew that half of them would be getting a placebo, the actual drug was *less* effective than in an open-label situation where 100 per cent of the participants knew that they were getting the real drug. It seems that in the first trial, many suspected that they were getting *merely* a placebo, which they imagined would not be effective, even if they were given the actual drug. Context matters: the belief in the power of the physician adds to the efficacy of the drug, or perhaps it's the corollary – knowing that you might be getting a placebo diminishes it.

By the twenty-first century the idea of the placebo is well established within scientific medicine, either as a technique or a bugbear. The law quickly tries to catch up. If it is the former, no problem, its efficacy is based on 'science' as well as patient response, but what if it is the latter: merely a medical fraud – medical malpractice hiding under the aegis of an untested theory? In 2006 the AMA condemned the use of 'deceptive placebos' without a patient's consent (evoking the basic ethical principle of informed consent established with the 1946 Doctors' Trial at Nuremberg and the 1976 Belmont Report on dealing with human subjects, which resulted from it). For the AMA the idea of bench-science evidence is at the core of its definition of a placebo: 'a substance provided to a patient that the physician believes has no specific pharmacological effect upon the condition being treated.'[128] And this triggered a similar discussion in the United Kingdom.[129] But of course, it would not be a placebo if the physician had the patient's consent.[130] 'So, suppose that a doctor gives a patient unmarked sugar pills and says, "A number of research studies suggest that these pills can help your pain." While the doctor has not uttered any factually false statements, assuming the patient accepts the pills under the conventional understanding that they contain active medication, the patient has nevertheless been deceived. In such cases, it would be incorrect to say that the patient was "informed of" and "agrees to" use the *placebo*, as the AMA requires.'[131]

Perhaps it wouldn't be a placebo if the physician truly believed the intervention to be effective. But what then is a placebo? We can think of the sugar water and saline injections as examples, but certainly more frequently we see antibiotics or vitamin supplements serving that purpose, and thus enriching the pharmaceutical industry and causing, perhaps, long-lasting harm through antibiotic resistance.

At the core of the AMA's concern, and here we can extrapolate this not only to the concern of professional organizations but to allopathic medicine in general, is whether deception is a moral error of the physician. Can one lie to one's patients, for what you believe to be their own good, or does this make you a quack? Even if a large minority, some 35 per cent of patients at mid-century were 'satisfactorily relieved by a placebo'.[132] Yet the most recent conversation about the morality of deception in the case of placebos has stressed 'their limited clinical utility and their implications for health, trust, and autonomy', and that 'in the vast majority of the cases the use of deceptive placebos is unjustifiable and thus unethical. Aside from a few exceptional cases, doctors have no good reason to use deceptive placebos.'[133] In other words, if they did work better, we should forgive their use in the twenty-first century, but as the author then concludes: 'we are all to some extent familiar with the benefits that situational deception may offer; prescribing impure placebos is very easy for doctors, and sometimes it may spare them a lot of time and effort.' And this was already, as we have seen, true before and at the very beginning of scientific medicine, if Oliver Wendell Holmes, Sr, and Frederick Simms are to be believed. Efficacy at all costs contradicts the ongoing fantasy of the benevolent physician whose motivation was and is solely ethical treatment, even if the treatment is rooted in deceiving the patient. Indeed, the debates about informing patients concerning the modalities of treatment extend to the use of placebos, as one study suggests: 'doctors may best benefit from placebo effects by influencing the patient's expectations through communication. An important principle is to give the patient information stating that a particular treatment is effective, as long as this is based on realistic optimism. A patient-centered style involving elements such as developing trust and respect, exploring the patient's values, speaking positively about treatments, and providing reassurance and encouragement might aid in activating placebo effects.' This, of course, vitiates the very use of placebos. Inform your patient that they must have 'an imagination of a specific outcome' and they will ask: why are you not giving me a 'real' treatment?[134]

The placebo thus confronts us with a differing perspective of the relationship between therapist and patient: 'those who deceive and those who are deceived tend to appraise the moral implications of

the same deceptive act in two dramatically different ways: the deceiv-
ers tend to justify and excuse their behavior, while the deceived tend
instead to magnify its negative implications.'[135] Unless, of course, the
patient's response is positive if the outcome matches their expectations. And here we return to not only why the placebo is employed
but equally what the expectations are when those of the therapist and
patients concur and when they are at odds. For 'when patients believe
that a therapy will work, their belief is capable of rendering it surprisingly efficacious; when doctors believe a therapy will work their
confidence is consistently transferred to the patient . . . If you change
the size or the colour of a pill, or the number of times a day it is administered, you alter its effectiveness. Patients who faithfully follow their
doctors' instructions do better than those who do not, even if the pills
they are being instructed to take are inert.'[136] Does the use or the avoidance of such an intervention put you as a practitioner over the ethical
line? Are you committing medical fraud (quackery) or merely malpractice? Patients, at least in the United States, cannot sue for fraud
if they discover that a placebo has been used while they believed that
some form of active intervention was taking place. But if they have
negative side-effects (say, to the supposedly inert substance used) they
can sue for malpractice. The law recognizes placebo therapy as therapy,
as when the Missouri Court of Appeals found that placebos are 'a recognized form of medical treatment' and quoted an expert witness who
said that you never tell a patient you are giving him a placebo because
'you are hoping that you will fool him.' The court then affirmed a lower
court's directed verdict against the plaintiff in question, expressing
doubts that he presented a fraud claim for being given a sugar pill to
treat his back pain. The court concluded that he more properly raised
a question of malpractice, not fraud.[137] Acupuncture straddled this
dilemma by rejecting the charge that it was 'merely' a placebo; it was
rather a scientifically validated therapy.

This has a long history. Alexander Wood (MD, University of
Edinburgh, 1839), the inventor of the modern hypodermic needle,
reported that he could cure the pain of neuralgia with injections of
morphine into the tender spot (1858). The relief these patients secured,
he claimed, was as much from the new scientific technology of the
injection as from the pharmacological effect of the drug.[138] This is
what we can label 'epistemic switches', a term Richard Wollheim
coined in relation to a thought experiment by the British philosopher

A. J. Ayer, which concerned a man whose knowledge of something was initially based on the testimony of others, until he found the source of it – unchanged in content – in his own memory. For Wollheim, an 'epistemic switch' referred to a change in the reasons for a true belief.[139] What if tricking the mind really does have the sort of efficacy that acupuncture promises?[140] And what if pain is one of the pathological symptoms that is well suited to such interventions as it is context specific?

White Coat Effects

Technology in the age of scientific medicine defined the boundary between the normal and the pathological. And this began to reshape the role of the physician during the late nineteenth and early twentieth centuries. Physicians became those specialists who had command of objective, technological modes of diagnosis and therapy. They, in complex ways, became an extension of their machines. The physician/novelist Abraham Verghese (MD, Madras University School of Medicine, 1980) observed that, while he was growing up, his 'uncle's doctor's bag' in India was 'almost like a trunk – a mobile office'. It was the world of the local, empathetic practitioner, who cared. Over time he added more and more technological innovations, and his 'bag' grew exponentially. The more the technology, the better the doctors, he claims: 'As technology advances and gets more portable, I see us bringing more tools to the bedside, and therefore spending more time with patients, instead of sending them hither and thither to diagnostic suites. The more time with the patient, the better.' But is the romance of the new technology merely a reflection of the technology that seems to improve but also isolates? More time staring at the records on the iPad and less time interacting with the patient may not be a utopian solution for the doctor, even with a 'modified messenger bag'.[141] And the more the technology, the less attention one does seem to pay to the patient.

Let us return to the 1930s as the assumptions about the scientific (bench-science) nature of evidence hardened. We find ourselves in Boston, USA, with the first true generation of cardiologists, such as Theodore Janeway (MD, College of Physicians and Surgeons, Columbia University, 1895; first full-time Professor of Medicine at Johns Hopkins School of Medicine) as well as the surgeon Harvey Cushing (MD,

Harvard School of Medicine, 1895; one of the first self-proclaimed
'cardiologists', as of 1912 teaching at Harvard). Our focus is on David
Ayman, trained at Harvard, both with a BA (1922) and an MD (1926),
and then for over a decade the head of the hypertension clinic at Beth
Israel Hospital in Boston as well as serving as a faculty member of the
Tufts School of Medicine.[142] In other words, well enough established
as a Jewish physician (who just missed the institution of Jewish quotas
at Harvard) in the post-Flexner world not only of scientific medicine
but the new yet no longer contested specialty of cardiovascular medicine and hypertension. He was a serious bench-based clinician in the
age which had, after the rediscovery of Mendelian genetics in 1900,
become fascinated with the not yet completely understood genetic aetiology of illness. The assumption at the time was that hypertension (after
the model of Huntington's disease) was thought to be inherited as a
single Mendelian dominant gene. But these earlier studies did not even
include blood pressure data, the basic building block of such a claim.
Ayman made meticulous measurements personally of each member
of three generations of a single family and of their mates. He subsequently published his blood pressure measurements of 1,524 members
of 277 families.[143] Real science in the age of real statistical argument.
Thus, in his meticulous way, he refuted the single-gene hypothesis.[144]

Yet Ayman seemed to be innately suspicious of the existing manner
of describing the very nature, diagnosis and treatment of hypertension,
a fact (combined with his Jewish identity) that probably led to his
overall exclusion during his career from the most prestigious teaching and research positions. Indeed by 1970 he had founded his own
independent cardiovascular clinic in Boston, where he practised until
the early 1980s.

In the late 1920s, he quickly realized that the science that claimed
a 'hypertension gene' was not much better than the drug treatments
offered to his patients. Indeed, in a paper published in 1930, he examined the widest range of interventions for symptoms associated with
essential hypertension. He argued that they are more easily relieved
when blood pressures were lowered, and that this relief may be
obtained using any of numerous drugs and methods. It is not probable, he thought, that each of these drugs has a specific action. 'It is
more reasonable to believe that there is a common and specific factor
associated with the administration of these drugs. I believe that this
common element is the enthusiastic giving or doing something to the

patient – it is treatment, regardless of its nature.'[145] His experiment was rather simple. He administered diluted hydrochloric acid to those presenting with hypertension, something that was not an accepted therapy and should have had absolutely no effect on the symptoms – but achieved an astounding 82 per cent rate of symptomatic relief. He recognized that, in his patients, their symptoms 'must be related definitely to a disorder in the psychic sphere; otherwise, all these methods (of suggestion) could hardly relieve the symptoms. There can be little doubt that the author's "treatment" is only a suggestion.'[146] A placebo? If so, some 25 years before Henry Beecher (MD, Harvard Medical School, 1932), who is generally credited with identifying the placebo effect on pain, replacing morphine treating wounded soldiers in the Second World War with saline solution, when he ran out of the former.[147]

Even more than that: following this claim was the second part of his article, which argued something even more revolutionary: that the technology reflected other variables than those supposedly being measured by the mercury sphygmomanometer. He noted that blood pressure was lower in the morning than in the evening, but that it was 'lower in a quiet room than in a noisy room. When someone enters a quiet room in which blood pressure was being recorded, the blood pressure may rise. If the patient suddenly becomes preoccupied with a disturbing thought, the blood pressure similarly may become elevated.'[148] He postulated even differences in seasons, a factor that was documented decades later.[149] Most importantly, he understood (and showed) that taking one's blood pressure at home rather than having it taken in the clinic setting appreciably lowered the readings.[150] Ayman describes what he labels the 'hypertensive personality', but sees these claims about context as ubiquitous to all of his patients.[151] All treatment can have repercussions (positive or negative), but the treatment needs to be a compact between the therapist and the patient.

Medicine does recognize, if marginally, the 'nocebo effect', when a patient fears a negative outcome if there is a belief that any given therapy will cause harm. Nocebo, a formation mimicking placebo, was coined by Walter Kennedy in 1961 (Latin *nocēbō*, 'I shall harm', from *noceō*, 'I harm').[152] This echoed a theme we have been following: the idea that the physician should 'do no harm.' In an odd way this threw the obligation back on the patient not even to imagine that harm could befall them through a prescribed therapy. The 'white coat' effect was read as something quite different. It seemed to measure the negative role of the physician in the mental life of the patient.[153]

'White coat hypertension' has been generally interpreted as an authority effect, but it is also a powerful negative placebo. Nocebo as a concept is an outlier in evidence-based medicine because of the massively positive mainstream medical bias regarding treatment effects that operates all around us. This assumes that people will respond to the physician's treatments, in part because they are predisposed to do so as part of the overall assumptions of scientific efficacy as well as the trust in the physician that these claims generate. But, as we know, for people with chronic, unremitting problems *made worse* by medical treatments, the negative bias effect of experience via 'expectation effects' are palpable, as in the case of Ayman's patients.

Now, Ayman's work was on the cusp of the takeover of medical diagnosis more and more by technologies. His image of the productive physician is that of the doctor with his 'black bag'. Thus he saw the home as a surrogate for the house call and the clinic as a poor replacement. He labels this 'the fact that the doctor is a form of standard pressor stimulus like breath-holding or cold. On removal of this stimulus and the determination of the blood pressure at home by a member of the household or the patient himself, the hypertensive effect of therapy becomes evident . . . It is our experience that a patient with essential hypertension can no more become non-reactive to the physician by repeated visits than he can become non-reactive to the pressor test of cold or breath-holding.'[154] So placebos can be negative as well as positive. We can manipulate the symptoms to exacerbate or reduce them by the very situations in which the patient and the therapist are to be found.

Dress Matters

The 'white coat effect' seems to prove the old social claim that we are what we wear. But it also showed that we react to what others wear too, for good or for ill, and not only in popular culture. The white coat effect is a reflex of the age of modern medicine. It is the other side of the coin from the placebo effect, which is generally defined as curative; the white coat effect is generally defined as exacerbating symptoms, yet it also functions in defining the line between patient and physician. Introduced as a laboratory coat, the dress of the bench scientist

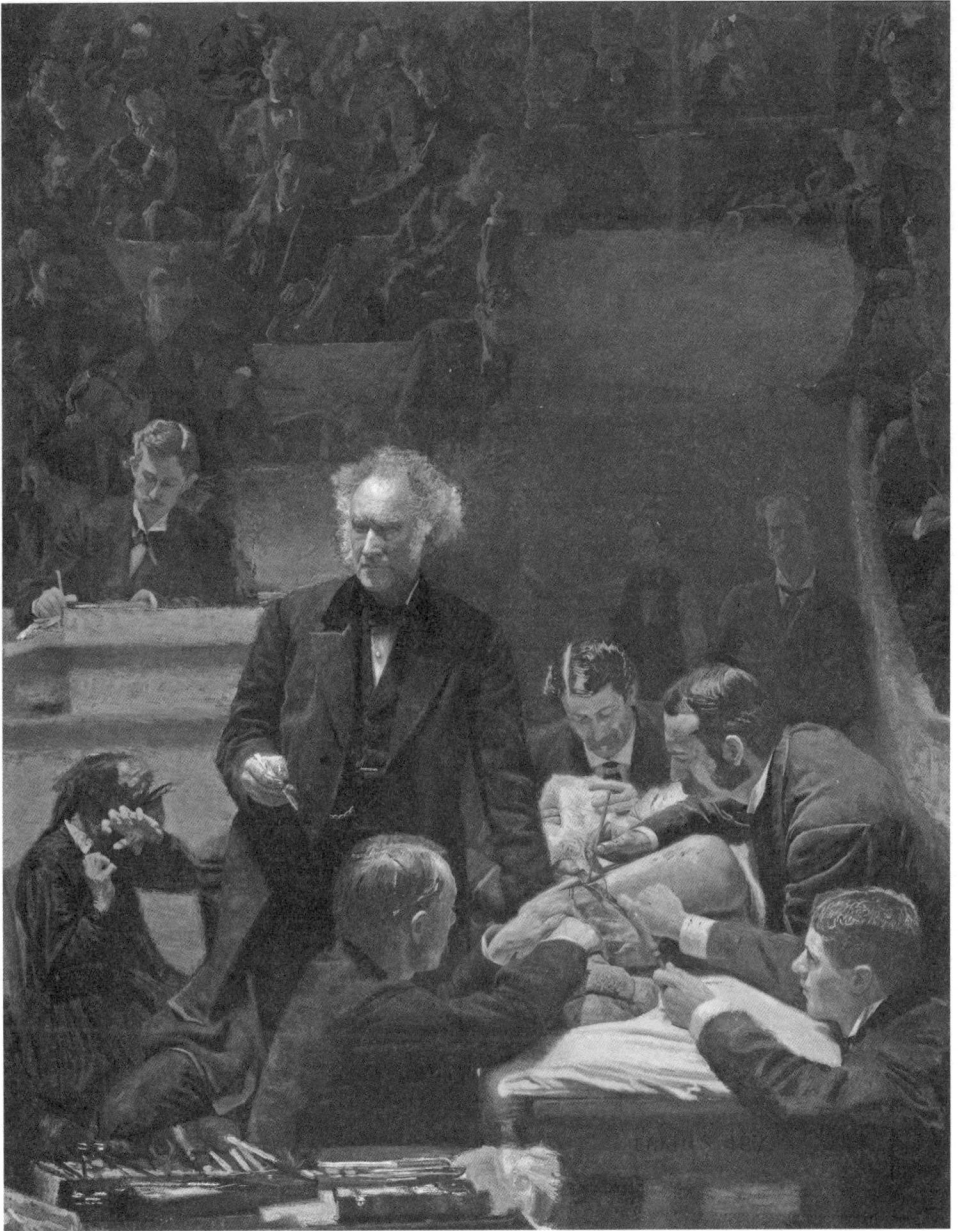

Thomas Eakins, *The Gross Clinic*, 1875, oil on canvas. Dr Samuel D. Gross, dressed in a black frock coat, is shown lecturing a group of Jefferson Medical College students and leading a clinic of five doctors operating on the left thigh of a patient. Included among the group is a self-portrait of Eakins, who is seen at the right-hand side of the painting, next to the tunnel railing, with a white cuffed sleeve sketching or writing. Seen over Gross's right shoulder is the clinic clerk, Franklin West, taking notes on the operation.

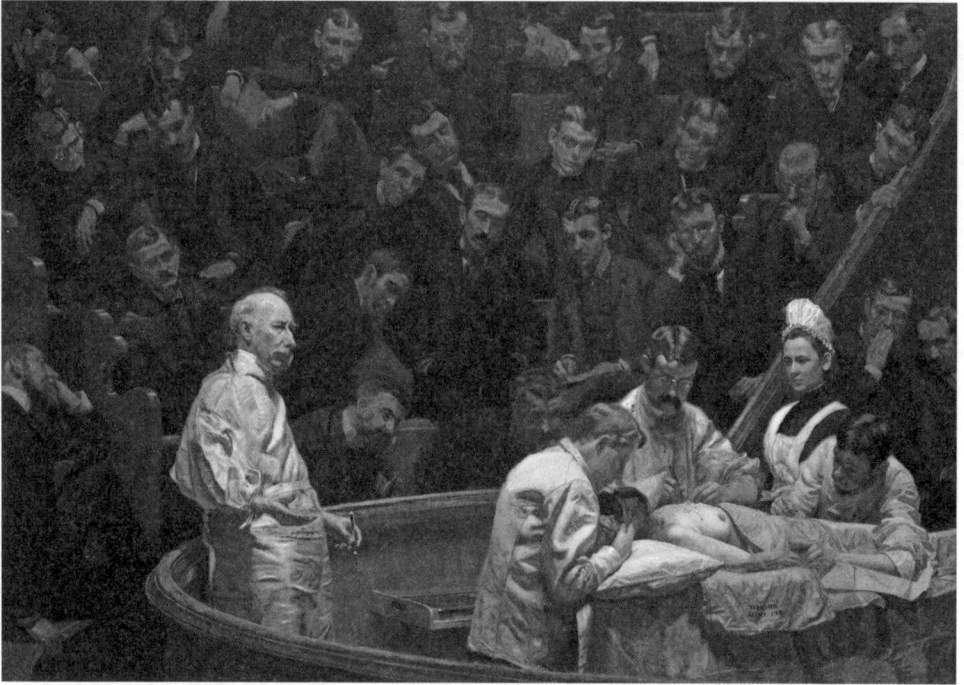

Thomas Eakins, *The Agnew Clinic*, 1889, oil on canvas. This painting depicts David Hayes Agnew, standing in the foreground to the left, in surgical scrubs performing a partial mastectomy. Also present are Drs J. William White, applying a bandage to the patient, Joseph Leidy, taking the patient's pulse, and Ellwood R. Kirby, administering anaesthetic. In the background is the operating room nurse, Mary Clymer.

needing to protect his suit from acid burns and stains, it became the visual sign of the clinical practitioner as much as the stethoscope well before the age of Flexner.[155] Lord Lister in his antiseptic surgical theatre simply 'took off his coat, turned up his shirt sleeves, pinned an ordinary unsterilized huckaback towel over his waistcoat (for his own protection not that of the patient) and washed his hands in 1 to 20 lotion, or even what he called "the strong lotion".[156] In 1883 the German surgeon Gustav Neuber (MD, University of Giessen, 1875), at the University of Kiel, following on Lister's work, first used a sterilized surgical cap and gown in his operating rooms but the tradition spread erratically, even in Germany.[157] Renowned surgeons of an older generation, such as our old friend (from Chapter One) Theodor Billroth (MD, University of Berlin, 1852), dismissed the introduction of surgeons washing their hands while wearing always fresh gowns and caps to facilitate antisepsis as 'Reinlichkeit bis zur Ausschweifung', 'cleanliness to excess'.[158]

Look at the portraits of local surgeons by the Philadelphia-based realist painter Thomas Eakins: in his portrait of Samuel Gross (MD, Jefferson Medical College, 1828) (1875), the surgeon with bloody fingers, he and everyone else in the operating theatre are wearing suits and ties.[159] In Eakins's portrait of David Hayes Agnew (MD, University of Pennsylvania Medical School, 1838) (1889) everyone is in white laboratory coats, except the surgical nurse, who is wearing a white apron over her nursing uniform.[160] We can also note that all are ungloved, as rubber gloves, manufactured by Goodyear Co., became commonplace only after the First World War, introduced initially by William Steward Halsted at Johns Hopkins to protect the surgeon from harsh sterilizing solutions. Daniel Webster Cathell (MD, State University of New York Downstate College of Medicine, 1865), whose vade mecum, *The Physician Himself*, rested on the desks of many medical students in multiple editions between 1882 and 1922, advised: 'Show aesthetic cultivation in your office arrangement, and make it look fresh, neat, clean and scientific.' Above all, one must avoid 'forcing on everybody the conclusion that you are, after all, but an ordinary person.'[161] At the same moment scientific reformers such as John Allen Hornsby (MD, Washington University, St Louis, MO, 1882), secretary of the Hospital Section of the AMA, set new national standards when he became, before the First World War, the director of the new Michael Reese Hospital in Chicago supported by the United Hebrew Charities. Hornsby, in his handbook entitled *The Modern Hospital*, the gold standard for what a twentieth-century hospital and its docs should look like, stated that all people connected with the healing process (including patients and visitors) were to be dressed in white, whereas the non-medical employees were to be given coloured uniforms.[162] Soon finer distinctions (Freud's narcissism of minor differences) limited this to the physician. The nurse's uniform, originating in the nun's habit, with her school cap, already identified her. But all, in the end, hark back to Hippocrates demanding of his pupils: 'On entering bear in mind your manner of sitting, reserve, arrangement of dress, decisive utterance, brevity of speech, composure, bedside manners, care, replies to objections, calm self-control to meet the troubles that occur, rebuke of disturbance, readiness to do what has to be done.'[163] You are what you appear to be, cloaked in the mantle of the physician.

Despite any anxiety generated by the presence of the physician in the clinic, white coats remain a consistent measure of trustworthiness.

Placebos swing both ways. Docs are supposed to look like quasi-scientists and that seems to be reassuring to patients and colleagues alike, but what that means in fashion terms has begun to shift in the twenty-first century. By 2005 'wearing professional dress (that is, a white coat with more formal attire) while providing patient care by physicians may favorably influence trust and confidence-building in the medical encounter.'[164] By 2013 a new variable had been introduced: 'Physicians in traditional dress were seen as most knowledgeable and most honest [and] . . . most caring.'[165] But to what semiotic signs were patients – present and prospective – responding? What was seen was that physicians were 'knowledgeable, trustworthy, caring, approachable and comfortable' and this was mitigated by gender, context of care (for example, inpatient v. outpatient) and geographical region.[166]

Yet the debate should focus, if this were the best of all possible worlds, on following *the* science, not following the perceptions of the patients. The UK National Health Service at that moment had already instituted a ban on laboratory coats that extended below the elbow, arguing, quite correctly, that shorter sleeves inhibited infections through facilitating hand decontamination. Thus the traditional white coat that marked the trust in the physician could also be a source of harm.[167] Needless to say these claims were contested, and five years

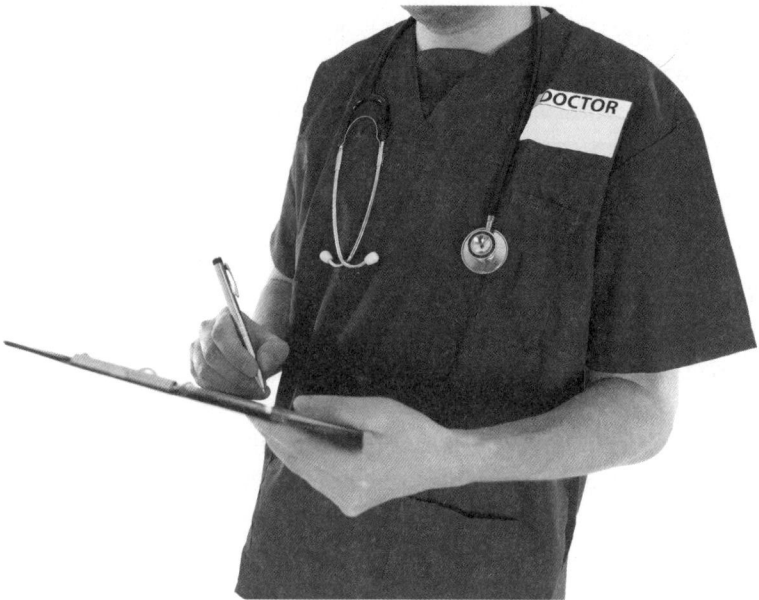

Modern scrubs.

after they were instituted a study showed that patients still 'preferred doctors to wear white coats . . . Patients disliked bare-below-the-elbow attire, scoring it lowest on the comfort and confidence scales.'[168] Maybe not just white coats but the expectation of the consistency of physical presentation took precedence.

White coats, the mark of the physician, had by the early twenty-first century slowly given way to 'scrubs', the dress of the surgeon. They take their name from the fact they are worn in a scrubbed, clean environment. With the introduction of antisepsis and anaesthesia, surgery became the highest-status medical specialty in the age of scientific medicine – which was defined in a patriarchal society as exclusively male.[169] A majority of those questioned in the survey did not identify women in scrubs as surgeons.[170]

Scrubs, like the lab coat, were initially white and unisex, and were hospital-issued and hospital-laundered, but this did not become common practice until the 1940s. 'Scrubs' were first suggested in 1894 by the Johns Hopkins gynaecologist Hunter Robb (MD, University of Pennsylvania, 1884), who stressed that

> it is safer and better that all should put on a complete change
> of costume rather than simply draw on a sterilized coat and
> pair of trousers over the ordinary clothes, as has been recom-
> mended by the German school. The former plan also offers
> many advantages, for not only are the warm out-door clothes
> exchanged for thin, cool garments, which are far better suited
> for the temperature of the operating-room, but the ordinary
> clothes run no risk of being soiled or of carrying away on them
> the disagreeable odor of the fumes of the anesthetic [when, it
> is implied, you go to your club after surgery].

They should be 'made in two separate parts, consisting of a shirt (or jacket) and a pair of trousers. The jacket can be made so as to button down either the front or the back, the former arrangement being prob-ably the more convenient. The trousers should not be long enough to allow the bottoms to drag on the floor.' He also suggested this attire is 'best made of some white material that can be easily and thoroughly washed.'[171] So very different from the bespoke, dark wool suits of the surgeon. White scrubs in the age of antisepsis had a secondary func-tion: if dirty, unlike street clothes, they signalled that the operating theatre was contaminated, with great cleanliness a selling point for all surgical facilities as time went by. But they did not come into widespread use in hospitals until the Second World War.

By the end of the twentieth century scrubs had morphed from white to green, as they were better able to function in the highly illuminated operating rooms. At the same moment, they suddenly began to be seen well beyond the confines of the operating theatre, as seen repeatedly in television doctors' dramas such as the American *Ben Casey* (1961–6) and the British *Casualty* (beginning in 1986). Notice that these featured male physicians. They also morphed into fashion statements already in the 1980s. 'The trendy costume is the surgical scrub suit, and they are disappearing from hospital storerooms by the thousand. You've probably seen the suit, with its slipover V-neck top and pull-on drawstring waist pants, during a hospital visit or on television doctors on "m-a-s-h", "General Hospital" or other shows . . . One way hospitals are cutting down on thefts is by actually selling the popular garb in their gift shops.'[172] The sight in the 1980s of 'young men dropping into their favorite club wearing hospital green scrubs clothes' triggered 'concern among hospitals from whom scrub suits or operating room wear was being pilfered'. And in some ways the status of the physician follows their clothing, as a group of young men found: '"three or four of us" wear scrub greens when . . . [we] visit local clubs . . . We have never intended to be taken for doctors . . . But at one of the clubs the band dubbed us "The Doctors".'[173] But that, of course, was in California, always ahead of the curve, but still just for guys.

Gender matters. When American patients were surveyed in 2015 about trustworthy dress 'for the female surgeon, white coat and scrubs were not different, however the white coat was preferred to business attire in four of seven categories.'[174] They needed an additional semiotic sign to be seen as more trustworthy. It was only in 1976 that sterile pants replaced sterile skirts for women in the operating room.[175] Yet in some clinical specialties '85 per cent of patients preferred scrubs to formal dress clothes. The preference for scrubs was higher in the endoscopic suites (89 per cent and 93 per cent) compared to the outpatient office (66 per cent). In addition, 82 per cent of patients said they felt more comfortable speaking with gastroenterology doctors wearing scrubs and 85 per cent of patients felt more confident about the skills of those gastroenterologists.'[176] During covid-19, the sight of doctors in 'scrubs (81 per cent) . . . [was] found to . . . [elicit a response that this was] the most acceptable physician attire'.[177] More, by the way, than masks and gloves and eye protection. While these surveys were done in the United States, little difference would be found elsewhere in the Global North, even where a certain licence in dress would be tolerated, as in the UK.

Scrubs had become a statement of the new medical cool. In the clinic, the white laboratory coat had begun to be replaced by coloured scrubs, but which colour also mattered, as male and female clinicians in blue scrubs were seen as the most caring across all age groups. Green marked you, especially if you were a young and female doc, as less caring. Some people felt that green scrubs looked janitorial, while others asserted that the black scrubs looked 'deathlike or like a mortician's uniform'.[178] I will remind you that in Japan, and elsewhere in Asia, the colour of death and mourning is white, not black, even though nurses early on, trained in institutions created by the British, wore white.

That is certainly not the reason that white scrubs vanish from the scene. Scrubs had become streetwear in the West; they had become hip. The COVID-19 pandemic saw 'the rise of athleisure, which extended the designer purview into the realm of stretchy, comfort clothing. It is not a great conceptual leap to believing that scrubs, which lie some-where between pajamas and performance clothes, deserve the same treatment'.[179] And by 2023 they were no longer monotone but featured bold floral patterns, checks or stripes; a fashion statement in the clinic and in the club. Certainly not white coats as they generated stress as well as comfort.

As David Ayman had noted, docs wearing lab coats represented a boundary between the clinic and its cold, impersonal technology and the supplicant patient. Recent American studies, however, show that today most patients want to be able to identify the physician and see the white coat as a marker for that role with all the positive qualities ascribed to it. Wear 'casual or slovenly dress' and your 'patient may respond in an inhibited manner, fail to volunteer information, refuse to carry out a recommended diagnostic or management program, fail to keep appointments, and be uncomfortable enough to seek help else-where. The rapport, so anxiously sought for with your patient, may be irretrievably lost'.[180] That the white coat or scrubs may also cause symptoms, as in hypertensive disease, has been well documented over almost a century. That this relates to the perception of the authoritative nature of the modern physician's role seems also to be a major factor. This seems to be contradictory to any feeling of 'friendliness' perceived by the patient, whether the doc was a male or a female.[181] But as Ayman noted, you may also increase their anxiety and thus their symptoms. You are damned if you do (you cause irremediable harm in increasing your patient's discomfort); you are damned if you don't (you lose rapport with your patient).

Acupuncture Again

This brings us back to the problem of acupuncture, evidence and context. And to the present state of acupuncture in British medicine. What if your back pain can be ameliorated by acupuncture but collective responses so necessary for evidence-based medicine cannot document this? Indeed, if your account is dismissed as *merely* anecdotal. What if the opposite of the white coat effect may well be part of your amelioration: that is acupuncture, and indeed CAM, is not quite evidence-based medicine, even with its modern practitioners' claims, but its efficacy may well lie in precisely a placebo effect that is heightened by the role of the scientific acupuncturist in a clinical setting?[182] But then it really is not medical science — just like allopathic medicine — as the creators of TCM and the advocates of acupuncture at the close of the twentieth century claimed, but rather a form of behavioural therapy.

By 2013 the NHS was spending approximately £25 million a year on acupuncture treatments for pain. Sceptics pointed out the continued lack of randomized, double-blind studies that would prove that, however the process took place, it was efficacious. Some noted the fact that the NHS was limiting sessions to about five minutes and that, at least, traditional acupuncturists took much longer with their clients. Could shorted clinical exposure account for the discrepancies between the claims of efficacy and its clinical reality? This was hard if not impossible to quantify.[183] But perhaps it was quantification that was at the core of the problem? Qualitative studies seemed to register improvement, but they *were* merely anecdotal, the statisticians claimed.

The Nordic Cochrane Centre in Copenhagen undertook a more detailed analysis, comparing sham (with needles that looked real but did not meaningfully puncture the skin or were placed randomly on the body) and real acupuncture, involving 3,025 patients. Researchers noted a small difference in efficacy between real and sham acupuncture, and a moderate difference between acupuncture and no acupuncture. They reported: 'A small analgesic effect of acupuncture was found, which seems to lack clinical relevance and cannot be clearly distinguished from bias. Whether needling at acupuncture points, or at any site, reduces pain independently of the psychological impact of the treatment ritual is unclear.' What would be desirable would be if 'researchers could try to separate the effects involved: the physiological effect of needling at acupuncture sites or at other sites and the psychological effect of the treatment ritual or of the patient-provider interaction more broadly.'[184] If it were merely 'psychological effect' of acupuncture, then this amelioration could be achieved by any form of intervention where the patient was convinced, they would have their pain relieved. Perhaps there were less expensive and shorter-term ones?

At the end of November 2016, the British National Institute for Health and Care Excellence (NICE) updated its guidelines for the management and treatment of low back pain and removed acupuncture as a recommended treatment.[185] This was based on a range of studies comparing 'varum' (real) acupuncture treatment to 'sham-acupuncture', an acupuncture-like treatment that also uses acupuncture needles but is not considered to be the equivalent to an inert placebo control. Now, we need to add there are various forms of acupuncture: some use shallow needles, some deep needles; others add further treatment at the time, such as heat lamps or manipulation. And there are alternative therapies, such as myofascial release therapy, that may use both deep and shallow 'dry needling' at the points of pain. These may not follow the patterns of Qi (life force) that underly the use of acupuncture in TCM and which occasion placing needles at some distance from the actual site of the pain. But Mark Baker, clinical practice director at NICE, said, 'Regrettably, there is a lack of convincing evidence of effectiveness for some widely used treatments. For example, acupuncture is no longer recommended for managing low back pain with or without sciatica. This is because there is not enough evidence to show that it is more effective than sham treatment.'[186] *Merely* a placebo?

Now, this case presents us with a set of dilemmas that we have seen before: what is evidence within medicine at any given moment? What happens when there is no consensus as to the efficacy of alternative views of therapy? What is treatment in general and what is a cure? The age of scientific medicine is, as Ian Hacking noted in detail many decades ago, the age of statistical reasoning in which 'the relationship between the data obtained . . . and [any] hypothesis about the efficacy of doctors, is not a causal one – it does not depend on any theory of medicine. It is an epistemological relationship independent of the particular subject matter.'[187] And indeed, all of the claims of science in this case are based on such logic. It does provide a sort of consensus response using ever larger numbers of subjects. (The bigger the 'n', the better the study, goes the mantra.) We see this in the creation of TCM, in the claims for the efficacy of 'modern' acupuncture. And in NICE's cost/benefit analysis. Statistical reasoning replaced the single case, the anecdote, in medicine. And yet what we find, over and over, is that when single cases are examined as to efficacy, they tend to illustrate, for good or for ill, some level of efficacy. Placebos and the 'white coat effect' enable patients, at least some of them, to deal with their immediate circumstances. I mentioned earlier that Ayman's work not only established the latter but dismissed the single gene theory of the aetiology of hypertension. Today, we find ourselves in a transitional moment in healthcare. We speak now of personalized genetic therapy for certain clusters of diseases, such as cancer. As was stated in 2014: 'The type and mode of gene therapy will be determined based on an individual's genomic constituents, as well as his or her tumor specifics, genetics, and host immune status, to design a multimodality treatment that is unique to each individual's specific needs.'[188] Here the individual and at least some of their constituent elements are considered. We think that this is an advancement of science, but it does not look at the complexity of diagnosis and treatment beyond the molecular. Our examination of the claims of CAM and acupuncture certainly would set the bar somewhat higher. The context of treatment, the affective response to diagnoses, setting and therapist; the social location of patient and physician; the claims and the belief in the claims of science, need to be added to the mix. The ever-shifting boundary between 'quackery' and 'medical science' means that the move from classes of illness back to individuals with illnesses does mean rethinking the absolute boundary implied by the technology of medicine and its claims.

5

Permanence and Change

As I was writing these case studies, a volume of *Daedalus*, the journal of the American Academy of Arts and Sciences, of which I am a member, appeared in my mailbox. The topic was 'Institutions, Experts and the Loss of Trust'. Perfect, I thought, as I opened the issue and hoped to find answers to the questions that are at the heart of my matter. The opening essay was one on 'The Discontents of Truth and Trust in the Twenty-First Century' by an eminent sociologist of science, Sheila Jasanoff, my former colleague at Cornell. Its point of departure was questions of belief and authority during the pandemic. She personified 'trust' in the figure of Anthony Fauci:

> Sometime in April 2020, a new icon of trust emerged on the American scene: Dr Anthony Fauci, director of the National Institute of Allergy and Infectious Diseases and chief medical advisor to the president. Born on Christmas Eve in 1940, Fauci was an unlikely folk hero. Yet the slogan 'In Fauci We Trust' sprouted on innumerable yard signs and pop culture merchandise like mugs and T-shirts. Dubbed the 'nation's top infectious disease expert', Fauci conducted countless press interviews while also appearing frequently at President Trump's side in his daily briefings on the pandemic . . . Fauci came to personify the caretaking ethos of the physician who has sworn an oath to put the patient's health foremost, in a moment when no one else in the federal administration seemed to offer coherence, competence, or caring. So seen, Fauci became the voice of

transcendent epistemic authority because his mission was that of the nation's healer, an embodiment of the view from every-where. Instructively, the CDC's [Centers for Disease Control and Prevention] efforts to restore trust through abstract appeals to science (the view from nowhere) in the first year of the Biden administration proved less persuasive than Fauci's pronouncements at the pandemic's height.[1]

What Jasanoff is illustrating is the double-whammy of investiture and nostalgia. Fauci becomes the 'good doctor' with the authority of both the state and the medical establishment. In retrospect, Fauci himself took on this role. In an interview in April 2023, after his retirement from the National Institutes of Health, he began by defining his role as 'a physician . . . That's my identity. I've taken care of thousands of patients in one period of my life during the early years of HIV. I believe that I have seen as much or more suffering and death as anybody has in most careers. I don't mean to seem preachy, but I don't want to see people suffer and I don't want to see people die.'[2] In his 2024 autobiography he amends this meaningfully: 'AIDS brought me into a world filled with suffering and death. I assumed the dual role of a physician-scientist and a domestic and global leader as NIAID direc-tor in the battle against HIV/AIDS.'[3] He was a public health specialist, not a local doc doing his rounds with a buggy and horse clutching his black bag; he was given authority, not by his claims on empathy and moral commitment to healing, but by the state, as he represents a state organ, the National Institutes of Health. Something that the members of Act-Up (AIDS Coalition to Unleash Power), such as Larry Kramer, made abundantly clear in the late 1980s even when they recognized his clearly empathetic personal response to the HIV crisis.

Expertise so grounded is celebrity status given by his position and those who granted it. Fauci is an expert, he knows the science as an immunologist and physician-scientist, but he is also an expert because of his degree (MD, Cornell Medical College, 1966), his employment (1980, chief of the National Institute of Allergy and Infectious Diseases Laboratory of Immunoregulation; 1984–2022, Director of NIAID) and the visibility of his science (especially in the realms of rheumatology and HIV/AIDS: 1983–2002, the thirteenth most-cited scientist among the 2.5 to 3 million authors in all disciplines throughout the world who published articles in scientific journals). He serves as one pole of the dichotomy that Jasanoff illustrates as undermining the very notion of expertise during the pandemic.

But there was an anti-Fauci in Jasanoff's narrative too: the 'bad' doc whose self-interest distorted his ability to 'follow *the* science'. For Jasanoff this was 'France's Didier Raoult [MD, Aix-Marseille Medical School, 1981], a charismatic, politically well-connected, and highly credentialed member of France's COVID-19 committee from Marseille . . . He won powerful support in France and elsewhere, although critics turned on him for deluding people who seemingly did not have the knowledge or capacity to disentangle good science from bad.'[4] Early on he advocated for hydroxychloroquine as a treatment for COVID-19, a therapy quickly labelled as ineffectual at best, quackery at worst. Status is tied to perceived expertise, something we have seen run through all our case studies. But expertise is always contingent on setting and its interpretation. While at any given point it is possible, indeed necessary, to define the boundary between the doc and the quack, the existence of such boundaries relies on a set of symbolic values, from investiture to social status to media presence, which generate, for good or for ill, 'trust'. Jasanoff concludes that 'experts must represent things in the world in ways that give voice to diverse standpoints, aggregate disparate opinions to produce a measure of objectivity, and find persuasive ways to bridge the gaps between available and ideal states of knowledge. Simply insisting on the authority of science without attending to the politics of reason and persuasion has proved not to restore trust in either knowledge or power.'[5] And we need to add loudly here: to acknowledge that such regimes are constantly in flux; that ambiguities need to be represented in any such system; and that 'science' is not a state but a process.[6] Fauci, in defence of his own necessary shifts in positions during the pandemic, stressed this in his 2024 autobiography, when he observed that 'the public expected definitive answers leading to immutable guidelines and recommendations. But this was impossible in a rapidly evolving situation.' And the reason for this was the notion of a fixity of science as 'people associate science with absolutes that are immutable, when in fact science is a process that continually uncovers new information. As new information evolves, the process of science allows for self-correction.'[7] And sometimes the very underpinnings of *the* science turn out to be problematic.[8]

'Above all,' Friedrich Nietzsche said about doing science, 'one should not wish to divest existence of its rich ambiguity.'[9] 'Walking

away from the politics of truth', a phrase that Jasanoff employs, is
what science, indeed especially medical science, as we have seen in
our case studies, does because of 'scientific' research and practice.
Each new truth modifies not only earlier assumptions but, even
more consequently for medicine, clinical practice, which in turn
includes the patient in every transformation. This is basically true
in physics also, but there is no 'patient' to fear or need to acknowledge the often-rapid shifts in diagnosis and treatment, never mind
aetiology, as in medicine. And here Rudolf Virchow in 1848 was
quite correct: medicine is politics, as it incorporates every aspect
of the state from regime to citizenry. And we can stress that that
is especially true of public health. Public health is at best one step
away from the laboratory and two steps away from the clinic. At
the very beginning of Baroness Heather Hallett's 2023 inquiry in
the United Kingdom about the course of COVID-19 and the Boris
Johnson/Matt Hancock government responses, Devi Sridhar (DPhil,
medical anthropology, 2006, Oxford University), who holds the chair
of global public health at the University of Edinburgh, tried to parse
out what she believed to be the different roles of the scientific and the
political realms. Science could 'rapidly collect data about a new patho-
gen, analyse it and provide factual advice to governments on the risks
that COVID-19 posed to human health, healthcare services and economic stability'. But, she concluded, 'what leaders decided to do with
that advice in terms of policy was 100 per cent political.' As Virchow
too had claimed a century before, she claimed: 'no scientist ever had
the executive power to make policy decisions. This was the responsibility of elected officials. And knowing my academic colleagues, none
of us would have wanted that power either.'[10]

Yet the reality is that by investing public health authorities, most
of whom are MDs, with the status that scientific medicine accrued to
itself beginning in the nineteenth century, the act of advising was,
of course, a highly charged political act. And we saw this over and
over again when government policy did not respond to the 'various
public health solutions to the challenge' or indeed even when they
did. Scientific medicine makes (or suggests) policy precisely to those
authorities that have invested them with the authority to do so. To
tease out, as Devi Sridhar does, how the scientists, working in their
lab coats at their proverbial benches, are completely dependent on the
political realm to create policy which does or does not mirror their

science, is at best naive, and at worst, given the very visibility of these scientists on daily television throughout the world during the pandemic, an attempt to shift whatever blame can be apportioned for acts responding to a dynamic public health crisis from themselves. Lab scientists, docs, public health authorities and those in the political realm dealing with the public's health are all complicit, as is each and every one of us, in a network that links the scientific, the medical and the political. And that network is as much affective as it is rational.

Ambiguity

If we acknowledge that ambiguity lies at the heart of medicine and medical praxis, that a necessary ambiguity triggers the placebo effect, for good or for ill, and that we often turn to medicine for answers to social ills and global phenomena, then the question of trust does become vital, in the sense that one needs to believe, as a physician and as a patient (and as a citizen), in the efficacy of the approach, the theory, the technology and the training. But always be prepared for the loss of trust on all sides when new verities are introduced. And this varies from problem to problem, from community to community, from time to time, as we saw and continue to see in the post-COVID-19 world, which is certainly not 'post'. Trust is a belief in the moral as well as the technical superiority of those granted power: power to heal, power to govern, power that we, as a society, grant them. But it is a chimera: the moral force posits the physician as the 'good doctor', whose calling is healing; the 'bad' doc does harm. This seems to be baked into the very notion of the professionalization of medicine, as the reformist headmaster at Rugby, Thomas Arnold, writes in 1836 to one of his students who had taken up medicine:

> It is a real pleasure to me to find that you are taking steadily to a profession, without which I scarcely see how a man can live honestly. That is, I use the term 'profession' in rather a large sense, not as simply denoting certain callings which a man follows for his maintenance, but rather a definite field of duty, which the nobleman has as much as the tailor, but which he has not, who having an income large enough to keep him from starving, hangs about on life, merely following his own caprices and fancies.[11]

We should remember that one of the new pedagogical ideals preached by Arnold was instilling 'kindness' in his students, a quality easily transmuted into 'empathy'. And being a professional in medicine is also defined by the notion that empathy is one of the hallmarks of medical professionalism.[12] After the horrors of the First World War Sir William Osler praised the ethos of empathy ascribed to Greek medicine as having amalgamated 'the love of humanity associated with the love of his craft! – *philanthropia* and *philotechnia* – the joy of working joined in each one to a true love of his brother'.[13] This was a fantasy of his age, seeing his world of scientific medicine likewise shaped by technical advances *and* moral principles. Greek healers were supposed to be motivated by their 'love of mankind'; the reality is that was less a calling than a job, less a belief system and more a social role. It was motivated, as was charged at the time, by love of money and glory, or indeed exemption from other forms of public service. Ancient physicians such as Galen sought to turn the tables, claiming that motivation mattered less than skill.[14]

Docs, such as Osler, who defined the age of scientific medicine needed to be seen as empathetic because technology was understood as distancing the physician from the patient, indeed, as we have seen, as reducing them to their symptoms. This became, in scientific medicine, one of the hallmarks of being a medical professional, which they believed separated them from all other professions. Sir Arthur Conan Doyle (BM/MB and CM, University of Edinburgh, 1881), a failed physician yet most successful author, writes a short story about a trained physician of his generation presenting to his younger colleagues what his generation conceived of as the moral centre of medicine. 'And besides, he is forced to be a good man. It is impossible for him to be anything else. How can a man spend his whole life in seeing suffering bravely borne and yet remain a hard or a vicious man? It is a noble, generous, kindly profession, and you youngsters have got to see that it remains so.'[15]

After the Holocaust and the horrors of Nazi medicine, after the corporatization of medical practice and the gradual alienation of the physician – through technology and time management – from the patient, beginning in the 1990s, medical institutions began trying to instil empathy into young physicians by any means possible. One pathway was the introduction of the medical humanities, which was claimed to 'humanize' the physician by teaching them compassion.

It became clear to all that this was not a failing of the individual but of the very assumption that empathy was inherent in the role of the healer. Jane Macnaughton (MA, MBChB, MRCGP, DRCOG, PhD in English), an obstetrician/gynaecologist and then director of the Institute for Medical Humanities at Durham, wrote already in 2009 that 'we cannot gain direct access to what is going on in our patient's head . . . Any mirroring of feeling will always differ quantitatively and qualitatively from that patient's experience. A doctor who responds to a patient's distress with "I understand how you feel" is likely, there-fore, to be both resented by the patient and self-deceiving.'[16] And, we can add, ineffectual. Here we can cite Talcott Parsons, as we did in our first chapter, who said that physicians as professionals are 'not in the usual sense "altruistic", nor [are] businessmen "egoistic". Indeed, there is little basis for maintaining that there is any important broad difference of typical motivation in the two cases, or at least any of sufficient importance to account for the broad differences in socially expected behaviour.'[17] But the reality, then and now, is that the context and meaning of both who heals and who is healed, who diagnoses and what is diagnosed, and how they are treated, is dependent on more variables than we can contemplate.

Yet the promise that young physicians are made, if only in the cinema and on television, is that they have a calling not a job. One case can suffice here. 'Keith Corl . . . was an idealist who quit a lucra-tive job in finance in his early 20s because he wanted to do something that would benefit people . . . Like many E.R. physicians, Corl viewed his job as a calling. But over time, his idealism gave way to disillusion-ment, as he struggled to provide patients with the type of care he'd been trained to deliver.'[18] The result of this double bind is what the psych-iatrist Jonathan Shay called a 'moral injury', looking at veterans with PTSD.[19] It is when the values that are the underlying assumptions of a profession, which define its investiture in an individual, are violated by the role that they assume in the profession. (This is a more focused reworking of Gregory Bateson's 1956 concept of the 'double bind'.) Moral injury is what alienates the physician from their practice, even though it is a small minority whose sense of alienation overwhelms their assumption of the social role of the healer. And this has been true from the creation of scientific medicine on, with its promise to answer questions which may well be unfathomable in their complexity. Patients remain lulled by this image, even as it collapses, for 'patients, many of whom naturally assume that their doctors are the ones who decide how much time to spend with them and what to charge them for care'. 'Doctors are increasingly the scapegoats of systemic problems within the health care system', Mona Masood (DO, Edward Via Virginia College of Osteopathic Medicine, 2011) a psychiatrist who established a support line for doctors shortly after the pandemic began, says, 'because the patient is not seeing the insurance company that denied them the procedure, they're not seeing the electronic medical records that are taking up all of our time. They're just seeing the doctor who can only spend 10 minutes with them in the room, or the doctor who says, "I can't get you this medication, because it costs $500 a month." And what ends up happening is we internalize that feeling.'[20]

And the situation in the British NHS, even with the absence of the direct financial question, remains parallel: patients see those in the white coats as standing between them and help, timelines for treatment increase and fewer and fewer patients can enter the system. (The Rishi Sunak government in May 2023 authorized pharmacists to cover the gap – something that the huge pharmaceutical conglomerates in the United States have long done.) In the People's Republic of China this has led to massive attacks on physicians in clinics and hospitals, for seeming cruelly to refuse treatment to the ill and the suffering.[21] They, not the Party, are seen as culpable.

Docs and Quacks

The debate about belief in a medicine that is both scientific and empathetic is underscored by the *Daedalus* volume that echoes a major shift in the claims about the social and political role in scientific medicine that occurred at the close of the twentieth century. The louder and more insistent the claim that in scientific medicine both efficacy and empathy could live side by side, indeed defined medical practice, the less both physicians and patients bought into this claim. Their experiences were radically different: alienation on the part of the practitioner and the patient's sense of being treated as a disease or a body part, not as a human being. I experienced this in my own career. After spending a year in residence at the Medical School at Cornell University, working on a project on the history of psychiatry, the then dean invited me in 1978 to join the faculty, as it was understood that medical students needed to be 'humanized'. This, although I ironically informed him that humanists were the least humane people teaching at any university, as they seemed mainly to quibble about parking spaces. I began a seventeen-year affiliation teaching the medical humanities. I was certainly not alone, not even in New York City, where the medical school was located, and where other humanists were suddenly drafted into schools of medicine.

Now, I was not completely naive. In 1975 the barbiturate-overdose deaths of Drs Stewart L. and Cyril C. Marcus, identical twins who were both faculty members at the Cornell Medical School, where they ran the infertility clinic, made the front pages of newspapers across the country. The immediate response was: how could such addicts not only continue to practise medicine, and more importantly, how could they continue to teach and research at one of the major schools of medicine in the United States? Evidently, something was amiss with their moral orientation. My function in the greater scope of things was to be proof that the medical school was answering the question of how you teach medical students to be better people and therefore better docs. Over the following decades, as this case became the stuff of popular culture, such as in David Cronenberg's film *Dead Ringers* (1988), my teaching seemed to fill a gap. By the way, in 1991, noting the collapse of the assumptions about scientific medical praxis, the AMA began a $1.75-million advertising campaign to polish up the image of the doctor, emphasizing the sort of good works that once were the specialties of film and television doctors. By then, however, Sinclair Lewis's literary and John Ford's cinematic hero Dr Martin Arrowsmith (Ronald Colman), whom we discussed in our opening chapter, had been replaced in the popular mind by Dr Judah Rosenthal (Martin Landau), an accessory to the murder of his mistress in Woody Allen's *Crimes and Misdemeanors* (1989).

In my subsequent career, I fulfilled this role at several other schools of medicine, all of which assumed, rightly or wrongly, that I would enrich their curricula by humanizing their students, perhaps by making them more empathetic to augment their scientific training. I too thought that perhaps I could help reorient them a bit to their new roles as medical students and then real-world practitioners, but never felt that I could make anyone a 'better', a more empathetic, person or doc. Most of the students at schools of medicine found that such courses were simply a waste of their time. They still wanted *the* science in *scientific* medicine to be foregrounded.

The answer to such claims in the age of COVID-19 was bizarre: making not the physician more empathetic but the image of science value neutral, Osler's old claim to objective medicine now prescribed as an answer to what is labelled an anti-science bias. It was argued that 'it is important that public health leaders not be seen as associated with one or the other political party. Public health agencies and advisory groups should be separated as much as possible from political decision-makers when making their public health recommendations.' And even odder that these now neutral arbiters of science in the public sphere must not only be neutral but simultaneously engaged: 'because of the political polarization by religion, race/ethnicity and region, it is important to have scientific spokespeople who are clearly identified with each demographic group across the country.' Here we reach a sort of apotheosis of fear about the loss of trust: 'because a substantial share of the public does not have confidence in scientists' advice, it is necessary for public health leaders to explain more fully the nature of the scientific findings that lead to their policy recommendations. It is not enough to say, "Scientists believe this, so here is what you should do."'[22] Because, of course, explaining means stating the unswerving, overdetermined, objective, underlying science that supports the public health interventions. A lot like the claims in the beginning of our age of scientific medicine that bench science provides truths about nature which can then be applied as verities in the clinic. If such information were truly to be transmitted, and in support of pure transparency, every claim would have to begin 'At the moment' and conclude with 'until we know more'. That is unacceptable if we believe that the physician (and by extension the physician as a public health expert) is endowed by training and certification and is invested by us, in terms of our own belief systems, with some greater ability (not knowledge) than mere mortals. Which of course they are not.

Ignoring *the* science is bad, following *the* science is good, seems a rather easy call. Unless you add the necessary caveats, which we have outlined in each of our cases: that science is not static, that what is good science at any moment can be very bad science the next. That what saves you might also kill you. And that the agents, the physicians and public health specialists, subscribing or denying the aetiology or efficacy of therapy, are necessarily inconsistent in their positions. It is not the state or its regulation that is in doubt but the investiture that these agents have as representatives of a transcendent truth. What

supervenes is not 'believing *the* science' but believing the social investment in science, the status we attribute to the scientist and therefore to
the science. Since we have so invested belief in our systems you have
only these two options: everyone is a quack, or no one is a quack. The
reality is that the dichotomy is false but, sadly, necessary. We live in
a world in which the fluidity of medicine and its contradictions run
against our own sense of vulnerability, whether a vulnerability because
of human fragility or human fear, death or taxes, illness or the state.
The irony, of course, is that we suffer and hope to ameliorate them as
much as possible.

It is the fact that we differentiate between the good doctors with
their calling to aid the sick (or at least to do no harm) and the time-
serving bureaucrats in the public health service, whose calling, as many
have said over and over, is to cover their claims. 'And unlike doctors
and nurses, whose heroic acts during the pandemic have been covered widely by the media, almost no attention has been paid to the
heroic deeds of public health officials who work for health depart-
ments administering vaccinations, COVID-19 tests, and contact tracing
in often dangerous settings, or to leaders who face threats of violence
simply for trying to serve the public.'[23] Such agents must be seen as
having a calling; not merely being employed in a profession. And the
reality was that it was those in public health across the world who
were excoriated because they could not get things right, could only
impose limits, could not make it all go away NOW. The claims of the
'healers', the physicians and the nurses, was that they were doing as
well as they could with limited information and limited resources,
under which, of course, the public health officials also suffered. People
banged their pots for the docs, the nurses, the food store workers, the
delivery people. They rarely banged their pots or applauded the epi-
demiologists, in the United States or elsewhere. Indeed, they often bore
the brunt of public's anathema.

The healers in the United States were and are virtually all employees
of mega-healthcare systems (some for-profit; some officially non-
profit, but still needing to make a profit). No lone practitioners visiting
the sick in the darkness of night bringing solace and cure. In Great
Britain, the National Health Service was no different, except perhaps
that, at least during COVID-19, the impact of decades of Conservative
attitudes towards the NHS showed that the institution was just as
unstable and unpredictable as the public health structures. Everyone

was overwhelmed by the systems in which they were employed. The post-COVID nurse and ambulance-driver strikes in 2022 bore witness to this in Great Britain and the United States. Indeed, they were acting not as individuals with a moral calling, but appropriately as employees of a mega-system. Just like the public health authorities. No quacks anywhere; only employees. Scientific medicine, with all its benefits and accomplishments, trails with it the problem which we have perhaps too richly illustrated in this volume: that there are many more variables that must be considered in clinical practice than the notion of a progressive, objective bench science (a claim that is also disputed by many of the bench scientists engaged in this process). And yet today we know that 'medicine is not a coherent whole. It is not a unity. It is, rather, an amalgam of thoughts, a mixture of habits, an assemblage of techniques. Medicine is a heterogeneous coalition of ways of handling bodies, studying pictures, making numbers, conducting conversations. Wherever you look, in hospitals, in clinics, in laboratories, in general practitioners' offices – there is multiplicity. There is multiplicity even in medicine's "core".[24] And that core is the notion of bench science that seems to underlie practice.[25] Medicine heals through innovation, but also through belief; medicine harms through innovation as well as belief. The line between the quack and the doc is amorphous but always present. Which is where we began and where, because of the reality of the world in which we function, we shall also end.

REFERENCES

Preface: A Road Map

1 Zain Asher, Nick Watt, Elizabeth Cohen, Salma Abdelaziz, Kyung Lah, Alison Kosik, Richard Quest, 'U.S. Hits 20 Million Cases as New COVID Strain Gains Ground; Markets Eye Georgia Runoff Elections Next Week; Thousands Gather to Celebrate New Year in Wuhan, China', CNN *International* (1 January 2021, aired 3–3.30 p.m. EST).

2 Ella Whelan, 'To Ban Talkradio for Criticising Lockdown Is to Suppress Healthy Debate Just When We Need It Most', *The Telegraph* (5 January 2021).

3 Venki Ramakrishnan, 'Following the Science', Royal Society blog (17 May 2020), https://royalsociety.org/blog/2020/05/following-the-science.

4 Anonymous review of T. Spencer Wells, 'Practical Observations on Gout and Its Complications', *Athenaeum*, MCCCLXXXVIII (3 June 1854), p. 684.

5 Eyal Press, 'The Moral Crisis of America's Doctors', *New York Times Magazine* (15 June 2023).

6 Rafael Lozano et al., 'Measuring Performance on the Healthcare Access and Quality Index for 195 Countries and Territories and Selected Subnational Locations: A Systematic Analysis from the Global Burden of Disease Study 2016', *The Lancet*, 391 (2 June 2018), pp. 2236–70.

7 Bridget M. Kuehn, 'COVID-19 Cuts Life Expectancy in Dozens of Countries', *JAMA*, 327 (18 January 2022), p. 209.

8 Michel Foucault, *Birth of the Clinic: An Archeology of Medical Perception*, trans. A. M. Sheridan Smith (New York, 1994), pp. 136ff.

9 Toby Gelfand, 'Gestation of the Clinic', *Medical History*, XXV (1981), pp. 169–80.

10 See the 1946 *cri de cœur* by F. Boenheim, 'Medical Education under Hitler', *Interne*, XII (1946), pp. 555–9.

11 On the problem of using Nazi medicine in ethical debates see Mathias Schütz and Harold Braswell, 'Ethicizing History: Bioethical Representations of Nazi Medicine', *Bioethics*, XXXVII (2023), pp. 1–10.

12 William Osler, *The Growth of Truth: As Illustrated in the Discovery of the Circulation of the Blood. Being the Harveian Oration Delivered at the Royal College of Physicians, London, October 18, 1906* (London, 1906), pp. 10–11.

13 Karl Popper, *Conjectures and Refutations: The Growth of Scientific Knowledge* (London, 1963), p. 38, fn. 3.

14 Karl Popper, *Objective Knowledge: An Evolutionary Approach* (Oxford, 1972), pp. 57–8.

15 Thomas S. Kuhn, *The Structure of Scientific Revolutions* [1962] (Chicago, IL, 1970), p. 1.

1 Confronting *the* Problem

1 Jay Katz, 'Why Doctors Don't Disclose Uncertainty', *Hastings Center Report*, XIV (1984), pp. 35–44, here, p. 40.
2 Irvine Loudon, 'Semmelweis and His Thesis', *Journal of the Royal Society of Medicine*, XCVIII (2005), p. 555.
3 There are hundreds of antiquarian books on the topic throughout the nineteenth and twentieth centuries, mainly written by retired physicians to underline the quality of the allopathic medicine in their age of scientific medicine. According to the statistics on *PubMed* (The National Library of Medicine's search engine) their peak intensifies from the 1850s to the 1920s, exactly the period of the establishment of modern allopathic medicine that we shall be examining. The best of the many modern, scholarly books on quackery stem from the pen of my late friend Roy Porter, such as his more popular one on *Quacks: Fakers and Charlatans in English Medicine* (Stroud, 2001), which followed up his *Health for Sale: Quackery in England, 1660–1800* (Manchester, 1989). Porter is the most important historian of medicine to write on this as a problem of social history. See his 'The Language of Quackery in England', in *The Social History of Language*, ed. Peter Burke and Roy Porter (Cambridge, 1987), pp. 73–103; William F. Bynum and Roy Porter, eds, *Medical Fringe and Medical Orthodoxy, 1750–1850* (London, 1987). See also E. S. Juhnke, *Quacks and Crusaders* (Lawrence, KS, 2002). Specifically on the United States see James H. Young, *The Toadstool Millionaires: A Social History of Patent Medicines in America before Federal Regulation* (Princeton, NJ, 1961); James H. Young, *The Medical Messiahs: A Social History of Health Quackery in Twentieth-Century America* (Princeton, NJ, 1992). On the representation of quackery see M. F. McLellan, 'Images of Physicians in Literature: From Quacks to Heroes', *The Lancet*, CCCXLVIII (1996), pp. 358–60; Sylvia Pamboukian, *Doctoring the Novel: Medicine and Quackery from Shelley to Doyle* (Columbus, OH, 2012). Most of the older studies assume that there is a discoverable, fixed line between the healer and the quack. I do not claim this.
4 Thomas Gieryn, 'Boundary-Work and the Demarcation of Science from Non-Science: Strains and Interests in Professional Interests of Scientists', *American Sociological Review*, XLVIII (1983), pp. 781–95.
5 Mark W. Weatherall, 'Making Medicine Scientific: Empiricism, Rationality, and Quackery in Mid-Victorian Britain', *Social History of Medicine*, IX (1996), pp. 175–94.
6 Stewart Gordon, ed., *Robes and Honor: The Medieval World of Investiture* (New York, 2001), pp. 1–15.
7 Ludwig Edelstein, 'The Professional Ethics of the Greek Physician', *Bulletin of the History of Medicine*, XXX (1956), pp. 391–419, here, p. 412, and Sergio Sconocchia, 'Greek Medicine in Scribonius Largus' Compositiones', in *'Greek' and 'Roman' in Latin Medical Texts*, ed. Brigitte Maire (Leiden, 2014), pp. 330–49, here, p. 334, on 'professio'.
8 Edelstein, 'Professional Ethics', p. 409.
9 Heinz Heinrich Gerth and C. Wright Mills, eds, *From Max Weber: Essays in Sociology* (London, 1970), p. 139.

10 Gerth and Mills, *From Max Weber*, p. 144.

11 R. H. Shryock, *Medical Licensing in America, 1650–1965* (Baltimore, MD, 1963).

12 Magali Sarfatti Larson, 'Professionalism: Rise and Fall', *International Journal of Health Services,* IX (1979), pp. 607–27, here, p. 611.

13 Eric L. Santner, *My Own Private Germany: Daniel Paul Schreber's Secret History* (Princeton, NJ, 1996), p. xii. Emphasis his.

14 H. Burger, 'The Doctor, the Quack, and the Appetite of the Public for Magic in Medicine', *Proceedings of the Royal Society of Medicine,* XXVII (1933), pp. 171–6, here, p. 172.

15 Eric Santner, *The Royal Remains: The People's Two Bodies and the Endgames of Sovereignty* (Chicago, IL, 2011), pp. 93, 52.

16 Ernst H. Kantorowicz, *The King's Two Bodies: A Study in Medieval Political Theology* (Princeton, NJ, 1985), p. 498.

17 Max Weber, *Theory of Social and Economic Organization*, trans. A. R. Anderson and Talcott Parsons (New York, 1947), p. 328.

18 Gerth and Mills, *From Max Weber*, p. 240.

19 Max Weber, *Economy and Society: A New Translation*, trans. Keith Tribe (Cambridge, 2019), p. 347.

20 Richard J. Miller, *Drugged: The Science and Culture behind Psychotropic Drugs* (Oxford, 2014), p. 9.

21 Gerth and Mills, *From Max Weber*, p. 251.

22 *The Novels of Daniel Defoe*, ed. W. R. Owens, P. N. Furbank and Liz Bellamy, VII: *Journal of the Plague Year* (1722), ed. John Mullen (London, 2017), pp. 46–7.

23 Augustin Belloste, *The Hospital-Surgeon; or, A New, Gentle, and Easie Way, to Cure Speedily All Sorts of Wounds, and Other Diseases Belonging to Surgery* (London, 1701), p. 248.

24 A. Ohry and J. Tsafrir, 'Running after Quacks and Mountebanks . . .', *Progress in Health Sciences,* II (2012), pp. 171–4.

25 William de Meij, *The Triumph of Truth and Good Sense; or, An Exposé of Quacks and Quackery* (London, 1834), p. 8.

26 Robert G. A. Dolby, 'Reflections on Deviant Science', *Sociological Review,* XXVII (1979), pp. 9–47, here, p. 41.

27 Granville P. Conn, 'State Medicine vs Fads', *Columbus Medical Journal,* XVI (1896), pp. 11–21, here, p. 11.

28 Bert Hansen, *Picturing Medical Progress from Pasteur to Polio: A History of Mass Media Images and Popular Attitudes in America* (New Brunswick, NJ, 2009).

29 T. Percival and C. D. Leake, eds, *Percival's Medical Ethics* (Baltimore, MD, 1927), pp. 104–5.

30 Erwin Liek, *The Doctor's Mission: Reflections, Reminiscences, and Revelations of a Medical Man*, trans. J. Ellis Barker (London, 1930), p. 252. Originally published as Erwin Liek, *Der Arzt und seine Sendung: Gedanken eines Ketzers* (Munich, 1926).

31 Paul Starr, *The Social Transformation of American Medicine* (New York, 1982), p. 23.

32 Nina Degele, 'On the Margins of Everything: Doing, Performing, and Staging Science in Homeopathy', *Science, Technology, and Human Values,* XXX, Special Issue: *Demarcation Socialized: Constructing Boundaries and Recognizing Difference* (2005), pp. 111–36.

33 David Wootton, *Bad Medicine: Doctors Doing Harm since Hippocrates* (Oxford, 2007), p. 37.

34 William G. Rothstein, *American Physicians in the Nineteenth Century: From Sects to Science* (Baltimore, MD, 1972).

35 Stephen Barrett and William T. Jarvis, *The Health Robbers: A Close Look at Quackery in America* (Buffalo, NY, 1993).

36 Michel Foucault, *The Archaeology of Knowledge*, trans. A. M. Sheridan Smith (New York, 1972), p. 199.

37 Reinhard Spree, *Health and Social Class in Imperial Germany: A Social History of Mortality, Morbidity, and Inequality*, trans. Stuart McKinnon-Evans and John Halliday (New York, 1988), pp. 176–7.

38 Jeremy Bentham, *Deontology Together with a Table of the Springs of Action and Article on Utilitarianism*, ed. Amnon Goldworth (Oxford, 1983), p. 50. See also Benjamin Spector, 'Jeremy Bentham, 1748–1832: His Influence upon Medical Thought and Legislation', *Bulletin of the History of Medicine*, XXXVII (1963), pp. 25–42.

39 Edith Lesky, *The Vienna Medical School of the Nineteenth Century*, trans. L. Williams and I. S. Levij (Baltimore, MD, 1976) as well as her 'American Medicine as Viewed by Viennese Physicians, 1893–1912', *Bulletin of the History of Medicine*, LVI (1982), pp. 368–76.

40 Theodor Billroth, *Über das Lehren und Lernen der medicinischen Wissenschaften an den Universitäten der deutschen Nation nebst allgemeinen Bemerkungen über Universitäten: Eine culturhistorische Studie* (Vienna, 1876), pp. 146–57. All quotes in the present book translated from German-language sources have been translated by the author unless otherwise stated.

41 W. O. [William Osler], 'Letter from Berlin', *Canada Medical and Surgical Journal*, XXII (1884), pp. 721–8, here, p. 728.

42 *The Medical Sciences in the German Universities: A Study in the History of Civilization*, trans. from the German of Theodor Billroth, with an Introduction by William H. Welch (New York, 1924), p. vi.

43 *Bentham's Theory of Legislation: Being Principes de Législation and Traités de Législation Civile et Pénale*, trans. and ed. Charles Milner Atkinson (Oxford, 1914), II, p. 296.

44 Rudolf Virchow, *Die medizinische Reform. Eine Wochenschrift* (Berlin, 10 July 1848), p. 2. See Laura Otis, *Müller's Lab* (Oxford, 2007), pp. 277ff., and Ian F. McNeely, *Medicine on a Grand Scale': Rudolf Virchow, Liberalism, and the Public Health* (London, 2002).

45 Bentham Manuscripts at University College London, Box 32, p. 168.

46 Fielding Hudson Garrison, *An Introduction to the History of Medicine*, 4th edn (Philadelphia, PA, 1966), p. 577. See also Anon., 'Professor Virchow on Quacks', *BMJ*, 1/2039 (1900), pp. 214–15.

47 Christoph Gradmann, 'Bazillen, Krankheit und Krieg: Bakteriologie und politische Sprache im deutschen Kaiserreich', *Berichte zur Wissenschaftsgeschichte*, XIX (1996), pp. 81–94.

48 Howard Waitzkin, 'The Micropolitics of Medicine: A Contextual Analysis', *International Journal of Health Services*, XIV (1984), pp. 339–78, here, p. 339.

49 Walter Bagehot, *Physics and Politics* [1872] (New York, 2007), p. 105.

50 George Cheyne, *Remarks on Two Late Pamphlets Written by Dr Oliphant, against Dr Pitcairn's Dissertations, and the New Theory of Fevers* (Edinburgh, 1702), p. 14.

51 Christoph Gradmann, 'A Spirit of Scientific Rigour: Koch's Postulates in Twentieth Century Medicine', *Microbes and Infection*, XVI (2014), pp. 885–92, here, p. 891.

52 T. Rivers, 'Viruses and Koch's Postulates', *Journal of Bacteriology*, XXIII (1937), pp. 1–12.

53 K. Codell Carter, *The Rise of Causal Concepts of Disease: Case Histories, the History of Medicine in Context* (Aldershot, 2003).

54 Austin Bradford Hill, 'The Environment and Disease: Association or Causation?', *Proceedings of the Royal Society of Medicine*, LVIII (1965), pp. 295–300.

55 Stanley Falkow, 'Molecular Koch's Postulates Applied to Microbial Pathogenicity', *Review of Infectious Diseases*, X (Suppl. 2) (1988), S274–6.

56 David Fredricks and David Relman, 'Sequence-Based Identification of Microbial Pathogens: A Reconsideration of Koch's Postulates', *Clinical Microbiology Reviews*, IX (1996), pp. 18–33.

57 Wilhelm Griesinger, 'Vorwort', *Archiv für Psychiatrie und Nervenkrankheiten* I (1868), pp. iii–viii, here, p. iii. See Edwin Clarke and L. S. Jacyna, *Nineteenth-Century Origins of Neuroscientific Concepts* (Berkeley, CA, 1987), pp. 133–8.

58 On gender and surgeons see Joan Cassell, *The Woman in the Surgeon's Body* (Cambridge, MA, 1998), pp. 240–45.

59 Starr, *Social Transformation of American Medicine*, p. 41.

60 'District Attorney Announces Civil Settlement with Nurse Practitioner for Unlawfully Advertising Herself as "Doctor"', www.slocounty.ca.gov (14 November 2022).

61 Daniel Wu, 'Should Nurses with PhDs be called Doctor? Lawsuit Targets California Rule', *Washington Post* (18 July 2023).

62 Edward M. Brown, 'Why Wagner-Jauregg Won the Nobel Prize', *History of Psychiatry*, XI (2000), pp. 371–82.

63 Jacalyn Duffin, 'Commemorating Excellence: The Nobel Prize and the Secular Religion of Science', in *Attributing Excellence in Medicine: The History of the Nobel Prize*, ed. Nils Hansson, Thorsten Halling and Heiner Fangerau (Amsterdam, 2019), pp. 17–38, here, p. 17.

64 Robert K. Merton, 'Recognition and Excellence: Instructive Ambiguities', in his *The Sociology of Science: Theoretical and Empirical Investigations*, ed. Norman W. Storer (Chicago, IL, 1973), pp. 419–37, here, p. 433.

65 Fabio De Sio, Nils Hansson and Ulrich Koppitz, 'John C. Eccles' Conversion and the Meaning of "Authority"', in *Attributing Excellence in Medicine*, ed. Hansson, Halling and Fangerau, pp. 143–74.

66 Duffin, 'Commemorating Excellence', p. 38. See also Harriet Zuckerman, 'The Sociology of the Nobel Prizes', *Scientific American*, CCXVII (1967), pp. 25–33, and her follow-up essay, 'Views: The Sociology of the Nobel Prize: Further Notes and Queries: How Successful Are the Prizes in Recognizing Scientific Excellence?', *American Scientist*, LXVI (1978), pp. 420–25; Colin Berry, 'The Nobel Scientists and the Origins of Scientific Achievement', *British Journal of Sociology*, XXXII (1981), pp. 381–91.

67 Lorraine Daston and Peter Galison, *Objectivity* (New York, 2010), p. 244.

68 See Carsten Timmermann, 'Weimar Medical Culture: Doctors, Healers, and the Crisis of Medicine in Interwar Germany, 1918–1933' (PhD Diss., University of Manchester, 1999), pp. 147–77.

69 Ludwig Edelstein, *The Idea of Progress in Classical Antiquity* (Baltimore, MD, 2019), p. 56.

70 On the reintroduction of the 'Hippocratic Oath' as a reflex of scientific medicine's claims see Elizabeth Williams, 'Hippocrates and the Montpellier Vitalists in the French Medical Enlightenment', in *Reinventing Hippocrates*, ed. David Cantor (Aldershot, 2002), pp. 157–77. On the history of the text see Ludwig Edelstein, *The Hippocratic Oath: Text, Translation, and Interpretation* (Baltimore, MD, 1943).

71 Wootton, *Bad Medicine*, p. 181.

72 Thomas Inman, *Foundation for a New Theory and Practice of Medicine* (London, 1860), p. 244. See also O. J. Eigsti and Pierre Dustin, Jr, *Colchicine in Agriculture, Medicine, Biology, and Chemistry* (Ames, IA, 1955).

73 See James H. Young, *Pure Food: Securing the Federal Food and Drug Act of 1906* (Princeton, NJ, 1989).

74 Anat Rosenberg, 'Exaggeration: Advertising, Law and Medical Quackery in Britain, *c.* 1840–1914', *Journal of Legal History*, XLII (2021), pp. 202–31.

75 Matthew Ramsey, 'Alternative Medicine in Modern France', *Medical History*, XLIII (1999), pp. 286–322.

76 E. Kossoy and A. Ohry, *The Feldshers* (Jerusalem, 1992), p. 6.

77 Adam Smith, *The Theory of Moral Sentiments* (London, 1892), p. 422.

78 Ibid., p. 367.

79 Roy Porter, *Quacks: Fakers and Charlatans in English Medicine* (Stroud, 2000), p. 16.

80 Ibid., p. 17.

81 Ibid., p. 208.

82 See Talcott Parsons, 'The Professions and Social Structure', in his *Essays in Sociological Theory* (New York, 1954), pp. 34–49; Gerald L. Geison, *Professions and Professional Ideologies in America* (Chapel Hill, NC, 1983), pp. 3–11; Jan Goldstein, 'Foucault among the Sociologists: The "Disciplines" and the History of the Professions', *History and Theory*, XXIII (1984), pp. 170–92.

83 Parsons, 'The Professions and Social Structure', p. 44.

84 Magali Sarfatti Larson, 'Professionalism: Rise and Fall', *International Journal of Health Services*, IX (1979), pp. 607–27, here, p. 624.

85 Eliot Freidson, *Profession of Medicine: A Study of the Sociology of Applied Knowledge* (Chicago, IL, 1970).

86 William J. Goode, 'Community within a Community: The Professions', *American Sociological Review*, XXII (1957), pp. 194–200.

87 'Notes', *Columbus Medical Journal*, XVI (1896), p. 141.

88 Peter A. Swenson, *Disorder: A History of Reform, Reaction, and Money in American Medicine* (New Haven, CT, 2021), p. 284.

89 Caroline Lockhart, *The Lady Doc* (Philadelphia, PA, 1912), pp. 158–9.

90 John Pattison, *Preface to Seventh Thousand [sic] of Cases of Cancer, Lupus, and Ulcers, Treated with Dr Pattison's New Remedy* (London, 1854), p. 66.

91 All references are to Elbert Hubbard, *The Doctors: A Satire in Four Seizures* (East Aurora, NY, 1922).

92 Ibid., p. 104.

93 Ibid., p. 107.

94 See J. C. Whorton, *Crusaders for Fitness: The History of American Health Reformers* (Princeton, NJ, 1982), pp. 205ff.

95 George Bernard Shaw, *The Doctor's Dilemma: A Tragedy* (London, 1906), pp. xxiv–v.

96 Erling Norrby, *Nobel Prizes and Life Sciences* (Singapore, 2010), p. 115.

97 H. S. Berliner, 'A Larger Perspective on the Flexner Report', *International Journal of Health Service*, V (1975), pp. 573–9.

98 Abraham Flexner, *I Remember: An Autobiography* (New York, 1940), p. 45.

99 Karl Ludmerer, *Let Me Heal: The Opportunity to Preserve Excellence in American Medicine* (New York, 2015), p. 14.

100 Abraham Flexner, *Medical Education in the United States and Canada: A Report to the Carnegie Foundation for the Advancement of Teaching, Bulletin No. 4* (New York, 1910), p. 8.

101 Ibid., p. 42.

102 Ibid., p. 166.

103 Ibid., p. 53.

104 William Osler, 'The Army Surgeon', *Medical News*, LXIV (1894), p. 318.

105 Flexner, *Medical Education*, p. 180.

106 W.E.B. Du Bois, *The Souls of Black Folk: Essays and Sketches* (Chicago, IL, 1904), p. 5.

107 Sander L. Gilman and Nancy Stepan, 'Appropriating the Idioms of Science: Some Strategies of Resistance to Biological Determinism', in *The Bounds of Race*, ed. Dominick La Capra (Ithaca, NY, 1991), pp. 72–103.

108 Deirdre Cooper Owens, *Medical Bondage: Race, Gender, and the Origins of American Gynecology* (Athens, GA, 2017).

109 Thomas N. Bonner, 'Searching for Abraham Flexner', *Academic Medicine*, LXXIII (1998), pp. 160–66.

110 Regina Morantz-Sanchez, *Sympathy and Science: Women Physicians in American Medicine* (Chapel Hill, NC, 1999).

111 Anne Taylor Kirschmann, *Vital Force: Women in American Homeopathy* (New Brunswick, NJ, 2003), p. 190.

112 Morris Fishbein, *Fads and Quackery in Healing: An Analysis of the Foibles of the Healing Cults* (New York, 1932), p. 95.

113 Philip Henry Pye-Smith, 'Medicine as a Science and Medicine as an Art', *The Lancet*, II (1900), pp. 309–12, here, p. 309.

114 D. J. Hamilton, 'The Study of Pathology', *BMJ*, II (1882), pp. 977–80, here, p. 977.

115 William C. Summers, 'On the Origins of the Science in *Arrowsmith*: Paul de Kruif, Felix d'Herelle, and Phage', *Journal of the History of Medicine and Allied Sciences*, XLVI (1991), pp. 315–32; Ilana Lowy, 'Immunology and Literature in the Early Twentieth Century: *Arrowsmith* and *The Doctor's Dilemma*', *Medical History*, XXXII (1988), pp. 314–32.

116 Ross McKibbin, 'Politics and the Medical Hero: A. J. Cronin's *The Citadel*', *English Historical Review*, CXXIII (2008), pp. 651–78; Sally Dux, '*The Citadel* (1938): Doctors, Censors and the Cinema', *Historical Journal of Film, Radio and Television*, XXXII (2012), pp. 1–17.

117 Reinhard Spree, 'The Impact of the Professionalization of Physicians on Social Change in Germany during the Late Nineteenth and Early Twentieth Centuries', *Historical Social Research/Historische Sozialforschung*, XV (1980), pp. 24–39.

118 Anon., 'Quacks in Germany', *BMJ*, I/2151 (1902), p. 734. For the number of 'quacks' in Germany at that time see Spree, *Health and Social Class in Imperial Germany*, p. 215.

119 Robert Jütte, *Geschichte der Alternative Medizin. Von der Volksmedizin zu den unkonventionellen Therapie von heute* (Munich, 1996), p. 232.

120 Abraham Flexner, *Medical Education in Europe: A Report to the Carnegie Foundation for the Advancement of Teaching* (Bulletin 5) (New York, 1912), pp. xiii, 316.

121 Reinhard Spree, 'Kurpfuscherei-Bekämpfung und ihre sozialen Funktionen während des 19. und zu Beginn des 20. Jahrhunderts', in *Medizinische Deutungsmacht im sozialen Wandel*, ed. Alfons Labisch and Reinhard Spree (Bonn, 1989), pp. 103–21.

122 Friedrich H. Moll and Matthis Krischel, 'Die Genese des Informed Consent im Kontext der medizinischen Forschungsethik 1900–1931', *Urologie*, LXII (2023), pp. 261–70.

123 Francis Dominic Degnin, 'Compassion and Medicine: Postmodern Ethics and the Physician-Patient Relationship (PhD Diss., Vanderbilt University, 2001), p. 1.

124 Roswitha Haug, 'Die Auswirkungen der NS-Doktrin auf Homöopathie und Phytotherapie: Eine vergleichende Analyse von einer medizinischen und zwei pharmazeutischen Zeitschriften' (Dr phil. Diss., Erlangen, 2009), p. 46.

125 Sabine Marx, 'Rethinking the Rise of Scientific Medicine: Trier, Germany, 1880–1914' (PhD Diss, Carnegie Mellon University, 2002), p. iii.

126 Ibid., p. 15.

127 Edward C. Halperin, 'The Jewish Problem in U.S. Medical Education, 1920–1955', *Journal of the History of Medicine*, LVI (2001), pp. 140–67.

128 Thomas Neville Bonner, *Iconoclast: Abraham Flexner and a Life in Learning* (Baltimore, MD, 2002), p. 223. See also his 'Abraham Flexner as Critic of British and Continental Medical Education', *Medical History*, XXXIII (1989), pp. 472–9.

129 U. Meyer, 'Pharmazeutische Industrie und "Neue Deutsche Heilkunde"', *Medizin, Gesellschaft, Geschichte*, XXIII (2004), pp. 165–82.

130 Haug, 'Die Auswirkungen der NS-Doktrin auf Homöopathie und Phytotherapie', p. 3.

131 Hans Wapler, 'Noch einmal *Similia similibus* als Leitgedanke in Politik und Medizin,' *Allgemeine Homöopathische Zeitung*, CLXXXI (1933), pp. 317–19, here, p. 318.

132 Matthias Wischner, *Kleine Geschichte der Homöopathie* (Essen, 2004), p. 62.

133 Alfred Haug, 'Die Reichsarbeitsgemeinschaft für eine Neue Deutsche Heilkunde (1935–1936)', *Würzburger medizinhistorische Mitteilungen*, II (1984), pp. 117–30, here, p. 117.

134 Ernst Klee, *Deutsche Medizin im Dritten Reich. Karrieren vor und nach 1945* (Frankfurt, 2001), p. 50.

135 Michael Kater, *Doctors under Hitler* (Chapel Hill, NC, 1989), p. 38.

136 Ludmerer, *Let Me Heal*, p. 26.

137 Eli Clare, *Brilliant Imperfection: Grappling with Cure* (Durham, NC, 2017), p. xvi.

138 Simon Garfield, MAUVE – *How One Man Invented a Colour That Changed the World* (London, 2000).

139 John Beer, 'Coal Tar Dye Manufacture and the Origins of the Modern Industrial Research Laboratory', *Isis*, XLIX (1958), pp. 123–31.

140 Carolyn Cobbold, *A Rainbow Palate: How Chemical Dyes Changed the West's Relationship with Food* (Chicago, IL, 2020).

141 Anthony S. Travis, 'Chemical Modeling: From Paul Ehrlich's Dyes to β-Blockers – a Brief History', *Journal of Computational Biology*, XXVI (2019), pp. 726–34.

142 Charles C. Mann and Mark L. Plummer, *The Aspirin Wars: Money, Medicine, and 100 Years of Rampant Competition* (New York, 1991). See also Walter Sneader, 'The Discovery of Aspirin: A Reappraisal', *BMJ*, CCCXXI (2000), pp. 1591–4.

143 Asha Persson, 'Incorporating Pharmakon: HIV, Medicine, and Body Shape Change', *Body and Society*, X (2004), pp. 45–67. This builds on Jacques Derrida, 'Plato's Pharmacy', in his *Dissemination*, trans. Barbara Johnson (Chicago, IL, 1981), pp. 63–171.

144 Plato, *Lysis. Symposium. Phaedrus*, ed. and trans. Christopher Emlyn-Jones and William Preddy, Loeb Classical Library, 166 (Cambridge, MA, 2022), p. 515.

145 Anon., 'Drug Addiction and Its Treatment', *The Lancet*, CC (1922), p. 137.

146 L. Cournot, 'Les tentatives de suicide par l'aspirine', *La Semaine des hôpitaux thérapeutique*, XXVI (1950), pp. 111–14.

147 For example, see S. O. Krasnoff and M. Bernstein, 'Acetylsalicylic Acid Poisoning, with a Report of a Fatal Case', *JAMA*, CXXXV (1947), pp. 712–14; J. C. Veltri and D. E. Rollins, 'A Comparison of the Frequency and Severity of Poisoning Cases for Ingestion of Acetaminophen, Aspirin, and Ibuprofen', *American Journal of Emergency Medicine*, VI (1988), pp. 104–7.

148 Hermann Schneider, *Kultur und Denken der Babylonier und Juden* (Leipzig, 1910), p. 663.

149 Robert Proctor, *The Nazi War on Cancer* (Princeton, NJ, 1999), p. 23.

150 Erwin Liek, 'Die Entseelung der Heilkunde', *Münchener Medizinische Wochenschrift*, LXXII (1925), pp. 1520–21.

151 Otto Weininger, *Sex and Character* (London, 1906), p. 315.

152 Eva-Maria Klasen, 'Die Diskussion über eine "Krise" der Medizin in Deutschland zwischen 1925 und 1935' (Dr phil. Diss., University of Mainz, 1984).

153 William Osler, *Aequanimitas with Other Addresses to Medical Students, Nurses and Practitioners of Medicine* (Philadelphia, PA, 1905), p. 301.

154 C. David Naylor, 'Grey Zones of Clinical Practice: Some Limits to Evidence-Based Medicine', *The Lancet*, CCCXLV (1995), pp. 840–42, here, p. 840.

155 Lee Peter Ruddin, 'You Can Generalize Stupid! Social Scientists, Bent Flyvbjerg, and Case Study Methodology', *Qualitative Inquiry*, XII (2016), pp. 797–812, here, p. 809.

156 Ibid., p. 804.

157 Ibid., p. 809.

158 Nikolas Rose, *Governing the Soul: The Shaping of the Private Self* (London, 1990), p. 7.

159 P. B. Medawar, *Advice to a Young Scientist* (New York, 1979), p. 50.

160 Gordon H. Guyatt, 'Evidence-Based Medicine', *ACP Journal Club*, CXIV (Suppl. 2) (1991), A-16; citation from David L. Sackett et al., 'Evidence Based Medicine: What It Is and What It Isn't', *BMJ*, CCCXII (1996), p. 71.

161 R. L. Sur and P. Dahm, 'History of Evidence-Based Medicine', *Indian Journal of Urology*, XXVII/4 (2011), pp. 487–9.

162 David Sackett, 'Why Did I Become a Clinician-Trialist?', *Journal of the Royal Society of Medicine*, CVIII (2015), pp. 325–30, here, p. 325.

163 Ibid., p. 330.

164 G. Guyatt et al., 'Evidence-Based Medicine: A New Approach to Teaching the Practice of Medicine', *JAMA*, CCLXVIII (1992), pp. 2420–25, here, p. 2421.

165 M. J. Barry and S. Edgman-Levitan, 'Shared Decision Making – The Pinnacle of Patient-Centered Care', *New England Journal of Medicine*, CCCLXVI (2012), pp. 780–81, here, p. 780.

166 M. Berkwits, 'From Practice to Research: The Case for Criticism in an Age of Evidence', *Social Science and Medicine*, XLVII (1998), pp. 1539–45, here, p. 1542.

167 William Godolphin, 'Shared Decision-Making', *Healthcare Quarterly*, XII (2009), e186–e190, here, e188.

168 Sander L. Gilman, '"Barbaric" Rituals?', in *Is Multiculturalism Bad for Women?*, ed. Joshua Cohen, Matthew Howard and Martha C. Nussbaum (Princeton, NJ, 1999), pp. 53–8.

169 N. J. Mackintosh et al., 'Interventions to Increase Patient and Family Involvement in Escalation of Care for Acute Life-Threatening Illness in Community Health and Hospital Settings', *Cochrane Database System Review*, XII (2020), CD012829.

170 Ariel L. Zimerman, 'Evidence-Based Medicine: A Short History of a Modern Medical Movement', *American Medical Association Journal of Ethics*, XV (2013), pp. 71–6.

171 C. David Naylor, 'Clinical Decisions: From Art to Science and Back Again', *The Lancet*, CCCLVIII (2001), p. 523.

172 James Giordano and Julia Pedroni, 'The Legacy of Albert Schweitzer's Virtue Ethics to a Moral Philosophy', in *Reverence for Life Revisited: Albert Schweitzer's Relevance Today*, ed. David A. Valone and David Ives (Cambridge, 2007), pp. 141–51, here, p. 143.

173 Edzard Ernst, 'Are We All Quacks?', *Archive of Family Medicine*, VI (1997), pp. 389–90, here, p. 390.

174 *Blackstone's Commentaries on the Laws of England*, Book the Third – Chapter the Eighth: Of Wrongs and Their Remedies, Respecting the Rights of Persons, https://avalon.law.yale.edu, accessed 19 July 2024.

175 *Blackstone's Commentaries on the Laws of England*, Book the Third – Chapter the Ninth: Of Injuries to Personal Property, https://avalon.law.yale.edu, accessed 19 July 2024.

176 *Blackstone's Commentaries on the Laws of England*, Book the Third – Chapter the Eighth: *Of Wrongs and Their Remedies, Respecting the Rights of Persons*, https://avalon.law.yale.edu, accessed 19 July 2024.

177 Adam Smith, *The Glasgow Edition of the Works and Correspondence of Adam Smith*, ed. Ernst Mossner and Ian Ross (Oxford, 1976–86), here, VI, p. 56.

178 Robert Knox, 'Anatomical Museums, Their Objects and Present Condition', *Medical Times*, XIV (1846), pp. 307–8, continued at 327–8, here, p. 307.

179 Theodore Silver, 'One Hundred Years of Harmful Error: The Historical Jurisprudence of Medical Malpractice', *Wisconsin Law Review*, IV (1992), pp. 1193–1242, here, p. 1194.

180 Fleming James, Jr, *The Law of Torts* (Boston, MA, 1956), pp. 602–20.

181 *Texas & Pacific Railway v. Behmyer* [1903], 189 U.S., pp. 468, 470.

182 *Albrighton v. Royal Prince Alfred Hospital* [1980] 2 NSWLR 542(CA), p. 562. I am indebted to Brian Hurwitz's survey 'How Does Evidence Based Guidance Influence Determinations of Medical Negligence?', *BMJ*, CCCXXIX (2004), p. 1024.

183 *Arland v. Taylor* [1955] O.R. 131 at p. 142.

184 *Blyth v. Birmingham Waterworks Co.* [1856], 11 Ex. 781 at p. 784.

185 A. P. Herbert, *The Uncommon Law* [1936] (London, 1952), p. 31.

186 Ibid., p. 130.

187 Silver, 'One Hundred Years of Harmful Error', p. 1196.

188 J. W. Brooke Barnett, 'Medical Malpractice: The American Disease. Is It Infectious?', *Medico-Legal Journal*, XLVIII (1980), pp. 63–75, here, p. 75.

189 Ibid., p. 65.

190 Ibid., p. 74.

191 Graham Virgo, 'Reconstructing Manslaughter on Defective Foundations', *Cambridge Law Journal*, LIV (1995), pp. 14–16.

192 *Jones v. Chidester* [1992] 610 A.2d 964. See Mary S. Newbold, 'Medical Malpractice Law – Pennsylvania's Two Schools of Thought Doctrine Revisited: Definition and Application Clarified – Underlying Goal Thwarted', *Temple Law Review*, LXVI (1993), pp. 613–28.

193 David S. Caudill and Lewis H. Larue, *No Magic Wand: The Idealization of Science in Law* (Lanham, MD, 2006), pp. xiiff.

194 *Daubert v. Merrell Dow Pharmaceuticals, Inc.* [1993] 590 U.S. 579, pp. 589–92. Not fixed but true, even though Justice Blackmun quoted from an *Amici Curiae* brief: 'Indeed, scientists do not assert that they know what is immutably "true" – they are committed to searching for new, temporary theories to explain, as best they can, phenomena.'

195 *Judicial Council of California Civil Jury Instructions* (2022 edn), www.justia.com, accessed 26 March 2023.

196 Michael H. Cohen, 'A Fixed Star in Health Care Reform: The Emerging Paradigm of Holistic Healing', *Arizona State Law Journal*, XXVII (1995), pp. 79–172, here, p. 103.

197 Ibid.

198 Karin Knorr Cetina, *Epistemic Cultures: How the Sciences Make Knowledge* (Cambridge, MA, 1999), pp. 29–32.

199 Stephanos Bibas, 'Bringing Moral Values into a Flawed Plea-Bargaining System', *Cornell Law Review*, LXXXVIII (2003), pp. 1425–32, here, p. 1429.

200 L. I. Resch, E. Ernst and J. Garrow, 'A Randomized Controlled Study of Reviewer-Bias against an Unconventional Therapy', *Journal of the Royal Society of Medicine*, XCIII (2000), pp. 164–7, here, p. 164.

2 Stomachs

1 C. O'Connor and J. O. Weatherall, 'False Beliefs and the Social Structure of Science: Some Models and Case Studies', in *Groupthink in Science: Greed, Pathological Altruism, Ideology, Competition, and Culture,* ed. D. M. Allen and J. W. Howell (Cham, Switzerland, 2020), pp. 37–48.

2 'It is never as severe as the pain of true peptic ulcer except when there is intermittent pylorospasm which produces an acute attack simulating perforated peptic ulcer or biliary colic.' Isidore William Held and Abraham Allen Goldbloom, *Peptic Ulcer* (Springfield, IL, 1946), p. 121.

3 Walter Pagel, 'Geschichte des runden Magengeschwürs: Beiträge zur historischen Pathologie und zur Geschichte der Diagnose I', *Sudhoffs Archiv für die Geschichte der Medizin*, XXV (1932), pp. 330–48.

4 Joshua O. Leibowitz, 'A Probable Case of Peptic Ulcer as Described by Amatus Lusitanus (1556)', *Bulletin of the History of Medicine*, XXVII (1953), pp. 212–16.

5 Joshua O. Leibowitz, 'Did Vesalius Suffer from Peptic Ulcer?', *Bulletin of the History of Medicine*, XXXII (1958), pp. 75–8.

6 Marcello Donato, *De medica historia mirabili libri sex* (Mantua, 1586), book IV, chap. 3, pp. 195–9.

7 Denis Gibbs, 'The Demon of Dyspepsia: Some Nineteenth-Century Perceptions of Disordered Digestion', in *Gastroenterology in Britain: Historical Essays,* ed. William F. Bynum (London, 1997), pp. 29–42.

8 R. James, *A Medical Dictionary* (London, 1745).
9 Anon., *The Edinburgh Practice of Surgery and Midwifery* (London, 1803), II, pp. 400–402.
10 W. Cullen and P. Reid, *First Lines of the Practice of Physic* (Edinburgh, 1816), II, pp. 39–51.
11 Elizabeth C. Gaskell, *The Life of Charlotte Brontë* (London, 1857), II, p. 310.
12 Samuel Gottlieb Vogel, *Sam. Gottl. Vogel's Handbuch der practischen Arzeneywissenschaft zum Gebrauche für angehende Aerzte* IV (Stendal, 1795), pp. 280–95.
13 W.A.N. Dorland, *The American Illustrated Medical Dictionary* (Philadelphia, PA, and London, 1900), p. 726.
14 Georg Ernst Stahl, *Dissertatio medica inauguralis vena portae porta malorum hypochondriaco-splenetico-suffocativo-hysterico-colico-haemorrhoidariorum* (Magdeburg, 1705), p. 45.
15 John Hunter, 'On the Digestion of the Stomach after Death', *Philosophical Transactions of the Royal Society of London*, LXII (1772), pp. 447–54, here, p. 450.
16 Matthew Baillie, *The Morbid Anatomy of Some of the Most Important Parts of the Human Body* (London, 1797), pp. 140–41.
17 William S. Haubrich, 'Cruveilhier of la maladie de Cruveilhier', *Gastroenterology*, CXV (1998), p. 12.
18 Roy Porter, 'Biliousness', in *Gastroenterology in Britain*, ed. Bynum, pp. 7–28, here, p. 23.
19 William Osler, *The Principles and Practice of Medicine Designed for the Use of Practitioners and Students of Medicine* (New York, 1892), p. 368.
20 See Anaïs Rameau and Albert Mudry, 'When Did Gastro-Esophageal Reflux Become a Disease? A Historical Perspective on GER(D) Nomenclature', *International Journal of Pediatric Otorhinolaryngology*, CXXXVII (2020), p. 110214.
21 Heinrich Quincke, 'Ulcus oesophagi ex digestione', *Deutsche Archiv für klinische Medizin*, XXIV (1879), pp. 72–9.
22 Simon X. M. Dong, Connie C. Y. Chang and Katelynn J. Rowe, 'A Collection of the Etiological Theories, Characteristics, and Observations/Phenomena of Peptic Ulcers in Existing Data', *Data Brief*, XIX (2018), pp. 1058–67.
23 Rudolf Virchow, 'Historische, Kritisches und Positives zur Lehre der Unterleibsaffektionen', *Archiv für pathologische Anatomie und Physiologie*, V (1853), pp. 281–375, here, pp. 282, 328.
24 Carl Schwarz, 'Über penetrierende Magen- und Jejunalgeschwüre', *Beiträge zur Klinischen Chirugurie*, LXVII (1910), pp. 96–128. See also S. Fatović-Ferenčić and M. Banić, 'No Acid, No Ulcer: Dragutin (Carl) Schwarz (1868–1917), the Man Ahead of His Time', *Digestive Diseases*, XXIX (2011), pp. 507–10.
25 Gibbs, 'The Demon of Dyspepsia', p. 35. See also Hisao Ishizuka, 'Carlyle's Nervous Dyspepsia: Nervousness, Indigestion and the Experience of Modernity in Nineteenth Century Britain', in *Neurology and Modernity: A Cultural History of Nervous Systems, 1800–1950*, ed. Laura Salisbury and Andrew Shail (London, 2010), pp. 81–96.
26 Thomas Trotter, *A View of the Nervous Temperament* (London, 1807), p. xv.
27 In an endnote filling out a page in *The Lancet*, LXXX (13 September 1862), p. 278.
28 Erasmus Darwin, *Zoonomia; or, The Laws of Organic Life* (London, 1794), p. 478.
29 J. Russell Reynolds, 'An Address on Specialism in Medicine', *The Lancet*, CXVIII/3033 (1881), pp. 655–8, here, p. 656.

30 Bartosz Michał Radomski, Dunja Šešelja and Kim Naumann, 'Rethinking the History of Peptic Ulcer Disease and Its Relevance for Network Epistemology', *History of Philosophy and the Life Sciences*, XLIII (2021), p. 113.

31 Samuel Hopkins Adams, 'The Great American Fraud: Patent Medicines, the Law, and the Public', *Colliers* (20 January 1912), p. 130.

32 Ibid.

33 James R. Zetka, Jr, *Surgeons and the Scope* (Ithaca, NY, 2003), p. 81.

34 William Beaumont, *Experiments and Observations on the Gastric Juice, and the Physiology of Digestion* (Plattsburgh, NY, 1833), pp. 107–8.

35 See in more detail Zetka, Jr, *Surgeons*, pp. 80–97.

36 J. M. Edmonson, 'History of the Instruments for Gastrointestinal Endoscopy', *Gastrointestinal Endoscopy*, XXXVII (1991) (Suppl.), S27–56.

37 P. Rathert, W. Lutzeyer and W. E. Goddwin, 'Philipp Bozzini (1773–1809) and the Lichtleiter', *Urology*, III (1974), pp. 113–18.

38 Ibid., p. 117.

39 Theodore Hieronymus Bast, *The Life and Times of Adolf Kussmaul* (New York, 1926), pp. 110–11.

40 Sander L. Gilman et al., *Hysteria: A New History* (Berkeley, CA, 1993), p. 392.

41 Adrian M. K. Thomas and Arpan K. Banerjee, *The History of Radiology* (Oxford, 2013), pp. 77–80.

42 Sarah M. Jordan, 'The Present Status of Peptic Ulcer', *New England Journal of Medicine*, CCIII (1930), pp. 917–20, here, p. 918.

43 William Brinton, *On the Pathology, Symptoms, and Treatment of Ulcer of the Stomach* (London, 1857), p. 95.

44 G. H. Lewes, *The Physiology of Common Life*, 2 vols (Edinburgh and London, 1859), I, p. 233.

45 Joel D. Howell, *Technology in the Hospital: Transforming Patient Care in the Early Twentieth Century* (Baltimore, MD, 1995), pp. 79–102.

46 Carl von Rokitansky, *A Manual of Pathological Anatomy*, 4 vols, trans. Edward Sieveking et al. (London, 1849), II, pp. 36–8.

47 William Gass, *Reading Rilke: Reflections on the Problems of Translation* (New York, 1999), p. 3.

48 Excerpted in Gert H. Brieger, ed., *Medical America in the Nineteenth Century: Readings from the Literature* (Baltimore, MD, 1972), pp. 198–200.

49 David Wootton, *Bad Medicine: Doctors Doing Harm since Hippocrates* (Oxford, 2007), p. 238.

50 S. J. Konturek, 'Gastric Secretion – from Pavlov's Nervism to Popielski's Histamine as Direct Secretagogue of Oxyntic Glands', *Journal of Physiological Pharmacology*, LV (2003), pp. 43–68.

51 'Report of the Medical Society of London', *The Lancet*, CLXXX (1912), pp. 1778–84.

52 Andrew Cunningham, 'Transforming Plague: The Laboratory and the Identity of Infectious Disease', in *The Laboratory Revolution in Medicine*, ed. Andrew Cunningham and Perry Williams (Cambridge, 1992), pp. 209–44, here, p. 239.

53 B.G.A. Moynihan, *Two Lectures on Gastric and Duodenal Ulcer: A Record of Ten Years' Experience* (Bristol, 1923), p. 19.

54 Paul Starr, *The Social Transformation of American Medicine* (New York, 1982), pp. 156–7.

55 *Merck Manual of Therapeutics and Materia Medica*, 6th and 7th edns (Rahway, NJ, 1934, 1940).

56 Frank Billings, 'Focal Infection: Its Broader Application in the Etiology of General Disease', *JAMA*, LVIII (1914), pp. 899–903, here, p. 899.

57 James W. Barton, MD, 'That Body of Yours', *The Kingston [NY] Daily Freeman* (23 December 1938), p. 4.

58 W. R. Burden and J. P. O'Leary, 'The Vagus Nerve, Gastric Secretions, and Their Relationship to Peptic Ulcer Disease', *Archives of Surgery*, CXXVI (1991), pp. 259–64.

59 Arthur Dean Bevan, 'Peptic Ulcer: Etiology, History and Surgical Treatment', *JAMA*, XCIV (1930), pp. 2043–6, here, p. 2043.

60 E. D. Palmer, 'Investigation of the Gastric Mucosa Spirochetes of the Human', *Gastroenterology*, XXVII (1954), pp. 218–20.

61 Richard Wollheim, 'On the Freudian Unconscious', *Proceedings and Addresses of the American Philosophical Association*, LXXVII (2003), pp. 23–35, here, p. 28.

62 Karl Abraham, 'Bericht über den VIII. Internationalen psychoanalytischen Kongress', *Internationale Zeitschrift für Psychoanalyse*, X (1924), pp. 211–44, here, pp. 217–18.

63 Cathy Carruth, *Unclaimed Experience: Trauma, Narrative and History* (Baltimore, MD, 1996), p. 30.

64 Sigmund Freud, *Beyond the Pleasure Principle* (1920), *The Standard Edition of the Complete Psychological Works of Sigmund Freud*, trans. and ed. James Strachey et al., 24 vols (London, 1953–74), XVIII, p. 12. See also Ernest Jones et al., eds, *Zur Psychoanalyse der Kriegsneurosen* (Vienna, 1919).

65 Desmond Curran and McDonald Critchley, 'German Neuropsychiatry with Reference to the *Kriegsmarine*', National Archives, Admiralty, and Ministry of Defence 213/76 (August 1946), p. 11. See also Ian Miller, 'The Mind and Stomach at War: Stress and Abdominal Illness in Britain, *c.* 1939–1945', *Medical History*, LIV (2010), pp. 95–110, and Edgar Jones, '"The Gut War": Functional Somatic Disorders in the UK during the Second World War', *History of the Human Sciences*, XXV (2012), pp. 30–48.

66 Joseph E. Crowell, *The Young Volunteer: The Everyday Experiences of a Soldier Boy in the Civil War*, 2nd edn (New York, 1906), p. 73.

67 Zachary Turpin, 'Introduction to Walt Whitman's "Manly Health and Training"', *Walt Whitman Quarterly Review*, XXX (2016), pp. 184–210, here, p. 186.

68 All quotations are from Mose Velsor [that is, Walt Whitman], 'Brief Sketch of a Day of Training, for the Use of Beginners', [26 September 1858] *Walt Whitman Quarterly Review*, XXX (2016), pp. 198–206.

69 George M. Beard, *American Nervousness: Its Causes and Consequences* (New York, 1881), p. 96. See Charles E. Rosenberg, 'George M. Beard and American Nervousness', in his *No Other Gods: On Science and American Social Thought* (Baltimore, MD, 1978), pp. 98–108.

70 Beard, *American Nervousness*, p. 27.

71 Ibid., p. 46.

72 Ibid., p. 44.

73 W. O. Huston, 'The American Disease', *Columbus Medical Journal*, XVI (1896), pp. 1–6, here, p. 1. See Gert H. Brieger, 'Dyspepsia: The American Disease? Needs and Opportunities for Research', in *Healing and History: Essays for George Rosen*, ed. Charles E. Rosenberg (New York, 1979), pp. 179–90.

74 Huston, 'The American Disease', p. 2.

75 Philip P. Wiener, 'G. M. Beard and Freud on "American Nervousness"', *Journal of the History of Ideas*, XVII (1956), pp. 269–74.

76 Sigmund Freud, *Civilization and Its Discontents* (1930), *The Standard Edition of the Complete Psychological Works of Sigmund Freud*, XXI, pp. 57–146.

77 Ibid., p. 83.

78 Ibid., p. 96.

79 Sigmund Freud, 'A Case of Successful Treatment by Hypnotism: With Some Remarks on the Origin of Hysterical Symptoms through "Counter-Will"' (1892), *The Standard Edition of the Complete Psychological Works of Sigmund Freud*, I, pp. 115–28.

80 J. Mason Good, *The Study of Medicine*, 4 vols (Boston, MA, 1823), I, p. 345.

81 Erika S. Schmidt, 'The Berlin Tradition in Chicago: Franz Alexander and the Chicago Institute for Psychoanalysis', *Psychoanalytic History*, XII (2010), pp. 69–83.

82 Franz Alexander, 'The Neurotic Character', *International Journal of Psychoanalysis*, XI (1930), pp. 291–311, here, p. 292.

83 Franz Alexander, *Psychosomatic Medicine: Its Principles and Applications* (New York, 1950), p. 134.

84 Franz Alexander, 'The Logic of Emotions and Its Dynamic Background', *International Journal of Psychoanalysis*, XVI (1935), pp. 399–413, here, p. 406.

85 Franz Alexander, 'Psychoanalysis and Medicine', *JAMA*, XCVI (1931), pp. 1351–8.

86 Franz Alexander, 'Functional Disturbances of Psychogenic Nature', *JAMA*, C (1933), pp. 469–73, here, p. 471.

87 Helen Flanders Dunbar, *Mind and Body: Psychosomatic Medicine* (New York, 1947), p. 55.

88 'The Notebooks of F. Scott Fitzgerald', www.fitzgerald.narod.ru, accessed 26 March 2023.

89 F. Scott Fitzgerald, *The Love of the Last Tycoon: A Western*, ed. Matthew J. Bruccoli (Cambridge, MA, 1993), p. 36.

90 Alexander, 'The Logic of Emotions', p. 407. See also Franz Alexander, 'A Case of Peptic Ulcer and Personality Disorder', *Psychosomatic Medicine*, IX (1947), pp. 320–30.

91 *Peptic Ulcer: Rise and Fall*, transcript of a witness seminar Held at the Wellcome Institute for the History of Medicine, London, on 12 May 2000, vol. XIV (London, 2002), p. 1.

92 On the history of stress see especially Mark Jackson, *The Age of Stress: Science and the Search for Stability* (Oxford, 2013).

93 Daniel T. Davies and A. T. Macbeth Wilson, 'Observations on the Life-History of Chronic Peptic Ulcer', *The Lancet*, CCXXX (1937), pp. 1353–60.

94 Pauline Langeluddecke, Kerry Goulston and Christopher Tennant, 'Type A Behaviour and Other Psychological Factors in Peptic Ulcer Disease', *Journal of Psychosomatic Research*, XXXI (1987), pp. 335–40.

95 Samuel C. Robinson, 'On the Etiology of Peptic Ulcer', *American Journal of Digestive Diseases*, II (1935), pp. 333–43, here, p. 343.

96 George Crile, *Diseases Peculiar to Civilized Man: Clinical Management and Surgical Treatment*, ed. Amy Rowland (New York, 1934), p. 100.

97 Joseph V. Brady, 'Ulcers in "Executive" Monkeys', *Scientific American*, CXCIX (1958), pp. 95–104. See also Robert Ader, 'The Role of Conditioning in Pharmacotherapy', in *The Placebo Effect: An Interdisciplinary Exploration*, ed. Anne Harrington (Cambridge, MA, 1997), pp. 138–65.

98 Theodor Adorno et al., *The Authoritarian Personality* [1950] (London, 2019), pp. 943, 963, 793.

99 C. Wright Mills, *White Collar: The American Middle Classes* [1951] (Oxford, 2002), pp. 98–9.

100 Paul Goodman, *Growing Up Absurd: Problems of Youth in the Organized Society* [1960] (New York, 2012), p. 85.

101 Abbie Hoffman, 'Media Freaking' [Lincoln Park, Chicago, 27 August 1968: 'Talking to the Yippies', taped by Charles Harbut], *Drama Review: TDR*, XIII/4 (1969), pp. 46–51, here, p. 46.

102 Alexander Mitscherlich and Margarete Mitscherlich, *The Inability to Mourn: Principles of Collective Behavior*, trans. Beverley R. Placzek (New York, 1975).

103 Ibid., p. 32.

104 Beard, *American Nervousness*, p. 44.

105 Mitscherlich, *The Inability to Mourn*, p. 33.

106 Alexander Mitscherlich, 'Ulcus ventriculi et duodeni – Schritte der Forschung', *Psyche*, XXI (1967), pp. 780–92.

107 Steffan Dörre, 'Epistemologische Neupositionierungen. Alexander Mitscherlich zwischen "naturwissenschaftlicher Methodik", Psychoanalyse und Psychosomatischer Medizin', *NTM: Zeitschrift für Geschichte der Naturwissenschaften, Technik und Medizin*, XXIX (2021), pp. 417–46.

108 Dagmar Herzog, *On Aggression: Psychoanalysis as Moral Politics in Post-Nazi Germany* (Florence, 2015), p. 3.

109 I am indebted to Mert Bahadır Reisoğlu, '*Gastarbeiterulcus* and Realism in Güney Dal: A Gastrointestinal Account of "*Gastarbeiterliteratur*"', *Seminar*, LIX (2023), pp. 24–43.

110 Joseph B. Kirsner, 'Hormones and Peptic Ulcer', *Bulletin of the New York Academy of Medicine*, XXIX (1953), pp. 477–504, here, p. 490.

111 Angela Zink and Johannes Korporal, 'Soziale Epidemiologie der Erkrankungen von Ausländern in der Bundesrepublik Deutschland', in *Zwischen zwei Kulturen – Was macht Ausländer krank?*, ed. Heribert Kentenich et al. (Berlin, 1984), pp. 24–41, here, p. 27.

112 Svetlana Boym, *The Future of Nostalgia* (Princeton, NJ, 2001), pp. 107–8.

113 Peter Sloterdijk, *Critique of Cynical Reason*, trans. Michael Eldred (Minneapolis, MI, 1987), p. 189.

114 R. Arnold, 'Epidemiologie, natürlicher Verlauf und sozioökonomische Bedeutung der Ulkuskrankheit', in *Der chronisch Kranke in der Gastroenterologie. Interdisziplinäre Gastroenterologie*, ed. H. Goebell, J. Hotz and E. H. Farthmann (Berlin, Heidelberg, 1984), pp. 34–47.

115 Fabian Bauer, 'Entwurzelung', in *Exil, Flucht, Migration: Konfligierende Begriffe, vernetzte Diskurse?*, ed. Bettina Bannasch, Doerte Bischoff and Burcu Dogramaci (Berlin, Boston, MA, 2022), pp. 62–71.

116 Günter Wallraff, *Ganz unten* (Cologne, 1985), p. 152.

117 Dr [Samuel] Cartwright, 'The Diseases of Negroes – Pulmonary Congestions, Pneumonia, etc.', *De Bow's Review*, XI (1851), pp. 209–13.

118 George M. Niles, 'A Therapeutic Comparison, Medicinal and Otherwise, as between the Caucasian and Afro-American', *Southern Medical Journal* (1 February 1913), pp. 127–9, here, p. 129.

119 Charles H. Garvin, 'Negro Health', *Opportunity* (November 1924), pp. 341–2, here, p. 342.

120 Andrew B. Rivers, 'Clinical Considerations of the Etiology of Peptic Ulcer', *Archive of Internal Medicine*, LIII (1934), pp. 97–119, here, p. 110.

121 J. Mason Good, *The Study of Medicine*, 4 vols (Boston, MA, 1823), I, p. 106.

122 Samuel C. Robinson, 'On the Etiology of Peptic Ulcer: An Analysis of 70 Ulcer Patients', *American Journal of Digestive Diseases and Nutrition*, II (1935), pp. 333–43, here, pp. 333, 342.

123 Bernie [Julia] Babcock, *The Daughter of a Republican* (Chicago, IL, 1900), p. 88.

124 Robinson, 'On the Etiology of Peptic Ulcer', p. 343.

125 U. G. Dailey, 'The Ulcer Patient', *Journal of the National Medical Association*, XXXVI (1944), pp. 129–30, here, p. 130.

126 Sander L. Gilman, *Freud, Race, and Gender* (Princeton, NJ, 1993).

127 Fredrick Steigmann, 'The Peptic Ulcer Syndrome in the Negro: Clinical and Statistical Evidence on Psychogenic as against Racial Factors in the Etiology of This Syndrome', *American Journal of Digestive Diseases and Nutrition*, III (1936), pp. 310–15.

128 H. A. Callis, 'Discrimination Neurosis', *Journal of the National Medical Association*, XLIV (1952), p. 464.

129 Robert Jackson and Bernard Harris, 'Study of Twenty Cases of Gastric and Duodenal Ulcer in the Negro', *Journal of the National Medical Association*, XXVI (1934), pp. 1–5, here, p. 3.

130 F. Stephan Carter, 'Peptic Ulcer in Africans', *BMJ*, I/5171 (13 February 1960), pp. 505–6, here, p. 506.

131 Such as Arline T. Geronimus, Jay A. Pearson, Erin Linnenbringer et al., 'Weathering in Detroit: Place, Race, Ethnicity, and Poverty as Conceptually Fluctuating Social Constructs Shaping Variation in Allostatic Load', *Milbank Quarterly*, XCVIII (2020), pp. 1171–1218.

132 Arline T. Geronimus, *Weathering: The Extraordinary Stress of Ordinary Life in an Unjust Society* (New York, 2023).

133 Georg Burgle, *Die Hysterie und die Strafrechtliche Verantwortlichkeit der Hysterischen: Ein praktisches Handbuch für Ärzte und Juristen* (Stuttgart, 1912), p. 19.

134 Wilhelm Erb, *Über die wachsende Nervosität unserer Zeit. Akademische Rede zum Geburtsfeste . . . Karl Friedrich am 22. November 1893* (Heidelberg, 1893), p. 22.

135 Emil Kraepelin, 'Zur Entartungsfrage', *Zentralblatt für Nervenheilkunde und Psychiatrie*, XIX (1908), pp. 745–51, here, p. 748.

136 Sander L. Gilman, 'Sexology, Psychoanalysis and Degeneration: From a Theory of Race to a Race to Theory', in *Degeneration*, ed. Sander L. Gilman and J. E. Chamberlin (New York, 1985), pp. 72–96.

137 Max Nordau, *Degeneration* (New York, 1895), p. 16. See Michael Berkowitz, *Max Nordau and the Early Zionist Movement, 1896–1905* (Madison, WI, 1983).

138 Nordau, *Degeneration*, p. 555.

139 Ibid., p. 423.

140 Ibid., p. 41.

141 William James, 'Degeneration and Genius', *Psychological Review*, II (1895), pp. 287–94; William Dean Howells, 'Degeneration', in *Howells as Critic*, ed. Edwin Cady (London, 1973), pp. 217–24. See also Dana Seitler, 'Degenerate America: Embodiment, Modernity and the Culture of Science (1890–1937)' (PhD Diss., University of Chicago, 2000).

142 Jeffery A. Marston, 'Tropical Life and Its Sequelæ', *The Lancet*, CXXXV (1890), pp. 588–90, here, p. 589.

143 J. Lawrence-Hamilton, 'Jewish Cattle Killing and Mosaic Meat', *Public Health*, VI (1893), pp. 122–3, here, p. 122.

144 T. Clifford Allbutt, 'Substance of the Address in Medicine', *The Lancet*, CXXXII (1888), pp. 246–50, here, pp. 247–8.

145 Maurice Fishberg, *The Jews: A Study of Race and Environment* (New York, 1911), pp. 309–10.

146 Raphael Patai, *The Jewish Mind* (Detroit, MI, 1996), p. 423.

147 Robert Jütte, *The Jewish Body: A History*, trans. Elizabeth Bredeck (Philadelphia, PA, 2021), pp. 141ff.

148 Charles Seligman Bernheimer, *The Russian Jew in the United States: Studies of Social Conditions in New York, Philadelphia, and Chicago; with a Description of Rural Settlements* (Philadelphia, PA, 1905), pp. 289, 313.

149 J. A. Pearson and A. T. Geronimus, 'Race/Ethnicity, Socioeconomic Characteristics, Coethnic Social Ties, and Health: Evidence from the National Jewish Population Survey', *American Journal of Public Health*, CI (2011), pp. 1314–21, here, p. 1315.

150 On the question of the malleability of concepts of racial difference in the American context see Matthew Frye Jacobson, *Whiteness of a Different Color: European Immigrants and the Alchemy of Race* (Cambridge, MA, 1998).

151 Herbert Wiener, 'The Concept of Psychosomatic Medicine', in *The History of Psychiatry and Medical Psychology*, ed. Edgar R. Wallace IV and John Gage (New York, 2008), pp. 485–518, here, p. 501.

152 Stewart Wolf, 'The Psyche and the Stomach: A Historical Vignette', *Gastroenterology*, LXXX (1981), pp. 605–14.

153 Walter B. Cannon, 'The Influence of Emotional States on the Functions of the Alimentary Canal', *American Journal of the Medical Sciences*, CXXXVI (1909), pp. 480–87, here, pp. 480, 487.

154 Ted Hunt, ed., *Selected Writings of Sir Arthur Hurst (1879–1944)* (London, 1969), pp. 5off.

155 Thomas R. Brown, 'Peptic Ulcer', in *A Text-Book of Medicine by American Authors*, ed. R. L. Cecil (Philadelphia, PA, 1927), pp. 245–56, here, p. 251.

156 E. W. Lipschutz, 'The Treatment of Peptic Ulcer Based on Its Etiology: A Survey of the Systemic Causes of the Disease', *Medical Journal and Record*, CXXVIII (1928), pp. 630–33, here, p. 632.

157 Sarah M. Jordan, 'The Present Status of Peptic Ulcer', *New England Journal of Medicine*, CCIII (1930), pp. 917–20, here, pp. 917–18.

158 Walter C. Alvarez, *Nervous Indigestion* (New York, 1930), p. 98. For a closer reading see Ian Miller, *A Modern History of the Stomach: Gastric Illness, Medicine and British Society, 1800–1950* (London, 2015).

159 C. T. Fitts et al., 'Acute Gastrointestinal Tract Ulceration: Cushing's Ulcer, Steroid Ulcer, Curling's Ulcer and Stress Ulcer', *American Surgeon*, XXXVII (1971), pp. 218–23.

160 Harvey Cushing, 'Peptic Ulcers and the Interbrain', *Surgery, Gynecology and Obstetrics*, LV (1932), pp. 1–34. See Gerald N. Grob, 'The Rise of the Peptic Ulcer, 1900–1950', *Perspectives in Biology and Medicine*, XLVI (2003), pp. 550–66.

161 Cushing, 'Peptic Ulcers and the Interbrain', p. 32.

162 Hans Selye, *The Stress of Life* (New York, 1956). See also S. Szabo, 'Hans Selye and the Development of the Stress Concept: Special Reference to Gastroduodenal Ulcerogenesis', *Annals of the New York Academy of Sciences*, DCCCLI (1998), pp. 19–27.

163 Hans Selye, 'A Syndrome Produced by Diverse Nocuous Agents', *Nature*, CXXXVIII (1936), p. 32.

164 *Peptic Ulcer: Rise and Fall*, p. 111.

165 I am greatly indebted to the thesis by Alexander Chapman Pollock, 'From
Dyspepsia to Helicobacter: A History of Peptic Ulcer Disease' (MD Thesis,
University of Glasgow, 2014), here, pp. 182ff.

166 B. W. Sippy, 'Gastric and Duodenal Ulcer: Medical Cure by an Efficient
Removal of Gastric Juice Corrosion', *JAMA*, LXIV (1915), pp. 1625–30. See also
Peptic Ulcer: Rise and Fall, p. 80.

167 Jordan, 'Present Status', pp. 917–18.

168 Howard W. Linn, 'An Analysis of Peptic Ulcer in South Australia, Based on a
Study of 1,027 Case Reports', *Medical Journal of Australia*, II (1933), pp. 649–58,
here, p. 658.

169 J. H. Baron and A. Sonnenberg, 'Hospital Admissions for Peptic Ulcers and
Indigestion in London and New York in the 19th and early 20th Centuries',
Gut, L (2002), pp. 568–70, here, pp. 568–9.

170 M. Susser and Z. Stein, 'Civilisation and Peptic Ulcer', *The Lancet*, I/7221 (1962),
pp. 115–19, here, p. 117.

171 J. I. Westbrook and R. L. Rushworth, 'The Epidemiology of Peptic Ulcer
Mortality, 1953–1989: A Birth Cohort Analysis', *International Journal of
Epidemiology*, XXII (1993), pp. 1085–92.

172 Leo Doyle, 'Peptic Ulcer', *Medical Journal of Australia*, II (1947), pp. 34–43,
here p. 34.

173 Philippa J. Martyr, *Paradise of Quacks: An Alternative History of Medicine in
Australia* (Sydney, 2002).

174 'Report of Committee of Inquiry into Claims of Cancer Cures by Mr J. Braund',
Medical Journal of Australia (29 May 1948), pp. 680–92, here, p. 681.

175 Ibid., p. 682.

176 Laura L. Dawes, '"Just a Quack Who Can Cure Cancer": John Braund, and
Regulating Cancer Treatment in New South Wales, Australia', *Medical History*,
LVII (2013), pp. 206–25, here, p. 211.

177 Ibid., p. 218.

178 Ibid.

179 'Report of the Queensland Royal Commission on Modern Methods for the
Treatment of Infantile Paralysis', *Medical Journal of Australia*, I/5
(29 January 1938), pp. 187–224.

180 Naomi Rogers, 'Sister Kenny Goes to Washington: Polio, Populism, and
Medical Politics in Postwar America', in *The Politics of Healing: Histories
of Alternative Medicine in Twentieth-Century North America*, ed. Robert D.
Johnston (New York and London, 2004), pp. 97–116, here, p. 112.

181 'Report of the Queensland Royal Commission', p. 220.

182 Ibid., p. 219.

183 D. Šešelja, C. Straßer, 'Heuristic Reevaluation of the Bacterial Hypothesis of
Peptic Ulcer Disease in the 1950s', *Acta Biotheoretica*, LXII (2014), pp. 429–54.

184 This 'official' history is to be found in J. R. Warren, 'Discovery of *H. pylori*
in Perth, WA', in *Helicobacter Pioneers: Firsthand Accounts from the Scientists
Who Discovered Helicobacters, 1892–1982*, ed. Barry Marshall (London, 2002),
pp. 151–64.

185 B. P. Billington, 'Gastric Ulcer: Age, Sex and a Curious Retrogression', *Australian
Annals of Medicine*, IX (1960), pp. 111–21; R. A. Douglas and E. D. Johnston,
'Aspirin and Chronic Gastric Ulcer', *Medical Journal of Australia*, XLVIII (1961),
pp. 893–7.

186 Melissa Sweet, 'SMUG AS A BUG: The Profile', *Sydney Morning Herald* (Australia) (2 August 1997).

187 B. J. Marshall and J. R. Warren, 'Unidentified Curved Bacilli in the Stomach of Patients with Gastritis and Peptic Ulceration', *The Lancet*, I/8390 (1984), pp. 1311–15.

188 B. J. Marshall and J. R. Warren, 'Unidentified Curved Bacilli on Gastric Epithelium in Active Chronic Gastritis', *The Lancet*, I/8336 (1983), pp. 1273–5.

189 'Nobel Laureate Marshall a Joker, Says Wife', *Agence France Presse – English* (4 October 2005).

190 J. S. Fordtran, 'The Psychosomatic Theory of Peptic Ulcer', in *Gastrointestinal Disease*, ed. M. H. Sleisenger and J. S. Fordtran (Philadelphia, PA, 1973), pp. 163–73.

191 Barry Marshall, 'Helicobacter Connections', *ChemMedChem*, I (2006), pp. 783–802, here, p. 789.

192 David Fredricks and David Relman, 'Sequence-Based Identification of Microbial Pathogens: A Reconsideration of Koch's Postulates', *Clinical Microbiology Reviews*, IX (1996), pp. 18–33, here, p. 20.

193 I. Kerridge, 'Altruism or Reckless Curiosity? A Brief History of Self-Experimentation in Medicine', *Internal Medicine Journal*, XXXIII (2003), pp. 203–7.

194 B. J. Marshall et al., 'Attempt to Fulfil Koch's Postulates for Pyloric *Campylobacter*', *Medical Journal of Australia*, CXLII (1985), pp. 436–9.

195 T. P. Rollason, J. Stone and J. M. Rhodes, 'Spiral Organisms in Endoscopic Biopsies of the Human Stomach', *Journal of Clinical Pathology*, XXXVII (1984), pp. 23–6.

196 Pollock, 'From Dyspepsia to Helicobacter', p. 234.

197 Barry Marshall, 'The Discovery That *Helicobacter pylori*, a Spiral Bacterium, Caused Peptic Ulcer Disease', in *Helicobacter Pioneers*, ed. Marshall, pp. 165–202, here, p. 201.

198 W. L. Peterson, 'Antimicrobial Treatment of Duodenal Ulcer? Hold Off for Now!', *Gastroenterology*, XCVII (1989), pp. 508–10.

199 Allan M. Brandt, *The Cigarette Century: The Rise, Fall, and Deadly Persistence of the Product That Defined America* (New York, 2007), pp. 149ff.

200 S. E. Hyman, 'Another One Bites the Dust: An Infectious Origin for Peptic Ulcers', *Harvard Review of Psychiatry*, I (1994), pp. 294–5.

201 A. Nomura et al., '*Helicobacter pylori* Infection and the Risk for Duodenal and Gastric Ulceration', *Annals of Internal Medicine*, CXX (1994), pp. 977–81.

202 K.E.L. McColl, '*Helicobacter pylori*, 1988–1998', *European Journal of Gastroenterology and Hepatology*, XI (1999), pp. 13–16.

203 John Bejakovic, 'A Return to Mad Men-Era Ulcer Gulch?' (19 April 2020), www.vulture.com.

204 Stephen Marsh, 'The Persistence of *Mad Men*' (23 March 2012), www.esquire.com.

205 S. M. Artaud-Wild et al., 'Differences in Coronary Mortality Can Be Explained by Differences in Cholesterol and Saturated Fat Intakes in 40 Countries but Not in France and Finland: A Paradox', *Circulation*, LXXXVIII (1993), pp. 2771–9.

206 R. Lordan et al., 'Dairy Fats and Cardiovascular Disease: Do We Really Need to Be Concerned?' *Foods*, VII (2018), p. 29.

207 Dong et al., 'A Collection of the Etiological Theories', p. 1060.

208 Morris Fishbein, *Fads and Quackery in Healing: An Analysis of the Foibles of the Healing Cults* (New York, 1932), p. 254.

209 Ibid., p. 205.

210 Helen Bynum, *Spitting Blood: The History of Tuberculosis* (Oxford, 2015), pp. 170–76.
211 G. Gasbarrini et al., 'A Population-Based Study of *Helicobacter pylori* Infection in a European Country: The San-Marino Study. Relations with Gastrointestinal-Diseases', *Gut*, XXXVI (1995), pp. 838–44.
212 J. Bruce Overmier and Robert Murison, 'Restoring Psychology's Role in Peptic Ulcer', *Applied Psychology Health and Well-Being*, V (2013), pp. 5–27, here, p. 5.
213 Bruno Latour, 'Give Me a Laboratory and I Will Raise the World', in *Science Observed: Perspectives on the Social Study of Science*, ed. Karin D. Knorr-Cetina and Michael Mulkay (London, 1983), pp. 141–69, here, p. 157.
214 P. A. Mackowiak, 'The Normal Microbial Flora', *New England Journal of Medicine*, CCCVII (1982), pp. 83–93.
215 Harvey Cushing, *The Life of Sir William Osler*, 2 vols (Oxford, 1925), II, pp. 215–16.
216 Martin J. Blaser, *Missing Microbes: How the Overuse of Antibiotics Is Fueling Our Modern Plagues* (New York, 2014), pp. 9, 113, 214, 115, 179, 105, 142.
217 Martin J. Blaser, 'Disappearing Microbiota: *Helicobacter pylori* Protection against Esophageal Adenocarcinoma', *Cancer Prevention Research*, I (2008), pp. 308–11.
218 Martin J. Blaser, 'Our Missing Microbes: Short-Term Antibiotic Courses Have Long-Term Consequences', *Cleveland Clinic Journal of Medicine*, LXXXV (2018), pp. 928–30, here, p. 928.
219 Ibid.
220 Zaira Aversa, et. al., 'Association of Infant Antibiotic Exposure with Childhood Health Outcomes', *Mayo Clinic Proceedings*, XCVI (2021), pp. 66–77.
221 M. J. Blaser, P. H. Chyou and A. Nomura, 'Age at Establishment of *Helicobacter pylori* Infection and Gastric Carcinoma, Gastric Ulcer, and Duodenal Ulcer Risk', *Cancer Research*, LV (1995), pp. 562–5.
222 E. A. Rauws et al., '*Campylobacter pyloridis*-Associated Chronic Active Antral Gastritis: A Prospective Study of Its Prevalence and the Effects of Antibacterial and Antiulcer Treatment', *Gastroenterology*, XCIV (1988), pp. 33–40.
223 R. Laxminarayan et al., 'Antibiotic Resistance – the Need for Global Solutions', *The Lancet Infectious Diseases*, 13 (2013), pp. 1057–98.
224 N. Stollman, '*Helicobacter pylori* Infection in the Era of Antibiotic Resistance', *Gastroenterology and Hepatology*, XII (2016), pp. 122–5.
225 B. Petschow et al., 'Probiotics, Prebiotics, and the Host Microbiome: The Science of Translation', *Annals of the New York Academy of Science*, MCCCVI (2013), pp. 1–17.
226 Angel Lanas and Francis K. L. Chan, 'Peptic Ulcer Disease', *The Lancet*, CCCXC (2017), pp. 613–24.
227 Christina Caron, 'This Nerve Influences Nearly Every Internal Organ. Can It Improve Our Mental State, Too?', *New York Times* (2 June 2022).
228 Ian Miller, 'The Gut-Brain Axis: Historical Reflections', *Microbial Ecology in Health and Disease*, XXIX (2018), art. 1542921.
229 Haruki Murakami, 'Speaking as an Unrealistic Dreamer', *Asia-Pacific Journal*, IX/29 (2011), www.tinyurl.com.
230 K. Yamanaka et al., 'Hemorrhagic Gastric and Duodenal Ulcers after the Great East Japan Earthquake Disaster', *World Journal of Gastroenterology*, XIX (2013), pp. 7426–32.
231 T. Kanno et al., 'Accommodation in a Refugee Shelter as a Risk Factor for Peptic Ulcer Bleeding after the Great East Japan Earthquake: A Case-Control Study of 329 Patients', *Journal of Gastroenterology*, L (2015), pp. 31–40.

232 S. Levenstein et al., 'Psychological Stress Increases Risk for Peptic Ulcer, Regardless of *Helicobacter pylori* Infection or Use of Nonsteroidal Anti-Inflammatory Drugs', *Clinical Gastroenterology and Hepatology*, XXIII (2015), pp. 498–506, here, p. 498.

233 Haruki Murakami, *The Wind-Up Bird Chronicle*, trans. Jay Rubin (New York, 2010), p. 223.

234 Overmier and Murison, 'Restoring Psychology's Role in Peptic Ulcer', p. 27.

3 Eyes

1 Karl Ludmerer, *Let Me Heal: The Opportunity to Preserve Excellence in American Medicine* (New York, 2015), p. 9.

2 Anon., 'Quack Oculists', *BMJ*, II (1893), p. 482.

3 Anon., 'Ophthalmic Quacks in America', *BMJ*, I (1907), pp. 892–3, here, p. 893.

4 Cyril H. Walker, 'Some Phases of Quackery in Relation to Diseases of the Eye', *Bristol Medico-Chirurgical Journal* XXXVIII/144 (1922), pp.129–42, here, p. 140.

5 Eric Jameson, *The Natural History of Quackery* (London, 1961), pp. 88–90.

6 Roy Porter, *Quacks: Fakers and Charlatans in English Medicine* (Stroud, 2001), pp. 73–4.

7 William Cheselden, 'An Account of Some Observations Made by a Young Gentleman, Who Was Born Blind, or Lost His Sight So Early, That He Had No Remembrance of Ever Having Seen, and Was Couched between 13 and 14 Years of Age', *Philosophical Transactions of the Royal Society*, XXXV (1727–8), pp. 447–8.

8 Porter, *Quacks*, p. 69.

9 Ibid., p. 68.

10 David M. Jackson, 'Bach, Handel, and the Chevalier Taylor', *Medical History*, XII (1968), pp. 385–93.

11 *The Posthumous Works of Robert Hooke, . . . Containing His Cutlerian Lectures, and Other Discourses, Read at the Meetings of the Illustrious Royal Society* (London, 1705), p. 127.

12 Andrzej Grzybowski and Charles N. J. McGhee, 'The Early History of Keratoconus prior to Nottingham's Landmark 1854 Treatise on Conical Cornea: A Review', *Clinical and Experimental Optometry*, XCVI (2013), pp. 140–45, here, p. 141.

13 Albrecht von Haller, 'Taylor quidam, famigeratus medicus ocularius', *Commercium litterarium ad rei medicae et scientiae naturalis incrementum institutum*, XLV (1734), pp. 353–4.

14 Porter, *Quacks*, p. 70.

15 Gerhard Ten Haaff, *Korte Verhandeling* (Rotterdam, 1761), pp. 16–17.

16 John Taylor, *The History of the Travels and Adventures of the Chevalier John Taylor, Ophthamiater*, 3 vols (London, 1761–2), I, p. 28.

17 J   ames Boswell, *The Life of Samuel Johnson, LL. D: Comprehending an Account of His Studies and Numerous Works*, 2 vols (London, 1791), II, p. 291.

18 *The Post Man and the Historical Account* ([London] 19 April 1701), p. 2.

19 Michael Irwin, ed., *The Life of Thomas Hardy, 1840–1928* (London, 2007), p. 157.

20 Rachel Ablow, *Victorian Pain* (Princeton, NJ, 2020), p. 23. See also Sander L. Gilman, 'Seeing Bodies in Pain', in *Health Humanities Reader*, ed. Therese Jones, Delese Wear and Lester D. Friedman (New Brunswick, NJ, 2014), pp. 171–86.

21 Stephanie J. Snow, *Blessed Days of Anaesthesia: How Anaesthetics Changed the World* (New York, 2008).

22 John B. West, 'Humphry Davy, Nitrous Oxide, the Pneumatic Institution, and the Royal Institution', *American Journal of Physiology: Lung Cellular and Molecular Physiology*, CCCVII (2014), L661–L667, here, L663.

23 Norman Kingsley, 'Has Legislation Cured Quackery?', *Transaction of the New York Odonatological Association* (1900), pp. 33–8, here p. 34.

24 Henry James, 'Notes', in his *The Sense of the Past* (New York, 1922), p. 296.

25 Theodor Ziolkowski, 'The Telltale Teeth: Psychodontia to Sociodontia', *PMLA*, XCI (1976), pp. 9–22, here, p. 15.

26 Guido Fischer, *Local Anesthesia in Dentistry*, trans. Richard Riethmüller (Philadelphia, PA, 1914), p. 31.

27 Martin S. Pernick, *A Calculus of Suffering: Pain, Professionalism and Anesthesia in Nineteenth-Century America* (New York, 1985), pp. 94–6.

28 D. Simpson, 'Simpson and "The Discovery of Chloroform"', *Scottish Medical Journal*, XXXV (1990), pp. 149–53.

29 Sigmund Freud, 'An Autobiographical Study' [1925], *The Standard Edition of the Complete Psychological Works of Sigmund Freud*, trans. and ed. James Strachey et al., 24 vols (London, 1953–74), XX, pp. 1–74, here, pp. 14–15.

30 Siegfried Bernfeld, 'Freud's Studies on Cocaine, 1884–1887', *Journal of the American Psychoanalytic Association*, I (1953), pp. 581–613, here, p. 588.

31 R. J. Defalque and A. J. Wright, 'The Short, Tragic Life of Robert M. Glover', *Anaesthesia*, LIX (2004), pp. 394–400.

32 Hortense Koller Becker, 'Carl Koller and Cocaine', *Psychoanalytic Quarterly*, XXXII (1963), pp. 309–73, here, p. 320.

33 Ibid., p. 324.

34 Ibid., p. 331.

35 Ibid., pp. 331–2.

36 Ibid., p. 336.

37 Eberhard Wolff, *Medizin und Ärzte im deutschen Judentum der Reformära: Die Architektur einer modernen jüdischen Identität* (Göttingen, 2014).

38 Leopold von Sacher-Masoch, 'Zwei Ärzte', in his *Jüdisches Leben* (Mannheim, 1892), pp. 287–98.

39 William Germano, *Eye Chart* (New York, 2017), pp. 5ff.

40 Freud, *Letters, Standard Edition*, LI: 208.

41 K. Hruby, 'Würde Dr Carl Koller 1885 aus Wien vertrieben?', *Wiener Klinische Wochenschrift*, XCVIII (1986), pp. 155–6, and Howard Markel, *An Anatomy of Addiction: Sigmund Freud, William Halsted, and the Miracle Drug Cocaine* (New York, 2011), pp. 24–7.

42 Mitchell G. Ash, 'Jewish Scientists and Scholars at the University of Vienna from the Late Habsburg Period until the Early Post-War Years', in *Jews and Science*, ed. Sander L. Gilman, Casden Institute Annual, XX (West Lafayette, IN, 2022), pp. 57–90.

43 E. Chan et al., 'Prevalence of Keratoconus Based on Scheimpflug Imaging: The Raine Study', *Ophthalmology*, CXXVIII (2021), pp. 515–52.

44 George Coats, 'The Chevalier Taylor', *Royal London Ophthalmic Hospital Reports*, XX (1915), pp. 1–92, here, p. 3.

45 John Taylor, *Description exacte de 243 différentes maladies auxquelles l'œil, ses enveloppes et ses parties contiguës sont exposées* (Angers, 1766), p. 13.

46 'Eine kegelförmige Gestalt der durchsichtigen conum, apice acuto, et basi diametro Hornhaut, deren Spiße scharf, der Grund aber corneæ æquali, dicitur dem Durchmesser der Hornhaut gleich ift, heißt Ochlodes', Johannis Taylor, *Nova nosographia ophthalmica; hoc est accurata receniso ducentorum et quadraginta trium affectuum, qui oculum humanum partesque vicinas ullo modo laedere aut ipsum visum adimere possunt* (Hamburg and Leipzig, 1766), p. 21.

47 Benedict Duddell, *A Supplement to the Treatise of the Diseases of the Horny-Coat of the Eye, and the Various Kinds of Cataract* (London, 1736), pp. 19–23, here, pp. 19–20.

48 Ibid., p. 22.

49 Porter, *Quacks*, pp. 73–4.

50 Sander L. Gilman, 'The Figure of the Black in the Aesthetic Theories of Eighteenth-Century Germany', *Eighteenth-Century Studies*, VIII (1975), pp. 373–91.

51 Lorraine Daston and Peter Galison, *Objectivity* (Cambridge, MA, 2021), p. 55.

52 Friedrich August von Ammon, 'Das Staphyloma Pellucidum Corneae als Morbus Congenitus bey drey Geschwistern, nebst einigen Reflexionen über die Natur dieser merkwürdigen Krankheit', *Isis von Oken*, II (1828), pp. 547–53, here, p. 547.

53 Ibid., p. 551.

54 James Wardrop, *Essays on the Morbid Anatomy of the Human Eye* (Edinburgh, 1808), pp. 119–21.

55 Commentary on G. B. Airey, 'On a Peculiar Defect in the EYE, and a Mode of Correcting It', *Edinburgh Journal of Science*, VII (1827), pp. 322–6, here, p. 325.

56 John Nottingham, *Practical Observations on Conical Cornea: And on the Short Sight, and Other Defects of Vision Connected with It* (London, 1854), p. 6.

57 J. R. Levine, 'The True Inventors of the Keratoscope and Photo-Keratoscope', *British Journal of the History of Science*, II (1965), pp. 324–42.

58 Marjorie Garber, *Academic Instincts* (Princeton, NJ, 2001), p. 67.

59 James H. Pickford, *On Conical Cornea* (Dublin, 1844), p. 31.

60 Lawrance Webster Fox, 'Conical Cornea: An Historical Review Together with a New Non-Operative Method of Treatment', *Ophthalmic Record*, XIII (1904), pp. 1–15, here, p. 7.

61 Henry Goode, 'On a Peculiar Defect of Vision', *Transactions of the Cambridge Philosophical Society*, VIII (1847), pp. 493–6, here, p. 495.

62 R. Martin, 'Cornea and Anterior Eye Assessment with Placido-Disc Keratoscopy, Slit Scanning Evaluation Topography and Scheimpflug Imaging Tomography', *Indian Journal of Ophthalmology*, LXVI (2018), pp. 360–66.

63 C. B. Courville, M. K. Smolek and S. D. Klyce, 'Contribution of the Ocular Surface to Visual Optics', *Experimental Eye Research*, LXXVIII (2004), pp. 417–25.

64 Wardrop, *Essays*, pp. xi–xii.

65 Ibid., p. 118.

66 Sir William Adams, 'On the Restoration of Vision, When Injured or Destroyed in Consequence of the Cornea Having Assumed a Conical Form', *Journal of Science and the Arts*, II (1817), pp. 402–17, here, p. 403.

67 Ibid., p. 404.

68 Ibid., pp. 406–7.

69 Ibid., p. 414.

70 Ibid., p. 408.

71 The average focusing power of the eye is approximately 64 dioptres – 2/3 from the cornea and 1/3 from the lens. In keratoconus the cornea alone can be so steep as to be 70 dioptres and more, making the eye VERY nearsighted. Remove a lens (mean power of approximately 18 dioptres) and the severe myopia is improved so the vision can be markedly better. Still poor due to corneal distortion, but better than pre-surgery. At least impressionistically.

72 Walter Baley, *Two Treatises concerning the Preseruation of Eie-Sight. The First Written by Doctor Baily Sometimes of Oxford: The Other Collected out of Those Two Famous Phisicions Fernelius and Riolanus* (Oxford, 1616), pp. 11–12.

73 Von Ammon, 'Das Staphyloma Pellucidum Corneae', p. 551.

74 H. Scott, MD, 'Some Remarks on the Arts of India, with Miscellaneous Observations on Various Subjects', *Journal of Science and the Arts*, II (1817), pp. 67–72, here, p. 69.

75 Nottingham, *Practical Observations*, p. 226. An engaging reading of Nottingham from a contemporary perspective is Akilesh Gokul, Dipika V. Patel and Charles N. J. McGhee, 'Dr John Nottingham's 1854 Landmark Treatise on Conical Cornea Considered in the Context of the Current Knowledge of Keratoconus', *Cornea*, XXXV (2016), pp. 673–8.

76 See Grzybowski and McGhee, 'The Early History of Keratoconus', pp. 143–4.

77 A. Rabagliati, 'Some Remarks on the Classification and Nomenclature of Diseases', *BMJ*, II (1881), pp. 114–17, here, p. 114.

78 Nottingham, *Practical Observations*, pp. xi–xii.

79 Ibid., pp. 170–71; Richard Middlemore, *A Treatise on Disease of the Eye and Its Appendages*, 2 vols (London, 1835), I, p. 532.

80 Mark J. Mannis, 'Keratoconus Therapy, Past, and Present', *American Journal of Ophthalmology*, CXLVII (2009), p. 1016.

81 Nottingham, *Practical Observations*, p. xiii.

82 J. Burdon-Sanderson and J. W. Hulke, eds, *The Collected Papers of Sir W. Bowman in Two Volumes* (London, 1892), I, p. xx.

83 William Bowman, 'On Conical Cornea and Its Treatment by Operation' (1859), in *The Collected Papers of Sir W. Bowman*, ed. Burdon-Sanderson and Hulke, II, pp. 271–82, here, p. 280.

84 Burdon-Sanderson and Hulke, eds, *The Collected Papers of Sir W. Bowman*, II, p. 276.

85 Johannes F. Horner, 'Zur Behandlung des Keratoconus', *Klinische Monatsblätter für Augenheilkunde*, V (1869), pp. 24–6.

86 L. M. Imbornoni, C.N.J. McGhee and M. W. Belin, 'Evolution of Keratoconus: From Diagnosis to Therapeutics', *Klinische Monatsblatt für Augenheilkunde*, CCXXXV (2018), pp. 680–88, here, p. 681.

87 Sander L. Gilman, 'Electrotherapy and Mental Illness: Then and Now', *History of Psychiatry*, XIX (2008), pp. 339–57.

88 Nottingham, *Practical Observations*, p. 16.

89 Ibid., p. 13.

90 Ibid., p. 25.

91 Ibid., p. 195.

92 Ibid.

93 Ibid., p. 185.

94 Ibid., p. 115.

95 William F. Bynum, 'The Great Chain of Being after Forty Years: An Appraisal', *History of Science*, XIII (1975), pp. 1–28.

96 Nottingham, *Practical Observations*, p. 4.

97 Ibid., p. 220.

98 Ibid., p. 217.

99 Robert Brudenell Carter, *Doctors and Their Work; or, Medicine, Quackery, and Disease* (London, 1903), p. 128.

100 David Wright, *Downs: The History of a Disability* (Oxford, 2011), pp. 9–10, 33–40.

101 J. Langdon H. Down, 'Observations on an Ethnic Classification of Idiots', *London Hospital Reports*, III (1866), pp. 259–62, here, p. 260.

102 Ibid., p. 261.

103 Ibid.

104 J. Langdon Down, *On Some of the Mental Affections of Childhood and Youth. The Lettsomian Lectures Delivered before the Medical Society of London in 1887 Together with Other Papers* (London, 1887), p. 280.

105 Ibid., p. 39.

106 August Siegrist, 'Zur Aetiologie des Keratokonous', *Bericht über die Versammlung der Ophthalmologischen Gesellschaft*, XXXVIII (1912), pp. 187–96, here, p. 190.

107 August Siegrist, 'Die Behandlung des Keratoconus', *Klinische Monatsblatt für Augenheilkunde*, LVI (1916), pp. 400–421.

108 No occurrence: F. Fimiani et al., 'Incidence of Ocular Pathologies in Italian Children with Down Syndrome', *European Journal of Ophthalmology*, XVII (2007), pp. 817–22; higher rates: M. B. Shapiro and T. France, 'The Ocular Features of Down's Syndrome', *American Journal of Ophthalmology*, XCIX (1985), pp. 659–63.

109 Theresa Akoto et al., 'The Underlying Relationship between Keratoconus and Down Syndrome', *International Journal of Molecular Science*, XXIII (2022), p. 10796.

110 Andrew Rados, 'Conical Cornea and Mongolism', *Archives of Ophthalmology*, XL (1948), pp. 454–78, here, p. 468.

111 B. Myers, 'Male Twins, One of Which is a Mongol', *Proceedings of the Royal Society of Medicine*, XVIII (1925), p. 69; L. B. Dickey, 'Mongolism in Both of Twins', *California and Western Medicine*, XXVI (1927), p. 344; A. Smith, 'A Note on Mongolism in Twins', *British Journal of Preventive and Social Medicine*, IX (1955), pp. 212–13. On keratoconus, an overview of familial patterns is to be found in Yaron S. Rabinowitz, 'Ectatic Diseases of the Cornea', in *Smolin and Thoft's The Cornea: Scientific Foundations and Clinical Practice*, ed. C. S. Foster, D. T. Azar and C. H. Dohlman, 4th edn (Philadelphia, PA, 2005), pp. 889–913, here, pp. 898–912.

112 A. R. Pearson et al., 'Does Ethnic Origin Influence the Incidence or Severity of Keratoconus?', *Eye*, XIV (2000), pp. 625–8; T. Georgiou et al., 'Influence of Ethnic Origin on the Incidence of Keratoconus and Associated Atopic Disease in Asians and White Patients', *Eye*, XVIII (2004), pp. 379–83; Maria A. Woodward, Taylor S. Blachley and Joshua D. Stein, 'The Association between Sociodemographic Factors, Common Systemic Diseases, and Keratoconus: An Analysis of a Nationwide Healthcare Claims Database', *Ophthalmology*, CXXIII (2016), pp. 457–65.

113 Sander L. Gilman, *Health and Illness: Images of Difference* (London, 1995), pp. 33–50.

114 F. Siegert, 'Der Mongolismus', *Ergebnisse der inneren Medizin und Kinderheilkunde*, VI (1910), p. 565; M. B. Gordon, 'Morphological Changes in the Endocrine Glands in Mongolian Idiocy', *Endocrinology*, XIV (1930), pp. 1–6.

115 James Harvey Young, *American Quackery: Collected Essays* (Princeton, NJ, 2014), p. 166.

116 Ibid., p. 220.

117 J. R. Mutch and M. B. Richards, 'Keratoconus Experimentally Produced by Vitamin A Deficiency', *British Journal of Ophthalmology*, XXIII (1939), pp. 381–7; Karen Schaeffer et al., 'Topographic Corneal Changes Induced by Oral Riboflavin in the Treatment of Corneal Ectasia', *Investigative Ophthalmology and Visual Science*, LIX (2018), p. 1413. See also E. Spoerl, M. Huhle and T. Seiler, 'Induction of Cross-Links in Corneal Tissue', *Experimental Eye Research,* LXVI (1998), pp. 97–103.

118 A. E. Sobel et al., 'Vitamin A Absorption and Other Blood Composition Studies in Mongolism', *American Journal of Mental Deficiency*, LXII (1958), pp. 642–56; R. M. Auld et al., 'Vitamin A Absorption in Mongoloid Children: A Preliminary Report', *American Journal of Mental Deficiency*, LXIII (1959), pp. 1010–13; Y. Hisbiyah et al., 'The Correlation between Vitamin D and Levels of IFN-γ, NF-κB, Thyroid Antibodies in Down Syndrome: Study in Indonesian Children', *Acta Bio-Medica*, XCIII (2022), e2022342.

119 F. C. Gomes et al., 'Vitamin D_3 Supplementation May Attenuate Morphological and Molecular Abnormalities of the Olfactory Bulb in a Mouse Model of Down Syndrome', *Tissue and Cell*, LXXVIII (2022), p. 101898.

120 Akoto et al., 'The Underlying Relationship', p. 10796.

121 An entire page is devoted to 'diseases reported in association with keratoconus', in Rabinowitz, 'Ectatic Diseases of the Cornea', p. 894.

122 Transcript of U.S. Defense Department Briefing: 'Secretary of Defense Donald Rumsfeld and Air Force General Richard Myers, Chairman, Joint Chiefs of Staff, briefed February 12 at the Pentagon . . . U.S. Department of Defense DoD News Briefing' (12 February 2002), https://usinfo.org/wf-archive, accessed 23 July 2024.

123 In general heat shrinks collagen and thus could flatten corneas. It is employed in contemporary practice followed by corneal cross-linking to 'lock in' the effect. Patients have now been followed for up to eleven years and they show stability, in sharp distinction to all other heat-based treatments. M. M. Sinjab et al., 'Outcomes of Conductive Keratoplasty Combined with Corneal Crosslinking in Advanced Ectatic Corneal Disease', *Clinical Ophthalmology*, XV (2021), pp. 1317–29.

124 Richard M. Pearson, 'An Appraisal of the Optics of the Hydrodiascope', *Contact Lens and Anterior Eye*, XXXI (2008), pp. 65–72.

125 Jacqueline Lamb and Tim Bowden, 'The History of Contact Lenses', in *Contact Lenses*, ed. Anthony J. Phillips and Lynne Speedwell (Amsterdam, 2019), pp. 2–17.

126 Frederic J. Haskin, 'Answers to Questions', *Oakland Tribune* (16 December 1930), p. 30.

127 Logan Clendening, MD, 'Invisible Spectacles Practical, Efficient', *Hammond [IN] Times* (2 February 1939), p. 57.

128 K. H. Weed and C. N. McGhee, 'Referral Patterns, Treatment Management and Visual Outcome in Keratoconus', *Eye*, XII (1998), pp. 663–8.

129 W. Sekundo and J. D. Stevens, 'Surgical Treatment of Keratoconus at the Turn of the Twentieth Century', *Journal of Refractive Surgery*, XVII (2001), pp. 69–73, here, p. 70.

130 Ibid., p. 73.

131 Hjalmar Schiotz, 'Ein Fall von hochgradigem Hornhautastigmatismus nach Staarextraction. Besserung auf operativem Wege', *Archiv für Augenheilkunde*, xv (1885), pp. 178–81.

132 'Dr Pond's Success', *Bangor [ME] Daily News* (17 October 1902), p. 3.

133 Eduard K. Zirm, 'Eine erfolgreiche totale Keratoplastik', *Archiv für Ophthalmologie*, LXIV (1906), pp. 580–93; a partial translation by Massimo Busin is available in *Refractive and Corneal Surgery*, v (1989), pp. 258–61.

134 Ramon Castroviejo, 'Keratoplasty for the Treatment of Keratoconus', *Transactions of the American Ophthalmological Society*, XLVI (1948), pp. 127–53.

135 Charles Wray, 'The Operative Treatment of Keratoconus (Conical Cornea)', *Proceedings of the Royal Society of Medicine (Section Ophthalmology)*, VII (1914), pp. 152–7, here, p. 152.

136 Ibid., p. 155.

137 Ibid., p. 156.

138 Ibid.

139 Charles Deval, *Chirurgie oculaire ou traité des opérations chirurgicales qui se pratiquent sur l'œil et ses annexes; avec un exposé succint des différentes altérations qui les réclament, ouvrage contenant la pratique opératoire de F. Jaeger et de A. Rosas* (Paris, 1844), p. 72.

140 Baron Alexis Boyer and Phillipe Boyer, *Traité des maladies chirurgicales et des opérations qui leur conviennent*, 5th edn, 6 vols (Paris, 1844–53), IV, p. 645.

141 Wray, 'The Operative Treatment of Keratoconus', p. 157.

142 Mannis, 'Keratoconus Therapy, Past, and Present', p. 1016.

143 H. J. Hettlich, K. Lucke and C. F. Kreiner, 'Light Induced Endocapsular Polymerization of Injectable Lens Refilling Materials', *German Journal of Ophthalmology*, I (1992), pp. 346–9.

144 E. Spörl et al., 'Erhöhung der Festigkeit der Hornhaut durch Vernetzung', *Ophthalmologe*, XCIV (1997), pp. 902–6; E. Schnitzler, E. Spörl and T. Seiler, 'Bestrahlung der Hornhaut mit UVLicht und Riboflavingabe als neuer Behandlungsversuch bei einschmelzenden Hornhautprozessen, erste Ergebnisse bei vier Patienten', *Klinische Monatsblatt für Augenheilkunde*, CCXVII (2000), pp. 190–93; G. Wollensak, E. Spörl and T. Seiler, 'Riboflavin/Ultraviolet-A-Induced Collagen Crosslinking for the Treatment of Keratoconus', *American Journal of Ophthalmology*, CXXXV (2003), pp. 620–27; G. Wollensak, E. Spörl and T. Seiler, 'Stress-Strain Measurements of Human and Porcine Corneas after Riboflavin-Ultraviolet-A-Induced Cross-Linking', *Journal of Cataract and Refractive Surgery*, XXIX (2003), pp. 1780–85.

145 N. Sharma et al., 'Collagen Cross-Linking in Keratoconus in Asian Eyes: Visual, Refractive and Confocal Microscopy Outcomes in a Prospective Randomized Controlled Trial', *International Ophthalmology*, XXXV (2015), pp. 827–32.

146 J. D. Marsack et al., 'Application of Topographical Keratoconus Detection Metrics to Eyes of Individuals with Down Syndrome', *Optometry and Vision Science*, XCVI (2019), pp. 664–9; K. J. Wroblewski et al., 'Long-Term Graft Survival in Patients with Down Syndrome after Penetrating Keratoplasty', *Cornea*, XXV (2006), pp. 1026–8.

147 T. Koller, M. Mrochen and T. Seiler, 'Complication and Failure Rates after Corneal Crosslinking', *Journal of Refractive and Corneal Surgery*, XXXV (2009), pp. 1358–62.

148 P. S. Hersh, A. Greenstein and K. L. Fry, 'Corneal Collagen Crosslinking for Keratoconus and Corneal Ectasia: One-Year Results', *Journal of Refractive and Corneal Surgery*, XXXVII (2011), pp. 149–60.

149 See Constance Chen, 'Current Surgical and Non-Surgical Treatment Options for Patients Diagnosed with Keratoconus' (MA Thesis, Boston University School of Medicine, 2022).

150 N. S. Vaidya et al., 'Pachymetric Assessment after EpiSmart® Epithelium-On Cross-Linking for Keratoconus and Post-Surgical Ectasia', *Clinical Ophthalmology*, XVI (2022), pp. 1829–35; R. J. Epstein et al., 'EpiSmart® Crosslinking for Keratoconus: A Phase 2 Study', *Cornea* (29 September 2022) (e-version).

151 R. S. Rubinfeld et al., 'Quantitative Analysis of Corneal Stromal Riboflavin Concentration without Epithelial Removal', *Journal of Refractive and Corneal Surgery*, XLIV (2018), pp. 237–42, and erratum in *Journal of Refractive and Corneal Surgery*, XLIV (2018), p. 523; R. S. Rubinfeld, C. Caruso and C. Ostacolo, 'Corneal Cross-Linking: The Science beyond the Myths and Misconceptions', *Cornea*, XXXVIII (2019), pp. 780–90; R. S. Rubinfeld et al., 'The Effect of Sodium Iodide on Stromal Loading, Distribution and Degradation of Riboflavin in a Rabbit Model of Transepithelial Corneal Crosslinking', *Clinical Ophthalmology*, XV (2021), pp. 1985–94.

152 F. Cifariello et al., 'Epi-Off versus Epi-On Corneal Collagen Cross-Linking in Keratoconus Patients: A Comparative Study through 2-Year Follow-Up', *Journal of Ophthalmology*, XXIX (2018), 4947983; S. M. Ng, B. S. Hawkins and I. C. Kuo, 'Transepithelial versus Epithelium-Off Corneal Crosslinking for Progressive Keratoconus: Findings from a Cochrane Systematic Review', *American Journal of Ophthalmology*, CCXXIX (2021), pp. 274–87.

153 P. Napolitano et al., 'Topographic Outcomes in Keratoconus Surgery: Epi-On versus Epi-Off Iontophoresis Corneal Collagen Cross-Linking', *Journal of Clinical Medicine*, XI (2022), p. 1785.

154 R. D. Stulting et al., 'Corneal Crosslinking without Epithelial Removal', *Journal of Refractive and Corneal Surgery*, XLIV (2018), pp. 1363–70, here, p. 1363.

155 Robert K. Merton, *On the Shoulders of Giants: A Shandean Postscript* (New York, 1965).

156 T. Seiler et al., 'Corneal Crosslinking without Epithelial Removal', *Journal of Refractive and Corneal Surgery*, XLV (2019), pp. 891–2.

157 Ibid., p. 891.

158 J. D. Bernal, *The Social Function of Science* (New York, 1939), pp. 150–51.

159 Seiler et al., 'Corneal Crosslinking', p. 891.

160 Ibid.

161 Ibid., p. 892.

162 R. Doyle Stulting et al., 'Reply', *Journal of Refractive and Corneal Surgery*, XLV (2019), pp. 892–3.

163 Ibid., p. 892.

164 Ibid.

165 Ibid., p. 893.

166 Ibid.

167 'CXL Ophthalmics Announces 32-Million Series A Investment Round Led by AXA, IM, Alts through Its Global Health Private Equity Strategy', www.businesswire.com, accessed 26 March 2023.

168 Jane S. Smith, *Patenting the Sun: Polio and the Salk Vaccine* (New York, 1990), p. 220.

169 Ibid., pp. 338ff.

170 R. H. Shryock, 'Freedom and Interference in Medicine', *The Annals*, CC (1938), pp. 32–59, here, p. 45.

171 Porter, *Quacks*, p. 68.

4 Backs

1 Mark Silvert, 'Acupuncture Wins BMA Approval', *BMJ*, CCCXXI (2000), p. 11.

2 Dennis Campbell, 'Back Sufferers to Receive Acupuncture on NHS', *The Observer* (24 May 2009).

3 British Medical Association, *Acupuncture: Efficacy, Safety and Practice* (Amsterdam, 2000).

4 R. A. Moore et al., 'BMA Approves Acupuncture', *BMJ*, CCCXXI (2000), p. 1220.

5 William Asscher, 'More on BMA's Approval of Acupuncture', *BMJ*, CCCXXII (2001), p. 45.

6 Mike Cummings, 'Acupuncture Techniques Should Be Tested Logically and Methodically', *BMJ*, CCCXXII (2001), p. 45.

7 The most sophisticated account of this approach remains Roger Cooter, ed., *Studies in the History of Alternative Medicine* (London, 1988).

8 *Select Committee on Science and Technology: Sixth Report on Complementary and Alternative Medicine* (21 November 2000), www.publications.parliament.uk.

9 Robert G. A. Dolby, 'Reflections on Deviant Science', *Sociological Review*, XXVII (1979), pp. 9–47, here, pp. 21–2, 24.

10 Y. Chae, Y.-S. Lee and P. Enck, 'How Placebo Needles Differ from Placebo Pills?', *Psychiatry*, IX (2018), p. 243.

11 F. Barlow et al., 'How the Psychosocial Context of Clinical Trials Differs from Usual Care: A Qualitative Study of Acupuncture Patients', *BMC Medical Research Methodology*, XI (2011), p. 79.

12 S. Lipton, 'Intractable Pain – the Present Position', *Annals of the Royal College of Surgeons England*, LXIII (1981), pp. 157–63, here, p. 158.

13 C. Paterson, 'Patients' Experiences of Western-Style Acupuncture: The Influence of Acupuncture "Dose", Self-Care Strategies and Integration', *Journal of Health Service Research Policy*, XII (2007), s1-39–45.

14 Enrique Ravina, *The Evolution of Drug Discovery: From Traditional Medicines to Modern Drugs* (New York, 2011), pp. 24ff.

15 D. M. Marcus and L. McCullough, 'An Evaluation of the Evidence in "Evidence-Based" Integrative Medicine Programs', *Academy of Medicine*, LXXXIV (2009), pp. 1229–34, here, p. 1229.

16 A. White and E. Ernst, 'A Brief History of Acupuncture', *Rheumatology*, XLIII (2004), pp. 662–3, here, p. 662.

17 I am indebted for this section to Zhou Xun, *The People's Health: Health Intervention and Delivery in Mao's China, 1949–1983* (Montreal, 2020).

18 Kim Taylor, *Chinese Medicine in Early Communist China, 1945–1963: A Medicine of Revolution* (New York, 2005), pp. 1–2, as well as Sean Hsiang-Lin Lei, *Neither Donkey nor Horse: Medicine in the Struggle over China's Modernity* (Chicago, IL, 2014).

19 Taylor, *Chinese Medicine in Early Communist China*, pp. 70–76.

20 Simon Ings, *Stalin and the Scientists: A History of Triumph and Tragedy, 1905–53* (New York, 2016).

21 Taylor, *Chinese Medicine in Early Communist China*, p. 53.

22 Ibid., p. 24.

23 James Reston, 'Now, about My Operation', *New York Times* (26 July 1971). See also James Reston, *Deadline: A Memoir* (New York, 1991), pp. 381–4.

24 Li-Gong Liu et al., 'The History of Acupuncture Anesthesia for Pneumonectomy in Shanghai during the 1960s', *Journal of Integrative Medicine*, XIV (2016), pp. 285–90.

25 Emerson Walden, 'Observations on Acupuncture and Reimplantation Surgery in the People's Republic of China', *Journal of the National Medical Association*, LXV (1973), pp. 14–16, here, p. 14.

26 W. Montague Cobb, 'The National Medical Association Delegation's Visit to the People's Republic of China', *Journal of the National Medical Association*, LXV (1973), pp. 3–7, here, p. 7.

27 Anon., 'Medical Missionary Society of China', *Boston Medical and Surgical Journal*, XI (1841), p. 176.

28 Lillian Africano, 'Acupuncture: Child of the Media', *The Nation* (31 May 1975), pp. 657–8.

29 David Colquhoun and Steven P. Novella, 'Acupuncture Is Theatrical Placebo', *Anesthesia and Analgesia*, CXVI (2013), pp. 1360–63, here, p. 1360.

30 Here quoted in Kelly Hacker Jones, 'Eastern Medicine, Western Bodies: Chinese Medicine in the Twentieth-Century United States' (PhD Diss., Stony Brook University, 2018), p. 100. See also Xun, *The People's Health*, pp. 275–80.

31 E. Grey Dimond, 'More Than Herbs and Acupuncture', *Saturday Review* (18 December 1971) pp. 17–19, here, p. 19.

32 Erasmus Darwin, *Zoonomia; or, The Laws of Organic Life* (London, 1794), p. 335.

33 Louis Victor Joseph Berlioz, *Mémoires sur les maladies chroniques, les evacuations sanguines et l'acupuncture* (Paris, 1816), p. 298.

34 Ibid., pp. 310–11. See also Roberta Bivins, 'The Needle and the Lancet: Acupuncture in Britain, 1683–2000', *Acupuncture in Medicine*, XIX (2000), pp. 2–14, as well as her *Acupuncture, Expertise, and Cross-Cultural Medicine* (London, 2001), p. 94.

35 The official index of members, *Plarr's Lives of the Fellows of the Royal College of Surgeons*, does not include him.

36 James Morss Churchill, *A Treatise on Acupuncturation; Being a Description of a Surgical Operation Originally Peculiar to the Japonese* [sic] *and Chinese, and by Them Denominated Zin-King, Now Introduced into European Practice, with Directions for Its Performance, and Cases Illustrating Its Success* (London, 1821), p. 22.

37 Ibid., p. 5.

38 James Morss Churchill, *Cases Illustrative of the Immediate Effects Acupuncturation: In Rheumatism, Lumbago, Sciatica, Anomalous Muscular Diseases, and in Dropsy of the Cellular Tissue, Selected from Various Sources, and Intended as an Appendix to the Author's Treatise on the Subject* (London, 1828), p. 2.

39 Sander L. Gilman, *Making the Body Beautiful: A Cultural History of Aesthetic Surgery* (Princeton, NJ, 1999), pp. 77–83.

40 'A Word of Defence in Favour of That Much Absurd and Long-Suffering People, the Medical Experimentalists, Usually Denominated Quacks', *Atlantic Monthly*, I (1824), p. 441. See Michael Devitt, 'From "Remedy Highly Esteemed" to "Barbarous Practice": The Rise and Fall of Acupuncture in Nineteenth-Century America' (PhD Diss., University of Missouri–Kansas City, 2014).

41 'Acupuncturation', *Ohio Medical Repository of Original and Selected Intelligence*, I (1826), p. 30.

42 George Bacon Wood, *A Treatise on Therapeutics, and Pharmacology or Materia Medica* (Philadelphia, PA, 1856), II, p. 740.

43 M. J. Morand, *Memoir on Acupuncturation, Embracing a Series of Cases, Drawn Up under the Inspection of M. Julius Cloquet, by M. Morand, Doctor of Medicine*, trans. Franklin Bache, MD (Philadelphia, PA, 1825).

44 Franklin Bache, 'Cases Illustrative of the Remedial Effects of Acupuncturation', *North American Medical and Surgical Journal*, I (1826), p. 311.

45 Oliver Wendell Holmes, 'The Contagiousness of Puerperal Fever', in his *Medical Essays, 1842–1882*, 2nd edn (Boston, MA, 1883), pp. 103–72.

46 All references are to Oliver Wendell Holmes, *The Poet at the Breakfast Table* (Boston, MA, 1886), p. 142.

47 Ibid.

48 Ibid., p. 143.

49 Oliver Wendell Holmes, *Currents and Counter Currents in Medical Science* (Boston, MA, 1861), p. 8.

50 William Osler, *The Principles and Practice of Medicine*, 1st edn (New York, 1892), pp. 282, 820.

51 Ilza Veith, 'Sir William Osler – Acupuncturist', *Bulletin of the New York Academy of Medicine*, LI (1975), pp. 393–9; M. H. Lipkovitz, 'Osler and Acupuncture', *JAMA*, CCXXV (1973), p. 749; L. Fernandez-Herlihy, 'Osler, Acupuncture and Lumbago', *New England Journal of Medicine*, CCLXXXVII (1972), p. 314.

52 William Osler, *Aequanimitas with Other Addresses to Medical Students, Nurses and Practitioners of Medicine* (Philadelphia, PA, 1905), p. 25.

53 Anon., 'Acupuncture and the Acuchiropractors', *JAMA*, CCXXIII (1973), pp. 682–3. See also Terri Anne Winnick, 'From Quackery to "Complementary" Medicine: The Integration of Alternative Therapies in the American Medical Profession' (PhD Diss., Indiana University, 2001).

54 William J. Curran, 'Acupuncture and the Practice of Medicine', *New England Journal of Medicine*, CCXCI (1974), pp. 1245–6.

55 Anne-Emanuelle Birn and Theodore M. Brown, eds, *Comrades in Health: U.S. Health Internationalists, Abroad and at Home* (New Brunswick, NJ, 2013), pp. 10ff., and Jane P. Brickman, 'Medical McCarthyism and the Punishment of Internationalist Physicians in the U.S.', in *Comrades in Health*, ed. Birn and Brown, pp. 82–96.

56 John Saar, 'A Prickly Panacea Called Acupuncture', *Life* (13 August 1971), pp. 33–5; Frances Lang, 'Acupuncture', *Ramparts*, X (October 1971), pp. 12–16; 'Medicine: Yang, Yin, and Needles', *Time* (9 August 1971), pp. 37–8.

57 Xun, *The People's Health*, p. 247.

58 Ibid., p. 244.

59 John Iliffe, *East African Doctors: A History of the Modern Profession* (Cambridge, 1998), p. 202.

60 Xun, *The People's Health*, pp. 277–8.

61 Ibid., p. 281.

62 Ibid.

63 David Joravsky, 'The Mechanical Spirit: The Stalinist Marriage of Pavlov to Marx', *Theory and Society*, IV (1977), pp. 457–77.

64 Paul Unschuld has critiqued this tendency as ahistorical and selective; it ignores those elements of Chinese medicine that do not fit the 'Western medicine is bad/

Eastern medicine is good' paradigm. See Paul Unschuld, *Medicine in China: A History of Ideas* (Berkeley, CA, 1985), pp. 1–2.

65 Elisabeth Hsu, 'The History of Chinese Medicine in the People's Republic of China and Its Globalization', *East Asian Science, Technology and Society: An International Journal*, II (2008), pp. 465–84, here, p. 480.

66 Richard Tomkins, 'The Retreat of Reason', *Financial Times – FT Magazine* (23 May 2009), p. 24.

67 Colquhoun and Novella, 'Acupuncture Is Theatrical Placebo', p. 1360.

68 Devra Davis, 'The History and Sociology of the Scientific Study of Acupuncture', *American Journal of Chinese Medicine*, III (1975), pp. 5–26, here, p. 16.

69 Editorial, 'Acupuncture', *JAMA*, CCXXIII (1973), pp. 77–8.

70 Bayard Taylor, *A Visit to India, China, and Japan, in the Year 1853* (New York, 1855), p. 285.

71 Kyla Schuller, *The Biopolitics of Feeling: Race, Sex, and Science in the Nineteenth Century* (Durham, NC, 2018), p. 148.

72 Xine Yao, *Disaffected: The Cultural Politics of Unfeeling in Nineteenth-Century America* (Durham, NC, 2021), pp. 171–207, here, p. 177.

73 I am indebted to the readings in Eric Hayot, *The Hypothetical Mandarin: Sympathy, Modernity, and Chinese Pain* (Oxford, 2009).

74 Peter Parker, *Statements Respecting Hospitals in China*, quoted by Hayot, *The Hypothetical Mandarin*, p. 120.

75 Cited by David Morris, *The Culture of Pain* (Berkeley, CA, 1991), p. 39.

76 The case material is reproduced from Hayot, *The Hypothetical Mandarin*, pp. 120ff.

77 Arthur Kleinman, *Social Origins of Distress and Disease: Depression, Neurasthenia, and Pain in Modern China* (New Haven, CT, 1986).

78 Hayot, *The Hypothetical Mandarin*, p. 123.

79 Sander L. Gilman, 'Lam Qua and the Development of a Westernized Medical Iconography in China', *Medical History*, XXX/1 (1986), pp. 57–69, and Stephen Rachman, 'Peter Parker's Patients', *Literature and Medicine*, XXIII/1 (2004), pp. 134–59.

80 Hayot, *The Hypothetical Mandarin*, p. 121.

81 Review in *Boston Medical and Surgical Journal*, XXXII (21 May 1845), p. 16, and cited in Lawrence Weschler, *Mr Wilson's Cabinet of Wonder* (New York, 1995), p. 140. Weschler cites the speculation that the author of the review was Oliver Wendell Holmes, Sr.

82 Oliver Wendell Holmes, *Medical Essays, 1842–1882* (Cambridge, MA, 1891), pp. 173, 390.

83 *Minutes of the Annual Meeting of the Medical Missionary Society in China; and Fifteenth Report of Its Ophthalmic Hospital at Canton for the Years 1848 and 1849* (Canton, 1848), p. 13.

84 Edward H. Hume, 'Peter Parker and the Introduction of Anesthesia into China', *Journal of the History of Medicine and Allied Sciences*, I (1946), pp. 670–74, here, p. 672.

85 William Hamilton Jeffreys and James L. Maxwell, *The Diseases of China: Including Formosa and Korea* (Philadelphia, PA, 1911), p. 8.

86 Ibid., p. 8.

87 Sunny Xiang, *Tonal Intelligence: The Aesthetics of Asian Inscrutability during the Long Cold War* (New York, 2020), p. 87.

88 Jeffreys and Maxwell, *The Diseases of China*, p. 8.

89 Xiang, *Tonal Intelligence*, p. 19.

90 Ibid., p. 10.
91 Jones, 'Eastern Medicine, Western Bodies', p. 120.
92 See Phoebe Friesen, 'Demystifying the Placebo Effect' (PhD Diss., City University of New York, 2018).
93 See Daniel E. Moerman, *Meaning, Medicine, and the 'Placebo Effect'* (Cambridge, 2002); Anne Harrington, ed., *The Placebo Effect: An Interdisciplinary Exploration* (Cambridge, MA, 1997); Harry A. Guess et al., eds, *The Science of the Placebo: Toward an Interdisciplinary Research Agenda* (London, 2002); Amir Raz and Cory Harris, eds, *Placebo Talks: Modern Perspectives on Placebos in Society* (Oxford, 2015).
94 Jacques Jouanna, *Greek Medicine from Hippocrates to Galen: Selected Papers*, ed. Philip van der Eijk (Leiden, 2012), p. 272.
95 Roy Porter, *Disease, Medicine and Society, 1660–1850* (London, 2009), p. 21. See also Roy Porter, 'Introduction', in *Patients and Practitioners: Lay Perceptions of Medicine in Pre-Nineteenth Century Society*, ed. Porter (Cambridge, 1986), pp. 1–22, here, also, p. 7.
96 Siddhartha Mukherjee, *The Laws of Medicine: Field Notes from an Uncertain Science* (New York, 2015), pp. 12–13.
97 I am indebted to Arthur K. Shapiro and Elaine Shapiro, *The Powerful Placebo: From Ancient Priest to Modern Physician* (Baltimore, MD, 1997), pp. 28–36ff.
98 A. Mervyn Davies, *Strange Destiny: A Biography of Warren Hastings* (New York, 1935), p. 373.
99 George Motherby, *A New Medical Dictionary; or, General Repository of Physic. Containing an Explanation of the Terms, and a Description of the Various Particulars Relating to Anatomy, Physiology, Physic, Surgery . . .* (London, 1785), p. 593.
100 Robert Hooper and John Quincy, *Quincy's Lexicon-Medicum* (London, 1802).
101 Walter Scott, *St Ronan's Well* [1823] (London, 1845), *Waverley Novels*, VIII, p. 462.
102 Anon., 'Surgical Lectures', *The Lancet*, I/8 (1823), pp. 253–60, here, p. 259.
103 Austin Flint, 'Natural History of Articulate Rheumatism', *American Journal of the Medical Sciences*, XLVI (1863), pp. 17–36, here, pp. 21–2.
104 W. R. Houston, 'The Doctor Himself as a Therapeutic Agent', *Annals of Internal Medicine*, XI (1938), pp. 1416–25, here, pp. 1417–18.
105 Christopher R. J. Milnes, *A History of Euphoria: The Perception and Misperception of Health and Well-Being* (New York, 2019), pp. 109ff.
106 I am indebted to Lindsey Marie Grubbs, 'The Politics and Poetics of Diagnosis in Nineteenth-Century American Literature and Medicine' (PhD Diss., Emory University, 2019).
107 Holmes, *Currents and Counter-Currents in Medical Science*, p. iv.
108 Oliver Wendell Holmes, *Homeopathy, and Its Kindred Delusions* (Boston, MA, 1842), pp. 69–70.
109 Stanley Joel Reiser, *Medicine and the Reign of Technology* (Cambridge, 1978), p. 72.
110 Ibid., p. 38.
111 Holmes, *Currents and Counter-Currents*, p. 295.
112 Ibid., p. 299.
113 J. Russell Reynolds, 'An Address on Specialism in Medicine', *The Lancet*, CXVIII/3033 (1881), pp. 655–8, here, p. 656.
114 Holmes, *Currents and Counter-Currents*, p. 392.

115 Frederick Simms, 'Homœopathy', *The Lancet*, CXXXVI (1890), p. 469.

116 Sigmund Freud, *The Future of an Illusion* (1927), *The Standard Edition of the Complete Psychological Works of Sigmund Freud*, trans. and ed. James Strachey et al., 24 vols (London, 1953–74), XXI, pp. 1–56, here, p. 56.

117 Alexander Wilder, 'Faith-Cure Becoming Scientific', *Ideal Magazine*, XIII (1900), pp. 222–6, here, p. 222.

118 Ibid., p. 224.

119 Erwin Liek, *The Doctor's Mission: Reflections, Reminiscences, and Revelations of a Medical Man*, trans. J. Ellis Barker (London, 1930), p. 52.

120 Howard Brody, 'The Lie That Heals: The Ethics of Giving Placebos', *Annals of Internal Medicine*, LXXXXVII (1982), pp. 112–18, here, p. 112.

121 *The Poems of Emily Dickinson*, ed. R. W. Franklin (Cambridge, MA, 2005), p. 95.

122 Holly Folk, *The Religion of Chiropractic: Populist Healing from the American Heartland* (Chapel Hill, NC, 2017).

123 N. W. Winkelman, Jr, and S. D. Saul, 'The Return of Suggestion', *Psychiatric Quarterly*, XLVIII (1974), pp. 230–38, here, pp. 232, 236.

124 Quoted ibid., p. 236.

125 Ibid., p. 232.

126 F. S. Berlin, R. Bartlett and J. D. Black, 'Acupuncture and Placebo: Effects on Delaying the Terminating Response to a Painful Stimulus', *Anesthesiology*, XLII (1975), pp. 527–31, here, p. 530.

127 Annelie Rosén, 'Placebo Effects in Health and Disease – How Expectations Shape Treatment Outcomes' (PhD Diss., Department of Clinical Neuroscience, Karolinska Institutet, Stockholm, 2016).

128 See Council on Ethical and Judicial Affairs, American Medical Association, Report 2-1-06, *Placebo Use in Clinical Practice* (2006) ('Physicians may use [a] placebo . . . for diagnosis or treatment only if the patient is informed of and agrees to its use'), www.ama-assn.org, accessed 26 March 2023.

129 D. K. Sokol, 'Can Deceiving Patients Be Morally Acceptable?', *BMJ*, CCCXXXIV (2007), pp. 984–98.

130 D. M. Shaw, 'Prescribing Placebos Ethically: The Appeal of Negatively Informed Consent', *Journal of Medical Ethics*, XXXV (2009), pp. 97–9.

131 Adam J. Kolber, 'A Limited Defense of Clinical Placebo Deception', *Yale Law and Policy Review*, XXVI (2007), pp. 75–134, here, p. 84.

132 Henry K. Beecher, 'The Powerful Placebo', *JAMA*, CLIX (1955), pp. 1602, 1604–5.

133 Marco Annoni, 'Exceptional Lies: The Ethics of Deceptive Placebos in Clinical Settings', *Bioetica e Pluralismo*, L (2015), pp. 5–22, here, pp. 14–16.

134 Martin Bystad, Camilla Bystad and Rolf Wynn, 'How Can Placebo Effects Best Be Applied in Clinical Practice? A Narrative Review', *Psychology Research and Behavior Management*, VIII (2015), pp. 41–5, here p. 41.

135 Beecher, 'The Powerful Placebo', p. 1604.

136 David Wootton, *Bad Medicine: Doctors Doing Harm since Hippocrates* (Oxford, 2007), p. 68.

137 Kolber, 'A Limited Defense', p. 128.

138 M. Kelly, 'Some Medical Myths', *World Medical Journal*, XI (1964), pp. 205–7, here, p. 206.

139 Richard Wollheim, 'Memory, Experiential Memory and Personal Identity', in *Perception and Identity: Essays Presented to A. J. Ayer*, ed. G. F. Macdonald (London, 1979), pp. 186–233, here, p. 199.

140 See Brian Hurwitz, 'Anecdotes: Epistemic Switching in Medical Narratives', in *Narrative Science: Reasoning, Representing and Knowing since 1800*, ed. Dominic J. Berry, Kim M. Hajek, Mary S. Morgan (Edinburgh, 2022), pp. 351–70.

141 Abraham Verghese, 'The Doctor's Bag for the New Millennium', *New York Times* (8 October 2012).

142 B. J. Materson and B. Leclercq, 'David Ayman, MD, an Early Investigator of Clinical Hypertension', *Journal of Clinical Hypertension*, VII (2005), pp. 218–23.

143 David Ayman, 'The Hereditary Aspect of Arteriolar (Essential) Hypertension: Study of Three Generations of a Family', *New England Journal of Medicine*, CCIX (1933), pp. 194–7.

144 David Ayman, 'Heredity in Arteriolar (Essential) Hypertension: A Clinical Study of the Blood Pressure of 1,524 Members of 277 Families', *Archives of Internal Medicine*, LIII (1934), pp. 792–802.

145 David Ayman, 'An Evaluation of Therapeutic Results in Essential Hypertension: I. The Interpretation of Symptomatic Relief', *JAMA*, XCV (1930), pp. 246–9, here, p. 247.

146 Ibid., p. 249.

147 Beecher, 'The Powerful Placebo', pp. 1602–6. A re-evaluation is to be found in G. S. Kienle and H. Kiene, 'The Powerful Placebo Effect: Fact or Fiction?' *Journal of Clinical Epidemiology*, L (1997), pp. 1311–18.

148 David Ayman, 'An Evaluation of Therapeutic Results in Essential Hypertension: I. The Interpretation of Blood Pressure Reductions', *JAMA*, XCVI (1931), pp. 2091–4, here, p. 2092.

149 P. J. Brennan et al., 'Seasonal Variations in Arterial Blood Pressure', *BMJ*, CCLXXXV (1982), pp. 919–23.

150 David Ayman and Archie Goldshine, 'Blood Pressure Determinations by Patients with Essential Hypertension: I. The Difference between Clinic and Home Readings before Treatment', *American Journal of Medical Science*, CC (1940), pp. 465–74.

151 Ayman, 'Evaluation of Therapeutic Results in Essential Hypertension: I. The Interpretation of Blood Pressure Reductions', p. 2093.

152 Walter P. Kennedy, 'The Nocebo Reaction', *Medical World*, XLV (1961), pp. 203–5.

153 A. Rosén et al., 'Surgeons' Behaviors and Beliefs regarding Placebo Effects in Surgery', *Acta orthopedica*, XCII (2021), pp. 507–12.

154 David Ayman and Archie Goldshine, 'Blood Pressure Determinations by Patients with Essential Hypertension: II. The Difference between Home and Clinic Readings during and after Treatment', *American Journal of Medical Science*, CCI (1941), pp. 157–61, here, p. 161.

155 D. W. Blumhagen, 'The Doctor's White Coat', *Annals of Internal Medicine*, XCI (1979), pp. 111–16.

156 John Godlee Rickman, *Lord Lister* (London, 1918), p. 460.

157 See Gustav Neuber, *Die aseptische Wundbehandlung in meinen chirurgischen Privathospitälern* (Kiel, 1886). See L. W. Adams et al., 'Uncovering the History of Operating Room Attire through Photographs', *Anesthesiology*, CXXIV (2015), pp. 19–24.

158 Ernst Georg Ferdinand Küster, *Geschichte der neueren deutschen Chirurgie* (Stuttgart, 1915), p. 46.

159 Michael Fried, 'Realism, Writing, and Disfiguration in Thomas Eakins's *Gross Clinic*, with a Postscript on Stephen Crane's Upturned Faces', *Representations*, IX (1985), pp. 33–104.

160 Bridget L. Goodbody, 'The Present Opprobrium of Surgery: The Agnew Clinic and Nineteenth-Century Representations of Cancerous Female Breasts', *American Art*, VIII (1994), pp. 33–52.

161 Daniel Webster Cathell, *The Physician Himself and What He Should Add to the Strictly Scientific* (Baltimore, MD, 1882), p. 56.

162 J. A. Hornsby and R. E. Schmidt, *The Modern Hospital: Its Inspiration, Its Architecture, Its Equipment, Its Operation* (Philadelphia, PA, 1913), pp. 543–5.

163 Hippocrates of Cos, II: *Prognostic. Regimen in Acute Diseases. The Sacred Disease. The Art. Breaths. Law. Decorum*, trans. W.H.S. Jones, Loeb Classical Library 148 (Cambridge, MA, 1923), p. 295.

164 S. U. Rehman et al., 'What to Wear Today? Effect of Doctor's Attire on the Trust and Confidence of Patients', *American Journal of Medicine*, CXVII (2005), pp. 1279–86.

165 S. Au, F. Khandwala and H. T. Stelfox, 'Physician Attire in the Intensive Care Unit and Patient Family Perceptions of Physician Professional Characteristics', *JAMA Intern Medicine*, CLXXII (2013), pp. 465–7.

166 C. M. Petrilli et al., 'Understanding Patient Preference for Physician Attire: A Cross-Sectional Observational Study of 10 Academic Medical Centres in the USA', *BMJ Open*, VIII (2018), e021239.

167 A. M. Treakle et al., 'Bacterial Contamination of Health Care Workers' White Coats', *American Journal of Infection Control*, XXXVII/2 (2009), pp. 101–5. The British debate is summarized in K. J. Griffin, D. J. Scott and N. Foster, 'Bare below the Elbows', *Annals of the Royal College of Surgeons of England*, XCIII (2011), p. 181.

168 M. Landry et al., 'Patient Preferences for Doctor Attire: The White Coat's Place in the Medical Profession', *Ochsner Journal*, XIII (2013), pp. 334–42, here, p. 342.

169 Ira Rutkow, *Empire of the Scalpel: The History of Surgery* (New York, 2022), and yet the employment patterns shift along with the other specialties as we shall see in our final chapter, see A. G. Charles and S. Ortiz-Pujols et al., 'The Employed Surgeon: A Changing Professional Paradigm', *JAMA Surgery*, CXLVIII (2013), pp. 323–8.

170 S. A. Aitken et al., 'The Importance of the Orthopaedic Doctors' Appearance: A Cross-Regional Questionnaire Based Study', *Surgeon*, XII (2014), pp. 40–46.

171 Hunter Robb, *Aseptic Surgical Technique* (Philadelphia, PA, 1894), pp. 47–8.

172 'Hospital Scrub Suits the Newest Fashion Craze', *Indiana Gazette* (9 October 1980), p. 40.

173 Chuck Palmer, 'Scrub Clothes May Cure Fashion Boredom, but the Trend is a Headache for Hospitals', *San Bernadino County Sun* (27 October 1981).

174 J. D. Jennings et al., 'Physicians' Attire Influences Patients' Perceptions in the Urban Outpatient Orthopaedic Surgery Setting', *Clinical Orthopaedics and Related Research*, CCCCLXXVI (2016), pp. 1908–18.

175 Nathan L. Belkin, 'Use of Scrubs and Related Apparel in Health Care Facilities', *American Journal of Infection Control*, XXV (1997), pp. 401–4, here, p. 402.

176 M. Clark et al., 'Patients' Perceptions of Gastroenterologists' Attire in the Clinic and Endoscopy Suite', *Annals of Gastroenterology*, XXXI (2018), pp. 237–40.

177 A. M. Omari et al., 'Patient Perception of Physician Attire in the Outpatient Setting during the COVID-19 Pandemic', *JAAOS: Global Research and Reviews*, V (2021), e21.00039.

178 A. Casey et al., 'Association between Patient Perception of Surgeons and Color of Scrub Attire', *JAMA Surgery*, CLVIII (2023), pp. 421–3.

179 Vanessa Friedman, 'Health Care Workers Deserve Fashion, Too', *New York Times* (9 June 2021).

180 I am indebted to Gary L. Brase and Jillian Richmond, 'The White-Coat Effect: Physician Attire and Perceived Authority, Friendliness, and Attractiveness', *Journal of Applied Social Psychology*, XXIV (2004), pp. 2469–81.

181 Joseph P. Kriss, 'On White Coats and Other Matters', *New England Journal of Medicine*, CCXCII (1975), pp. 1024–5.

182 T. Hubkova, 'Lifestyle Approaches to White Coat Hypertension', *American Journal of Lifestyle Medicine*, XI (2016), pp. 29–32.

183 David Derbyshire, 'Why Acupuncture Is Giving Sceptics the Needle', *The Observer* (26 July 2013).

184 Matias Vested Madsen, Peter C. Gøtzsche and Asbjørn Hróbjartsson, 'Acupuncture Treatment for Pain: Systematic Review of Randomised Clinical Trials with Acupuncture, Placebo Acupuncture, and No Acupuncture Groups', *BMJ*, CCCXXXVIII (2009), a3115.

185 National Institute for Health and Care Excellence, *Low Back Pain and Sciatica: Draft Guidance* (March 2016), www.nice.org.uk.

186 Jacqui Wise, 'NICE Recommends Exercise and Not Acupuncture for Low Back Pain', *BMJ*, CCCLII (2016), 10.1136.

187 Ian Hacking, *The Emergence of Probability: A Philosophical Study of Early Ideas about Probability, Induction and Statistical Inference*, 2nd edn (Cambridge, 2006), p. 105.

188 Magid H. Amer, 'Gene Therapy for Cancer: Present Status and Future Perspective', *Molecular Cell Therapy*, II (2014), p. 27.

5 Permanence and Change

1 Sheila Jasanoff, 'The Discontents of Truth and Trust in the Twenty-First Century', *Daedalus*, CLI (2022), pp. 25–43, here, pp. 37–8.

2 David Wallace-Wells, 'Dr Fauci Looks Back: "Something Clearly Went Wrong"', *New York Times Magazine* (24 April 2023).

3 All quotations are from the e-book version of Anthony Fauci, *On Call: A Doctor's Journey in Public Service* (New York, 2024).

4 Jasanoff, 'The Discontents of Truth', p. 31.

5 Ibid., p. 39.

6 Garland E. Allen, 'The Role of Experts in Scientific Controversy', in *Scientific Controversies: Case Studies in the Resolution and Closure of Disputes in Science and Technology*, ed. Hugo Tristram Engelhardt and Arthur Leonard Caplan (New York, 1987), pp. 169–202.

7 Fauci, *On Call*.

8 Allen, 'The Role of Experts in Scientific Controversy'.

9 Friedrich Nietzsche, *The Gay Science*, trans. Walter Kaufmann (New York, 1974), p. 335, § 373.

10 Devi Sridhar, 'Don't Blame Scientists for What Went Wrong with Covid – Ministers Were the Ones Calling the Shots', *The Guardian* (13 June 2023).

11 A. P. Stanley, *Life of Thomas Arnold, DD* (London, 1910), p. 288.

12 Daniel Duman, 'The Creation and Diffusion of a Professional Ideology in Nineteenth Century England', *Sociological Review*, XXVII (1979), pp. 113–38.

13 William Osler, *The Old Humanities and the New Science* (Boston, MA, and New York, 1920), p. 64.
14 Ludwig Edelstein, 'The Professional Ethics of the Greek Physician', *Bulletin of the History of Medicine*, XXX (1956), pp. 391–419, here, p. 407.
15 Arthur Conan Doyle, 'The Surgeon Talks', in his *Round the Red Lamp: Being Facts and Fancies of Medical Life* (New York, 1896), pp. 296–307, here, p. 307.
16 Jane Macnaughton, 'The Dangerous Practice of Empathy', *The Lancet*, CCCLXXIII (2009), pp. 1940–41, here, p. 1941.
17 Talcott Parsons, 'The Professions and Social Structure', in his *Essays in Sociological Theory* (New York, 1954), p. 44.
18 Eyal Press, 'The Moral Crisis of America's Doctors', *New York Times Magazine* (15 June 2023).
19 Jonathan Shay, 'Moral Injury', *Psychoanalytic Psychology,* XXXI (2014), pp. 182–91.
20 Press, 'Moral Crisis'.
21 Q. Yang et al., 'Measuring Public Reaction to Violence against Doctors in China: Interrupted Time Series Analysis of Media Reports', *Journal of Medical Internet Research*, XXIII (2021), e19651.
22 Robert J. Blendon and John M. Benson, 'Trust in Medicine, the Health System and Public Health', *Daedalus*, CLI (2022), pp. 67–82, here, p. 77.
23 Ibid., p. 77.
24 Marc Berg and Annemarie Mol, 'Differences in Medicine: An Introduction', in *Differences in Medicine: Unraveling Practices, Techniques, and Bodies*, ed. Marc Berg and Annemarie Mol (Durham, NC, 1998), p. 3.
25 Thomas P. Duffy, 'The Flexner Report: 100 Years Later', *Yale Journal of Biology and Medicine*, LXXVII (2011), pp. 269–76.

FURTHER READING

Bosk, Charles L., *Forgive and Remember: Managing Medical Failure* (Chicago, IL, 2003)

Bourke, Joanna, *The Story of Pain: From Prayer to Painkillers* (Oxford, 2014)

Braude, Hillel D., *Intuition in Medicine: A Philosophical Defense of Clinical Reasoning* (Chicago, IL, 2012)

Clare, Eli, *Brilliant Imperfection: Grappling with Cure* (Durham, NC, 2017)

Cooter, Roger, ed., *Studies in the History of Alternative Medicine* (London, 1988)

—, ed., *A Cultural History of Medicine*, 6 vols (London, 2021)

Dieppe, Paul, *Healing and Medicine: A Doctor's Journey towards Their Integration* (London, 2023)

Gilman, Sander L., *Difference and Pathology: Stereotypes of Sexuality, Race, and Madness* (Ithaca, NY, 1985)

—, *Disease and Representation: Images of Illness from Madness to AIDS* (Ithaca, NY, 1988)

Gordon, James S., *Transforming Trauma: The Path to Hope and Healing* (New York, 2019)

Greenberg, Daniel S., *Science for Sale: The Perils, Rewards, and Delusions of Campus Capitalism* (Chicago, IL, 2007)

Hoberman, John, *Black and Blue: The Origins and Consequences of Medical Racism* (Chapel Hill, NC, 2009)

Hurwitz, Brian, *Clinical Guidelines and the Law: Negligence, Discretion and Judgment* (Boca Raton, FL, 1998)

Makari, George, *Of Fear and Strangers: A History of Xenophobia* (New York, 2021)

Micale, Mark, and Paul Lerner, eds, *Traumatic Pasts: History, Psychiatry, and Trauma in the Modern Age, 1870–1930* (Cambridge, MA, 2001)

Otis, Laura, *Müller's Lab* (Oxford, 2007)

Pernick, Martin S., *A Calculus of Suffering: Pain, Professionalism and Anesthesia in Nineteenth-Century America* (New York, 1985)

Porter, Roy, *Health for Sale: Quackery in England, 1660–1800* (Manchester, 1989)

—, *Quacks: Fakers and Charlatans in English Medicine* (Stroud, 2001)

Ravina, Enrique, *The Evolution of Drug Discovery: From Traditional Medicines to Modern Drugs* (New York, 2011)

Savitt, Todd, *Race and Medicine in Nineteenth- and Early-Twentieth-Century America* (Kent, OH, 2007)

Schama, Simon, *Foreign Bodies: Pandemics, Vaccines and the Health of Nations* (New York, 2023)

Schuller, Kyla, *The Biopolitics of Feeling: Race, Sex, and Science in the Nineteenth Century* (Durham, NC, 2018)

Starr, Paul, *The Social Transformation of American Medicine* (New York, 1982)

Wailoo, Keith, *Pain: A Political History* (Baltimore, MD, 2014)

Watson, Katherine, *Medicine and Justice: Medico-Legal Practice in England and Wales, 1700–1914* (London, 2020)

Wootton, David, *Bad Medicine: Doctors Doing Harm since Hippocrates* (Oxford, 2007)

Xine, Yao, *Disaffected: The Cultural Politics of Unfeeling in Nineteenth-Century America* (Durham, NC, 2021)

Young, James Harvey, *The Medical Messiahs: A Social History of Quackery in Twentieth-Century America* (Princeton, NJ, 1992)

Zhou, Xun, *The People's Health: Health Intervention and Delivery in Mao's China, 1949–1983* (Montreal, 2020)

ACKNOWLEDGEMENTS

As is evident from this book, I am indebted to the extraordinarily wide range of existing literature that has focused on the case material I am presenting. The medical literature, broadly understood, that I am employing was made available and accessible by the librarians at Emory University, who were not only willing to ferret out odd essays in remote places but to send me, in Washington during the lockdown, volumes they were able to borrow for me. I have presented bits and pieces of this volume both virtually and more recently 'live' to very mixed audiences who always asked questions that I could not answer. I am also truly indebted to my friends – at least they were my friends when I asked them to read the manuscript, to comment on the text. Linda and Michael Hutcheon, George Makari, Brian Hurwitz and Sharrona Pearl were gracious in providing me with critical readings for which I am grateful. Marina Gilman listened with the forbearance of one who had suffered through my obsessive recounting of earlier books with an equanimity that was overwhelming.

PHOTO ACKNOWLEDGEMENTS

The author and publishers wish to express their thanks to the sources listed below for illustrative material and/or permission to reproduce it. Some locations of artworks are also given below, in the interest of brevity:

From Theodore H. Bast, *The Life and Time of Adolf Kussmaul* (New York, 1926): p. 102; from James Morss Churchill, *A Treatise on Acupuncturation; Being a Description of a Surgical Operation Originally Peculiar to the Japonese* [sic] *and Chinese, and by Them Denominated Zin-King . . .* (London, 1821), photo Wellcome Library, London: p. 247; from O. Haab, *Atlas of the External Diseases of the Eye: Including a Brief Treatise on the Pathology and Treatment*, 2nd edn (Philadelphia, PA, New York and London, 1903), photo Wellcome Library: p. 188; History of Medicine (IHM), National Library of Medicine, Bethesda, MD: p. 252; Medical Historical Library, Harvey Cushing/John Hay Whitney Medical Library, Yale University, New Haven, CT: pp. 25, 94, 177; National Galleries of Scotland, Edinburgh: p. 179; National Gallery of Art, Washington, DC: p. 43; Osler Library of the History of Medicine, McGill University, Montreal: p. 57; The Penn Art Collection, University of Pennsylvania, Philadelphia: p. 280; Philadelphia Museum of Art, PA: p. 279; from Simon Snell, *A Practical Guide to the Examination of the Eye: For Students and Junior Practitioners* (Edinburgh, 1898): p. 195; Wellcome Collection, London: pp. 47, 72, 99, 105 (CC BY 4.0), 158, 174, 180, 241, 258, 282 (photo Adrian Wressell, Heart of England NHS Foundation Trust, CC BY 4.0); from *Wiener klinische Wochenschrift*, IX/6 (6 February 1896), photo University of Illinois Urbana-Champaign: p. 103.

INDEX

riboflavin (vitamin B2) 214, 223, 225–7
Richardson's ether spray 183–4
Richet, Charles 101
Riis, Jacob 45
Rilke, Rainer Maria 109
Ritter, Johann 223
Rivers, Andrew B. 136
Rivers, Harrison David 140
Robb, Hunter 283
Robinson, Samuel C. 136–7
Rockefeller Institute for Medical
    Research 54
Rokitansky, Carl von 31, 108–9, 112, 146
Röntgen, Wilhelm 104, 113–14
Roosevelt, Eleanor 155
Rose, Nikolas 78
Rosebury, Theodore 167
Rosen, Samuel 252
Rowlandson, Thomas 174
Royal College of General Practitioners
    235–6
Royal College of Physicians (RCP) 39
Royal College of Surgeons (RCS) 39–40,
    84, 218
Royal Dental Institute 182
Royal Medical Association 185
Royal Society of Edinburgh 197
Royal Society of Medicine 218–19
Royal Society of Physicians 200–201
Royal Society of Surgeons 201
Rubinfeld, Roy 226–9, 231–3
Rumsfeld, Donald 214–15
Rush, Benjamin 249
Russell, Rosalind 155
Russian Empire 141

Sabin, Albert 232–3
Sacher-Masoch, Leopold von 186
Sachs, Hanns 120
Sackett, David 79–80
St Martin, Alexis 100–101, 156
Saint Yves, Charles 178
salicylic acid 71
Salk, Jonas 232–3
Sanford, Nevitt 126
Santner, Eric 21–3
Scheimpflug images 230
Schering (Pharmaceuticals) 68
Schiener, Christoph 194
Schiotz, Hjalmar 217

schizophrenia 189
Schleiermacher, Friedrich 30
Schneider, Hermann 74–5
Schreiber-Grabitz, Brigitte 132
Schwarz, Dragutin (aka Carl) 97, 151
sciatica 251
science 13–14
    definition of 60
    deviant 238
    and evidence-based medicine
        76–82
    following the 7–9, 13–14, 298–9
    in medicine 30, 36–8, 297
    of medicine 79
    race theory 22, 64–5, 135–46,
        206–211
    secular religion of 41–2
    as vocation or calling 20
scientific evidence 239–45
scientific journals 91
scientific medicine 17–18, 31–2, 48–9,
    82, 230, 233–4, 297, 300
scientific method 229–30
scientific physicians 46–54, 65–6
scientific pragmatism 19
scientist (term) 18
scientists vs quacks 17–18, 173–234
Scott, Walter 264
Scribonius Largus 19–20
scrubs 14, 282–5
SDS (Students for a Democratic Society)
    128
seasonal affective disorders (SAD) 223
Second World War 116
Seiler, Theo 221–4, 228–33
self-experimentation 159–60
self-hypnosis 256–7
Selye, Hans 149–50
Semmelweis, Ignaz 17–18
Semon, Felix 212–13
Seneca 22–3
serum therapy 42
Seventh-Day Adventist Church 53
Sewall, Thomas 99
Seyle, Hans 140
sham acupuncture 286–7
shaman 23–4
Shapiro, Sidney 81
Shaw, George Bernard 53
Shay, Jonathan 295–6

tinidazole 160
Tissot, Samuel August 95
tobacco
    abuse 136, 149
    and 'science' 161
    as therapy 204
tombstone trials 81
Traditional Chinese Medicine (TCM)
    28–9, 239–45, 253–5, 270, 287
transferability 77
transference 148
translational medicine 222–3
transparency 34
transplantation, corneal 218, 221
Trattler, William B. 233
trauma 171–2
trisomy 21, 208, 211–12, 215
tropical medicine 36
Trotter, Thomas 97–8, 174
Trudeau, Edward Livingston 107
trust 51, 66, 83, 269–71, 278, 289–91,
    293
truth-telling 64, 238, 267, 289, 292
tsunamis 172
tuberculin skin test 164
tuberculosis 36, 77–8, 108–9, 164
'Turkish ailment' (*Türkenkrankenheit*)
    133–5
Tuskegee Syphilis Experiment 139
'Type A' behaviour 125

ulcers
    Curling's 148–9
    war 116
ultraviolet (UV) light 223–7
United Kingdom (UK) 10, 74
    medical degrees 40
    see National Health Service (NHS)
United States (USA) 10, 74, 80
    Chinese Exclusion Act (1882) 257
    Civil War 116
    Hartmann Era 131–2
    healers 299–300
    Medicaid fraud 89
    medical degrees 39–40
    medical practice 86–7
    medical schools 49–50, 54–62
    Missouri Court of Appeals 274
    National Committee for Quality
        Assurance 169

National Institutes of Health (NIH)
    160–61, 226–7, 290
National Jewish Population Survey
    145
Pure Food and Drug Act 45–6, 74
    scientific physicians 49–54
United States Supreme Court 88–9
University College London 19
University of Berlin 19, 42
University of Edinburgh 51, 194, 292
University of Greifswald 36
University of Kansas 245
University of New York (New York
    University) 51
University of Pennsylvania 57, 75–6,
    249
University of Toronto 76, 234
University of Virginia 19, 160
University of Zurich 221
U.S. Department of Agriculture 46
USSR (Soviet Union) 222, 232, 242
utilitarianism 30

vaccines 42, 164, 232–3
vagal surgery 112
vagotomy 112, 150
vagus massage oil 170
vagus nerve 108, 170–71
van Swieten, Gottfried 95
Vereniging tegen de Kwakzalverij
    (Society against Quackery) 44
Verghese, Abraham 275
Vesalius 93
Vienna and medicine 31–2
Vietnam War 128
Vinciguerra, Paolo 233
Virchow, Rudolf 31, 33–5, 60, 62–4, 97,
    141, 250, 292
visceral neuralgia 143
Vitalism 95
vitamin A 214
vitamin B 213–14
vitamin B$_2$ (riboflavin) 214, 223, 225–7
vitamin B$_{12}$ 213–14
vitamin D 214
vitamin hypothesis 213
vitamin 'P' 213–14
vitamin supplements 213, 272–3
von Ammon, Friedrich August 192,
    199–200, 222